Praise for *Sleep Paralysis: Historical, Psychological, and Medical Perspectives*

"Sleep specialists are well aware of the subject of sleep paralysis because it is a member of the so-called narcolepsy tetrad. However, the exact mechanism by which strong emotion precipitates sleep paralysis in victims of narcolepsy is still unclear.

Not well known by the general public is that sleep paralysis occurs as an isolated phenomenon in otherwise normal individuals. Because most individuals are unaware that this is a normal part of REM sleep, the inability to move is incredibly terrifying. Given that prior knowledge of this phenomenon would avoid a long period of fear and worry for some individuals, it is my fervent hope that Dr. Sharpless and Dr. Doghramji's book will be at the top of the best seller list."

—William Dement, MD, PhD, Professor, Psychiatry and Behavioral
Sciences, Stanford Center for Sleep Sciences and Medicine

"This book provides the most comprehensive coverage of ' o date. In addition to presenting an excellent summary of ʼ ιis strange and fascinating phenomenon, Sharpl ʻe further investigation is required. This volume w ːtitioners treating those who suffer from sleep pa "

—Christopher Fren ʻchology
Research ., ʋf London

"This is a very welcome and important con ι ̤ ̤ ̤ιɪe study of sleep paralysis. There is a growing literature on this fascinating phenomenon, and the volume does an admirable job of summarizing and synthesizing material."

—Devon E. Hinton, MD, PhD, Associate Professor of Psychiatry,
Massachusetts General Hospital, Harvard Medical School

"The only current book discussing sleep paralysis from a clinical, psychological, and medical perspective, Dr. Sharpless and Dr. Doghramji take a balanced multifaceted approach to understanding complex sources of sleep paralysis and associated experiences. The book provides an accessible overview of cultural, historical, mythic, and psychological aspects of sleep paralysis phenomena before turning to a strong focus on clinical aspects. A thorough treatment of the topic and a quick reference for researchers and clinicians."

—James A. Cheyne, PhD, Professor Emeritus,
Department of Psychology, University of Waterloo

"One of the great mysteries of sleep is the paralysis associated with REM sleep. This volume does an outstanding job in demystifying this phenomenon. It puts sleep paralysis in a historic perspective and sleep physiology framework, as well as the perspective of sleep disorders. Both the general public and sleep clinician can appreciate it. This volume unravels one of the great mysteries of sleep and its disorders."

—Thomas Roth, PhD, Director Sleep
Disorders and Research Center, Henry Ford Hospital

"In this fine collaboration, Sharpless and Doghramji explore the long history of a frightening intermittent sleep disorder we now recognize as one of the symptoms of the narcolepsy tetrad. The authors recognize a larger group who experience sleep paralysis as an isolated phenomenon. These present differently in different historical and cultural contexts from being possessed through witchcraft to being kidnapped by space invaders. Beyond the enjoyment of reading this book, the authors offer detailed treatment programs for those suffering from this disorder and extensive references to encourage further diagnostic recognition and treatment outcome research."

—Rosalind Cartwright, PhD,
FAASM Professor Emeritus, Rush University Medical Center

SLEEP PARALYSIS

Historical, Psychological, and Medical Perspectives

Brian A. Sharpless, PhD
Washington State University
Karl Doghramji, MD
Thomas Jefferson University

OXFORD
UNIVERSITY PRESS

OXFORD
UNIVERSITY PRESS

Oxford University Press is a department of the University of
Oxford. It furthers the University's objective of excellence in research,
scholarship, and education by publishing worldwide.

Oxford   New York
Auckland   Cape Town   Dar es Salaam   Hong Kong   Karachi
Kuala Lumpur   Madrid   Melbourne   Mexico City   Nairobi
New Delhi   Shanghai   Taipei   Toronto

With offices in
Argentina   Austria   Brazil   Chile   Czech Republic   France   Greece
Guatemala   Hungary   Italy   Japan   Poland   Portugal   Singapore
South Korea   Switzerland   Thailand   Turkey   Ukraine   Vietnam

Oxford is a registered trademark of Oxford University Press
in the UK and certain other countries.

Published in the United States of America by
Oxford University Press
198 Madison Avenue, New York, NY 10016

Library of Congress Cataloging-in-Publication Data
Sharpless, Brian A., author.
Sleep paralysis : historical, psychological, and medical perspectives / Brian A Sharpless,
Karl Doghramji.
p. ; cm.
Includes bibliographical references and index.
ISBN 978-0-19-931380-8
I.   Doghramji, Karl, author. II.   Title.
[DNLM: 1. Sleep Paralysis. WL 108]
QP425
612.8'21—dc23
2014043380

I dedicate this book to my parents, Linda and Gary, for their unwavering support over the years; to my mentors, Jacques Barber, Thomas Borkovec, James Martin, and Larry Michelson for their ongoing intellectual inspiration; and to Howard Allan Stern for teaching me to never shy away from exploring the unusual vicissitudes of human experience.

Brian A. Sharpless

I dedicate this book to my wife Laurel, son Mark, and daughter Leah, for their loving encouragement and support.

Karl Doghramji

CONTENTS

FOREWORD

Given the talents and acumen of Brian Sharpless and Karl Doghramji, two first-rate clinician scholars in psychology and psychiatry, respectively, it is not surprising that this volume on sleep paralysis should present a deep and broad array of historical, psychological, and medical perspectives on one of the most "unusual vicissitudes of human experience," as Dr. Sharpless terms it in his dedicatory to the volume.

In the parlance of contemporary neuroscience, the field of sleep research and sleep disorders medicine understand sleep paralysis to be characterized by conscious awareness in conjunction with temporary muscle atonia, occurring during sleep onset (hypnogogic) or sleep offset (hypnopompic). These are the essential features of the clinical phenotype. It may represent the product of a "dysregulation of the timing and consolidation of REM (rapid eye movement) sleep," as the authors have put it. Sleep paralysis is typically accompanied by a feeling of suffocation, fear (sometimes unto death), and often by hallucinations (across multiple sensory modes), including an alien presence of something sitting on one's chest ("incubus" and "succubus" have been used in ancient medicine to describe this alien presence). Sleep paralysis provides both a remarkable window into the functioning of the central nervous system, especially during transitions between sleep and wakefulness, as well as an opportunity to understand how it has grasped the human imagination for centuries. Drs. Sharpless and Doghramji tell a fascinating story, weaving a panorama of science and art.

Sleep Paralysis tells how different cultures over millennia have interpreted the phenomenon of sleep paralysis. Thus, many legends have been influenced by the experience of sleep paralysis, including themes of alien abduction and shadow people, malevolent presence, and mortal terror. Some cultures may be primed to experience sleep paralysis as a nocturnal smothering from a malevolent presence (succubus). The authors document many vivid depictions of sleep paralysis predating formal medical naming and diagnosis. Their excursions into fictional literature are particularly interesting, with rich citations from the work of such authors as Herman Melville, Guy de Maupassant, and F. Scott Fitzgerald. They also take the reader through early medicine, documenting debates over causes, health implications, and treatment of "nightmares." Throughout, the book is richly annotated with classical and scientific references, and with case studies from ancient and modern literature.

Sleep Paralysis provides a comprehensive description of current research into the epidemiology, pathophysiology, diagnosis, assessment, and treatment of the phenomenon. In clinical practice, sleep paralysis is usually not an isolated phenomenon and usually occurs in the context of other disorders, such as narcolepsy-cataplexy. The authors identify the need for accurate prevalence rates, especially for isolated sleep paralysis. They provide extensive description of its co-occurrence with a range of medical and psychopathological conditions, underscoring the need for more research into risk factors for sleep paralysis and how such risks are mediated. They conclude that as of now there is no accepted, integrated theory of etiology. Like many behavioral phenotypes, it would not be surprising to learn that its etiology is indeed heterogeneous and its response to interventions no less so.

The authors are superbly qualified to offer perspectives on contemporary clinical practice. They conclude that much work remains to be done to determine and validate the most appropriate diagnostic criteria (especially for isolated sleep paralysis). While acknowledging the lack of a current gold standard instrument, they provide a useful semi-structured interview for assessment, emphasizing that many disorders and symptoms can mimic sleep paralysis. After a discussion of folk remedies to prevent and disrupt sleep paralysis, the authors provide a review of evidence from contemporary intervention research. They conclude that there is no well-established pharmacological treatment of isolated sleep paralysis and that there are similarly limited outcome data from behavioral and psychosocial treatments. They provide an interesting approach to intervention embodied in cognitive behavioral psychotherapy. Throughout, as wise clinicians, the authors emphasize the need for careful clinical assessment and differential diagnosis as a prerequisite to intelligent intervention to help persons who experience distress and impairment from sleep paralysis, whether isolated or co-occurring with other disorders.

The reader comes away from this volume with a sense of surprise at what a tight grip on human imagination sleep paralysis has held for millennia. The literary and artistic explorations of sleep paralysis documented here are nothing short of amazing. At the same time, the opportunities for understanding the functioning of the brain, provided by sleep paralysis, are richly documented with appropriate attention to a multifaceted research agenda. We owe a debt of gratitude to Brian Sharpless and Karl Doghramji for their magnificent integration of humanistic and scientific medicine. Such integration is, sadly, all too rare these days, but is one of the many strengths of sleep research and sleep disorders medicine captured so elegantly in this compendium from two of our best exemplars of the scholarly, humanistic, and scientific clinician.

Charles F. Reynolds III, M.D.
UPMC Endowed Professor in Geriatric Psychiatry,
University of Pittsburgh
Past Chair, DSM-5 Sleep Wake Disorders Workgroup (2007–2013)

ACKNOWLEDGMENTS

We would both like to acknowledge our gratitude to Oxford University Press for their dedication to this project, and would especially like to thank David D'Addona, Sarah Harrington, Jean Lee, Courtney McCarroll, and Craig Panner for their help and support.

Brian A. Sharpless: I would like to express gratitude to my colleagues and students at Washington State University, the University of Pennsylvania, and Pennsylvania State University (you know who you are). Desmond Oathes, Matt Rothrock, Jamie Weaver, Jason Baker, the Wachters, Sandra Testa, Elinor Beck, Deborah Seagull, and F.Z. Moop all provided help, fun, friendship, and *indefatigable* support over the years that will always be remembered. I would also like to thank the numerous individuals with sleep paralysis who directly contributed to this volume. Last, but certainly not least, I would like to thank Karl Doghramji for helping to make this book a very fun project.

Karl Doghramji: My thanks to Brian Sharpless, for being such a wonderful co-author and a joy to work with; and to my patients whose lives are the subject of this work.

Sleep Paralysis

CHAPTER 1

What Are Sleep Paralysis and Isolated Sleep Paralysis?

SLEEP PARALYSIS IN CONTEXT

Since the first hominid opened its eyes in a start to realize that what it was experiencing was not actually "real," but instead immediately dissipated upon awakening, sleep and dreaming have been mysterious subjects. How can one explain the multitude of occurrences, both delightful and terrifying, that occur with the cessation of normal conscious activity that is the onset of sleep? Early humans must have been able to use their own subjective experiences to understand that the act of sleep is not only necessary for healthy functioning, but an indicator of overall health as well. Thus, disruptions to sleep, and especially anomalous experiences that *occurred during sleep*, would have been both noteworthy and important.

Indeed, sleep (both non–rapid eye movement [NREM] and rapid eye movement [REM] types) comprises two of the three fundamental states through which all human and mammalian brains regularly cycle. The other, wakefulness, is the state that can bring analytical reasoning to bear for the purpose of understanding the other two. Dreams occurring during REM sleep have possessed a particularly powerful draw for the waking mind, with many attempts to understand, interpret, and decode their secrets.

It is perhaps not surprising that sleep and dreaming have played large roles in myth and legend for thousands of years (viz., with written records of dreams dating back to early Sumerian [3100 B.C.]

writings). Some writers have gone so far as to claim that dreams, not being recognized as dreams, were core contributors to numerous religious and supernatural beliefs. For instance, the philosopher Thomas Hobbes claimed that, "From this ignorance of how to distinguish dreams, and other strong fancies, from vision and sense, did arise the greatest part of the religion of the gentiles in time past, that worshipped satyrs, fawns, nymphs, and the like; and now-a-days the opinion that rude people have of fairies, ghosts, and goblins, and of the power of witches" (Hobbes, 1929, p. 17). Although some may disagree with the broad scope of Hobbes' claim, the potential role of dreams in these matters would not be negligible. Placing oneself back into a pre-scientific worldview in which narratives of otherworldly and powerful beings hold sway, the power of dreams, and especially *vivid* dreams, is easy to comprehend.

Along with the ways in which dreams have been incorporated into various explanatory belief systems, efforts were also made to utilize dreams in more instrumental fashions. "Oneiromancy," or the systematic use of dreams as a means to divine the future or interpret the will of the gods, was found in many different times and places. Presumably, the vivid nature of dreams combined with their oftentimes fantastical and provocative contents prompted efforts to "decode" them. The result of these efforts was a number of functional (and not so functional) interpretations. Such interpretations held the potential to shape human and world events, and in fact did so. For example, both Alexander the Great and Hannibal Barca reportedly utilized their dreams to make military decisions (e.g., Livius, 1903; O'Brien, 1992). During the 13th century, Pope Innocent III had a dream in which he saw the Church of St. John Lateran collapsing upon itself. Right before destruction, a small peasant (viz., St. Francis) was seen holding it up, and straightening it (Nigg, 1975). This dream led the Pope to approve the Franciscan order. More recently, a dream of Adolf Hitler's during World War I (1917) resulted in him leaving the trench he was stationed in immediately before it was struck by a shell. The resulting explosion killed all of his comrades (Anderson, 1995). Clearly, history would be much different had these particular dream interpretations not occurred.

Thus, dreams can certainly be persuasive and influential. However, most dreamers are aware of the sharp disjuncture between these nocturnal events and their waking, conscious awareness. This may not be the case, however, when a person is experiencing the phenomenon of sleep paralysis.

WHAT IS SLEEP PARALYSIS?

Sleep paralysis is the experience of either falling asleep or waking up and finding oneself unable to move. With the exception of the eyes, no other voluntary muscle movements are possible during this state except for respiration. As demonstrated in subsequent chapters, the majority of sleep paralysis episodes are experienced as unpleasant, often harrowing ordeals that may eventuate in significant consequences for the unfortunate sufferer that may also persist beyond the cessation of paralysis.

Along with distress from unexpected atonia, the majority of sleep paralysis episodes are accompanied by hypnagogic (i.e., when falling asleep) or hypnopompic (i.e., when awakening) hallucinations (see chapter 6). These hallucinations typically consist of threatening presences and odd sensations that possess the subjective veracity of normal waking perception. Therefore, in sleep paralysis one has waking consciousness *alongside* the atonia and bizarre images of typical REM sleep. This combination of seemingly incompatible states of experience can be extremely disorienting, even in relatively healthy individuals. As discussed further in chapters 3 and 10, these fairly unique characteristics of sleep paralysis hold promise as a potentially naturalistic explanation for otherwise anomalous beliefs in fantastical creatures and paranormal situations across different times and cultures. Indeed, several current (and fairly widespread) paranormal beliefs in the 21st century Western world may be associated with sleep paralysis (e.g., abductions by extraterrestrial aliens, shadow people).

In spite of the provocative ways in which the associated features of sleep paralysis manifest, it is a relatively well-described, REM-based biological phenomenon. These aspects are noted in chapters 6 and 10. However, in spite of these biological underpinnings, a number of psychological, behavioral, and cultural factors may be responsible for making sleep paralysis more likely to occur. These same factors bear relevance for the particular manner in which episodes are subjectively experienced, interpreted, and potentially treated.

SLEEP PARALYSIS, ISOLATED SLEEP PARALYSIS, AND FEARFUL ISOLATED SLEEP PARALYSIS

Sleep paralysis is commonly found in several medical conditions. For instance, episodes of sleep paralysis, along with excessive daytime sleepiness, cataplexy, and hypnagogic hallucinations, comprise what is often termed the "narcoleptic tetrad." Thus, it is often prudent to follow up patient complaints of sleep paralysis with additional questions in order to determine whether or not the patient is suffering from undiagnosed narcolepsy. Sleep paralysis can also be triggered by acute intoxication from a variety of substances (e.g., alcohol), hypokalemia (i.e., low serum potassium levels), or as a side effect of withdrawal from certain prescribed medications (e.g., selective serotonin reuptake inhibitors, tricyclic antidepressants, benzodiazepines).

When sleep paralysis occurs in the absence of medical/situational conditions, or when it is not better accounted for by the presence of another disorder (e.g., a seizure or another sleep disorder), it is customarily termed "isolated sleep paralysis." A subtype of isolated sleep paralysis has also been proposed recently (Sharpless et al., 2010). Specifically, when isolated sleep paralysis is accompanied by clinically significant levels of distress and/or fear, it is termed "fearful isolated sleep paralysis" (see chapters 6 and 11).

SLEEP PARALYSIS IN CONTEMPORARY DIAGNOSTIC SYSTEMS

Although isolated sleep paralysis can be coded in current diagnostic schemes, its prominence varies widely according to the specific system. In most recent cases, it has been classified as a *parasomnia*.

The term "parasomnia" derives from the Greek prefix *para* (alongside of) and the Latin word *somnus* (sleep). Thus, parasomnias can be broadly defined as unwanted and/or distressing events/experiences that occur during, after, or upon entry into sleep (*International Classification of Sleep Disorders* [ICSD]—3rd ed. [American Academy of Sleep Medicine, 2014]). They often consist of experiences resulting from some degree of overlap between the various sleep states. Two major classification systems, the *Diagnostic and Statistical Manual of Mental Disorders* (DSM-4, American Psychiatric Association, 2000) and the *International Classification of Diseases* (ICD-10 World Health Organization, 2008), neither agree on the number nor the specific sorting of the parasomnias.

The DSM-4-TR (American Psychiatric Association, 2000) has the fewest entries, and only includes a total of four potential parasomnia diagnoses (i.e., sleepwalking, sleep terrors, nightmare disorder, and parasomnia not otherwise specified). In contrast, the ICD-10 (World Health Organization, 2008) includes a total of 10 diagnostic choices delineated into three categories. Specifically, there are 1) disorders of arousal (from NREM sleep) such as sleep terrors, 2) parasomnias usually associated with REM sleep such as nightmare disorder, and 3) a group of other parasomnias such as exploding head syndrome and sleep enuresis. The ICSD-2 (American Academy of Sleep Medicine, 2005) contains the same tripartite classification as ICD-10.

Regarding DSM-IV-TR (American Psychiatric Association, 2000), no individual code exists for isolated sleep paralysis. Instead, this phenomenon, along with diagnoses such as REM sleep behavior disorder, can only be documented as a "parasomnia not otherwise specified" (code 307.47). Diagnostic criteria are unfortunately quite vague. In ICD-10 (World Health Organization, 2008), recurrent isolated sleep paralysis is a codable entity (G47.53) found in the "parasomnias usually associated with REM sleep" group.

In the newly released DSM-5 (American Psychiatric Association, 2013) and ICSD-3 (American Academy of Sleep Medicine, 2014) manuals, the sleep disorders have been renamed as the "sleep–wake disorders." Regarding the former, a number of modifications to the previous DSM-IV diagnoses were made that are not discussed further here. Interestingly, sleep paralysis is not mentioned in this diagnostic module at all. It is neither assigned a specific diagnostic code nor retained in the criteria for narcolepsy. A patient suffering from clinically significant isolated sleep paralysis would now be diagnosed with "other specified sleep–wake disorder" (code 307.49) or "unspecified sleep–wake disorder" (code 307.40). As for the new ICSD, the category of recurrent isolated sleep paralysis has been retained (G47.51), but has been modified to require clinically significant distress (see chapter 11).

STRUCTURE

Throughout the remainder of this book we justify our belief in the importance of sleep paralysis using several contemporary intellectual perspectives (e.g., history, folklore, psychology, and medicine). Specifically, we first situate the phenomenon of sleep paralysis in broad historical contexts, and find that it had a prominent role to play not only in mythology, art, and literature, but in early medicine as well. We find that sleep paralysis was the original *Nightmare*, and quite different from the scary, but somewhat weak and anemic "scary dream" that this word connotes today (e.g., Sharpless, 2014).

Second, we synthesize the available empirical literatures on isolated sleep paralysis for such topics as prevalence, associated features, and the known relations to other forms of pathology. Building upon these foundations, we then review and critically evaluate the many etiological theories that have been proposed.

Third, the clinical aspects of isolated sleep paralysis are discussed. Specifically, we summarize the difficulties one faces when assessing isolated sleep paralysis, and provide information we view as critical for accurate differential diagnosis. Next, data on the treatment of chronic cases of isolated sleep paralysis are reviewed, and are shown to be quite limited. However, we end this monograph by describing a new psychosocial treatment for clinically significant cases of isolated sleep paralysis (viz., a brief cognitive behavioral approach) and also provide tentative medication guidance for clinicians interested in working with these individuals. Finally, we provide an adherence measure for our proposed treatment for use in research settings.

REFERENCES

American Academy of Sleep Medicine. (2005). *International classification of sleep disorders: Diagnostic & coding manual* (2nd ed.). Darien, IL: American Academy of Sleep Medicine.

American Academy of Sleep Medicine. (2014). *International classification of sleep disorders: Diagnostic and coding manual* (3rd ed.). Darien, IL: American Academy of Sleep Medicine.

American Psychiatric Association. (2000). *Diagnostic and statistical manual of mental disorders: DSM-IV-TR* (4th text rev. ed.). Washington, DC: American Psychiatric Association.

American Psychiatric Association. (2013). *Diagnostic and statistical manual of mental disorders* (5th ed.). Arlington, VA: American Psychiatric Association.

Anderson, K. (1995). *Hitler and the occult*. Amherst, NY: Prometheus Books.

Hobbes, T. (1929). *The leviathan*. London: Oxford University Press.

Livius, T. (1903). *The history of Rome, Volume 2*. (D. Spillan, C. Edmunds Trans.). London: Geoge Bell and Sons.

Nigg, W. (1975). *Francis of Assisi* (W. Neil Trans.). Oxford, UK: Franciscan Herald Press.

O'Brien, J. M. (1992). *Alexander the Great: The invisible enemy*. London: Routledge.

Sharpless, B. A. (2014). Changing conceptions of the nightmare in medicine. *Hektoen International: A Journal of Medical Humanities (Moments in History Section)*, Retrieved from: http://www.hektoeninternational.org.

Sharpless, B. A., McCarthy, K. S., Chambless, D. L., Milrod, B. L., Khalsa, S. R., & Barber, J. P. (2010). Isolated sleep paralysis and fearful isolated sleep paralysis in outpatients with panic attacks. *Journal of Clinical Psychology, 66*(12), 1292–1306. doi: 10.1002/jclp.20724; 10.1002/jclp.20724

World Health Organization. (2008). *International statistical classification of diseases and related health problems* (10th rev. ed.). New York: World Health Organization.

CHAPTER 2

Should Sleep Paralysis Be More Frequently Assessed in Research Studies and Clinical Practice?

The enjoyment of comfortable and undisturbed sleep is certainly to be ranked amongst the greatest blessings which heaven has bestowed on mankind; and it may be considered as one of the best criterions of a person enjoying perfect health.
—John Waller, 1816

As described in chapter 1, sleep paralysis is a relatively well-known phenomenon. Not only sleep experts, but also cross-cultural researchers and folklorists are interested in this experience. A literature base has begun to develop in all of these specialties, and several cross-discipline books have been published (e.g., Adler, 2011; Hufford, 1982). Sleep paralysis has also periodically captured the attention of the lay public through popular press articles and television documentaries. This is perhaps not surprising given the provocative nature of its paradigmatic symptoms (i.e., paralysis and associated hallucinations) and frequent connections to the paranormal. However, in spite of the preceding, sleep paralysis is not typically assessed in most forms of clinical practice. Even in research studies there is relatively little consideration of this phenomenon unless sleep paralysis is the actual focus of investigation.

A number of factors likely contribute to this state of affairs. For instance, there may be a general lack of awareness of sleep paralysis and how it specifically manifests in patients. In fact, sleep paralysis is not mentioned in the sleep disorder sections of many abnormal psychology textbooks.

Further, in countries such as the United States and Canada where the DSM-5 (American Psychiatric Association, 2013) is widely used, some may not know that recurrent and problematic isolated sleep paralysis can be coded as an "unspecified sleep–wake disorder" or that "recurrent isolated sleep paralysis" is an actual code in the ICD-10 (World Health Organization, 2008) and ICSD-3 (American Academy of Sleep Medicine, 2014). And whereas there are resources available to facilitate diagnosis (see chapter 12), modules for the assessment of sleep paralysis are not found in the major structured diagnostic interviews for Axis-I disorders (e.g., *Structured Clinical Interview for DSM-5*, First, Williams, Karg, & Spitzer, in press; the *Anxiety and Related Disorders Interview Schedule*, ADIS, Brown & Barlow, 2014).

Therefore, it is easily possible that one could conduct a multi-hour interview with a patient and never be prompted to assess for sleep paralysis or, for that matter, many other specific types of sleep disturbance. This lack of attention raises an important question: Should sleep paralysis be more routinely assessed? Given the practical fact that time with patients is always limited, and also the fact that there are ever-increasing pressures to condense the intake process, this is certainly a reasonable question. As demonstrated in the following and in subsequent chapters, however, there appear to be a number of compelling reasons that warrant an increased frequency of assessment.

SLEEP PARALYSIS HAS HIGHER THAN EXPECTED PREVALENCE RATES

One important reason that warrants an increased frequency of assessment is that sleep paralysis is more common than many researchers and clinicians may think. The latest research indicates that sleep paralysis is not a rare event (see chapter 7). Although lifetime prevalence rates for the general population are less than 8%, much higher rates are found among students, with the highest rates found in psychiatric patients. Reasons for these disparities in prevalence are being slowly elucidated, as are the relationships among sleep paralysis, culture, ethnicity, medical conditions, and certain psychiatric diagnoses.

Sleep paralysis may not be limited to humans. The first author witnessed an episode of apparent sleep paralysis in a six-year-old, purebred Staffordshire terrier. The dog was prescribed 50 mg of diphenhydramine (Benadryl) by his veterinarian and, perhaps not surprisingly, experienced a side effect of drowsiness. At one point his eyes suddenly opened and began darting around the room, seemingly in an acute state of fear. His owner and the writer went to check on him and found that he was unable to move despite several efforts on their part. The paralysis lasted approximately four minutes, and was quite upsetting to the terrier. This happened multiple times during the course of treatment.

SLEEP PARALYSIS IS ASSOCIATED WITH OTHER MEDICAL CONDITIONS

Routine assessment of sleep paralysis may also prompt clinicians to assess for associated, and often more serious, neuropsychiatric conditions. Although most practitioners would thoroughly assess for the presence of narcolepsy upon disclosure of sleep paralysis episodes, assessing for other conditions may be less automatic and ingrained. For instance, sleep paralysis may also occur in the context of seizure disorders and substance abuse.

SLEEP PARALYSIS MAY BEAR A RELATIONSHIP TO CERTAIN TYPES OF PSYCHOPATHOLOGY

Sleep paralysis is also important to our basic knowledge of psychopathology. Although it is well known to occur in the context of the medical conditions noted in the preceding section, sleep paralysis has also been found to be associated with specific symptoms (e.g., anxiety sensitivity), certain psychiatric diagnoses (e.g., post-traumatic stress disorder), and with higher levels of psychiatric comorbidity (as reviewed in chapters 8 and 9). Although sleep disturbances in general have been shown to increase the risk for other physical and mental ailments (e.g., Ford & Kamerow, 1989), the causal sequence and specific nature of these relationships between sleep paralysis and other disorders have yet to be clarified. The implications (treatment or otherwise) for patients who experience sleep paralysis in the context of these more well-known conditions is similarly unclear. Therefore, a great deal of information about psychopathology may result from more thorough explorations of these relationships. Knowledge about etiology, common pathways to the expression of distress, and possibly even treatment recommendations could result from such endeavors.

SLEEP PARALYSIS, IN SOME CASES, MAY BE CONSIDERED TO BE A FORM OF PSYCHOPATHOLOGY

The study of sleep paralysis also possesses relevance for psychopathology in a more direct manner. Namely, the distressing nature of sleep paralysis episodes (e.g., fear from atonia and hallucinations plus their idiosyncratic appraisals) potentially places it within the realm of psychopathology. Although this has not yet received much empirical attention, limited data indicate that a minority of individuals (especially those with psychiatric conditions) can experience repetitive and problematic episodes of sleep paralysis (see chapter 6). As it is so rarely assessed in clinical settings, the ultimate extent of these more severe cases of sleep paralysis is unclear.

However, additional evidence of distress and impairment can be found in the cross-cultural literatures. It seems noteworthy that the peculiar and distressing nature of sleep paralysis phenomena prompted various attempts at treatment across time, place, and culture (see chapter 14). The ubiquity of these treatment attempts, some of them quite elaborate, makes it fairly unlikely that sleep paralysis was viewed as a benign or superfluous event. On the contrary, this folk psychological evidence of the troubling nature of sleep paralysis, albeit indirect, is consistent with empirical findings.

TREATMENTS FOR SLEEP PARALYSIS ARE NOT CURRENTLY WELL ARTICULATED

Sleep paralysis may impact on functioning and health in a number of negative ways, and these vary markedly from patient to patient. Treatment approaches are neither clearly described nor, apart from psychopharmacology, readily available to most individuals. Thus, at the present time there are relatively few options available in a practitioner's armamentarium for those individuals suffering from more severe and recurrent cases of sleep paralysis.

SLEEP PARALYSIS POSSESSES CULTURAL IMPORTANCE

Sleep paralysis as a rapid eye movement (REM)–based biological phenomenon does not appear to be "bound" to any particular culture or ethnicity, but rates among groups can and do differ (see chapter 7). Although all evidence points to it being a fairly universal occurrence, culture seems to impact the ways in which sleep paralysis episodes are described, understood, and rationalized. We and others would argue that the particular appraisal of sleep paralysis (especially the atonia, fear, and hallucinations), as well as the subsequent cultural elaboration of these appraisals, possess more than just a passing historical interest. In contrast to many other symptoms and disorders, these elaborate cultural/historical backdrops have been important foci for many of the sustained discussions of sleep paralysis (e.g., Hufford, 1982). Specifically, one of the most interesting aspects of sleep paralysis is its potential role as a naturalistic explanation for certain supernatural and paranormal beliefs. Many aspects of these beliefs bear a striking resemblance to sleep paralysis phenomena (see chapter 3). Regardless, given the multitude of interpretations that have been overlaid onto sleep paralysis, the study of these various interpretations may yield important information about particular cultures and their concerns.

Therefore, it seems reasonable to conclude that these sleep paralysis interpretations can, in effect, be treated as cultural "artifacts." Artifacts in this sense are objects or ideas that, when properly embedded in their historical/cultural context, can transmit information about that context (e.g., Cushman, 1996). Although all of psychopathology and nosology could conceivably be considered in this manner, the ambiguous nature of the sleep paralysis experience makes it a particularly good resource. Thus, the study of these—for lack of a better term—"projective" aspects of sleep paralysis, could potentially serve as a vehicle to important cross-cultural knowledge.

ASSESSING FOR SLEEP PARALYSIS MAY AVOID MISDIAGNOSIS AND OVERPATHOLOGIZING

Not considering sleep paralysis as a clinical possibility may eventuate in misdiagnosis, and in some cases may lead assessors to overestimate a patient's level of illness. These possibilities are most easy to envision when patients present in either a state of acute distress or if a cultural disconnect between patient and assessor is present.

It is well known that patients often seek treatment in the wake of upsetting life events or the intensifications of already-existing symptomatology. In the specific case of sleep paralysis, a patient may arrive at a hospital emergency department or therapist's office in a very agitated state. When this agitated individual begins to describe seemingly supernatural or paranormal events to a provider (e.g., believing that he or she was vertically levitated by a "tractor beam" or suffocated by a small, malevolent being), it is easy to see how these descriptions could be misconstrued as either the result of substance abuse or evidence of a recent psychotic break. Although hopefully uncommon, cases such as these have been described in the literature (e.g., Douglass, Hays, Pazderka, & Russell, 1991; Gangdev, 2004; Shapiro & Spitz, 1976). Complicating this already murky picture is the fact that realistic sleep paralysis hallucinations can occur during the day when the patient is either napping or more generally sleepy. Without a relatively thorough history taking and/or a broader assessment of reality testing, misdiagnosis could result (also see chapter 13).

Some (e.g., de Jong, 2005) have speculated that misinterpretations of sleep paralysis episodes may result in false allegations of sexual abuse. Although no thoroughly verified cases of this were found in our litera- ture review, Hays (1992) and Stein, Solvason, Biggart, and Spiegel (1996) noted several case studies that are consistent with this possibility. As described in more detail in chapter 6, one of the three common hallucina- tions (i.e., the incubus subtype) involves feeling as if someone (or some- thing) is on top of you and placing pressure on your chest. This "entity" is commonly experienced as tearing/clawing at your clothing, and may even force unwanted sexual acts upon you. The vividness of these hallucinatory experiences could conceivably lead a person to attribute real-world verac- ity to this imaginal episode, especially if the person is already troubled in other ways (e.g., existing psychosis or certain personality disorder traits). In general, the comorbidity of sleep paralysis episodes with any psychotic disorder may confuse the overall symptomatic picture if they are not rec- ognized as distinct conditions (Gangdev, 2006).

When working with individuals from different cultures, there may exist baseline tendencies to either overestimate or underestimate pathol- ogy (e.g., Gray-Little, 2009). Given its oftentimes provocative expression and the heterogeneity of cultural elaboration, *overestimation* appears to be more likely with sleep paralysis. One need look no further than the panic disorder literature to view another example in which cultural presenta- tions of specific symptoms may result in misestimates of psychopathol- ogy. For example, patients from Nigeria often report an unusual (from a Westerner's standpoint) interoceptive sensation when experiencing anxi- ety, depression, or panic attacks. Their acute distress is often reported as feeling as if parasites or ants are moving under the skin or "in the head" (Paniagua, 2000). This sensation is also found in a culture-bound syn- drome called *Ode Ori*. Such presentations of panic are clearly much rarer in the West, and may be misconstrued as incipient psychosis. This actual scenario arose a few years ago when the first author supervised a graduate student diagnostician. The patient was a Nigerian man in his early twenties, and during the initial administration of the ADIS the patient described periods of intense anxiety and the *Ode Ori* symptoms mentioned in the preceding. As the patient's age fell within the range that psychotic symptoms often first manifest in males, it was necessary to spend time disentangling cultural elaborations of distress from potential psychotic phenomena. Given the heterogeneity of cultural expressions (some of which may involve the activities of ghosts and witches), a diagnostician confronted with sleep paralysis could be similarly tempted to attribute greater levels of psychopathology than would be warranted. And, clearly, treatment recommendations would be radically different depending upon the specific case conceptualization (i.e., reassurance and psychoeducation vs. antipsychotic medications and supportive therapy).

ASSESSMENT OF SLEEP PARALYSIS MAY NORMALIZE A POTENTIALLY FRIGHTENING EXPERIENCE

Although the majority of reasons described so far have focused on the *avoidance* of negative and potentially harmful outcomes such as misdiagnosis, there are also positive reasons to assess sleep paralysis. Persons who experience sleep paralysis are often quite confused by the episodes. For many (especially those who experience vivid and disturbing hallucinations), a fear may exist that they are losing contact with reality, having a "breakdown," "going crazy," or are otherwise "abnormal" (e.g., Neal, Rich, & Smucker, 1994). Some may be so troubled that they do not disclose the event to family or friends, and are left to wonder alone about the ramifications this experience might have for their lives and mental health.

These fears can often be allayed through a frank (and non–jargon-based) discussion and colloquial demystification of the phenomenon with a concerned professional. The very act of screening for sleep paralysis often results in feelings of relief (e.g., Otto et al., 2006; Sharpless et al., 2010). As one example, when conducting an intake interview with a nervous 56-year-old woman presenting with a lengthy trauma history, administration of sleep paralysis screening questions visibly impacted her. The patient's reaction was initially one of surprise, and when she came to understand that sleep paralysis was not a purely idiosyncratic experience, her mood visibly brightened. She then proceeded to ask a number of follow-up questions and was much more relaxed throughout the remainder of the interview. In many cases both relief and a strengthening of the therapeutic alliance are the immediate results of these discussions.

CONCLUSIONS

In closing, a great deal about sleep paralysis remains unknown. However, a research base is developing that indicates that, at least in certain cases and contexts, there is a strong justification for assessing it more frequently in both clinical and research settings. The next chapter presents the historical precursors to our current understanding of sleep paralysis.

REFERENCES

Adler, S. (2011). *Sleep paralysis: Night-mares, nocebos, and the mind-body connection.* Newark, NJ: Rutgers University Press.

American Academy of Sleep Medicine. (2014). *International classification of sleep disorders: Diagnostic and coding manual* (3rd ed.). Darien, IL: American Academy of Sleep Medicine.

American Psychiatric Association. (2013). *Diagnostic and statistical manual of mental disorders* (5th ed.). Arlington, VA: American Psychiatric Association.

Brown, T. A., & Barlow, D. H. (2014). *Anxiety and related disorders inverview schedule for DSM-5: Lifetime version.* New York: Oxford University Press.

Cushman, P. (1996). *Constructing the self, constructing America: A cultural history of psychotherapy.* Boston: Da Capo Press.

de Jong, J. T. V. M. (2005). Cultural variation in the clinical presentation of sleep paralysis. *Transcultural Psychiatry, 42*(1), 78–92. doi: 10.1177/1363461505050711

Douglass, A. B., Hays, P., Pazderka, F., & Russell, J. M. (1991). Florid refractory schizophrenias that turn out to be treatable variants of HLA-associated narcolepsy. *The Journal of Nervous and Mental Disease, 179*(1), 12–17.

First, M. B., Williams, J. B. W., Karg, R. S., & Spitzer, R. L. (in press). *Structured clinical interview for DSM-5 disorders: Patient edition.* New York: Biometrics Research Department.

Ford, D. E., & Kamerow, D. B. (1989). Epidemiologic study of sleep disturbances and psychiatric disorders: An opportunity for prevention? *Journal of the American Medical Association, 262*(11), 1479–1484.

Gangdev, P. (2004). Relevance of sleep paralysis and hypnic hallucinations to psychiatry. *Australasian Psychiatry, 12*(1), 77–80. doi: 10.1046/j.1039-8562.2003.02065.x

Gangdev, P. (2006). Comments on sleep paralysis. *Transcultural Psychiatry, 43*(4), 692–694. doi: 10.1177/1363461506066992

Gray-Little, B. (2009). The assessment of psychopathology in racial and ethnic minorities. In J. N. Butcher (Ed.), *Oxford handbook of personality assessment* (pp. 396–414). New York: Oxford University Press.

Hays, P. (1992). False but sincere allegations of sexual assault made by narcotic patients. *The Medico-Legal Journal, 60*(4), 265–271.

Hufford, D. (1982). *The terror that comes in the night: An experience-centered study of supernatural assault traditions.* Philadelphia: University of Pennsylvania Press.

Neal, A. M., Rich, L. N., & Smucker, W. D. (1994). The presence of panic disorder among African American hypertensives: A pilot study. *Journal of Black Psychology, 20*(1), 29–35.

Otto, M. W., Simon, N. M., Powers, M., Hinton, D., Zalta, A. K., & Pollack, M. H. (2006). Rates of isolated sleep paralysis in outpatients with anxiety disorders. *Journal of Anxiety Disorders, 20*(5), 687–693. doi: 10.1016/j.janxdis.2005.07.002

Paniagua, F. A. (2000). Culture-bound syndromes, cultural variations, and psychopathology. In I. Cuellar, & F. A. Paniagua (Eds.), *Handbook of multicultural health* (p. 142). San Diego: Academic Press.

Shapiro, B., & Spitz, H. (1976). Problems in the differentiatial diagnosis of schizophrenia. *American Journal of Psychiatry, 133*(11), 1321–1323.

Sharpless, B. A., McCarthy, K. S., Chambless, D. L., Milrod, B. L., Khalsa, S., & Barber, J. P. (2010). Isolated sleep paralysis and fearful isolated sleep paralysis in outpatients with panic attacks. *Journal of Clinical Psychology, 66*(12), 1292–1306. doi: 10.1002/jclp.20724

Stein, S. L., Solvason, H. B., Biggart, E., & Spiegel, D. A. (1996). A 25-year-old woman with hallucinations, hypersexuality, nightmares, and a rash. *American Journal of Psychiatry, 153*, 545–551.

World Health Organization. (2008). *International statistical classification of diseases and related health problems* (10th rev. ed.). New York: World Health Organization.

CHAPTER 3

The History of Sleep Paralysis in Folklore and Myth

... I going well to bed, about the dead of the night felt a great weight upon my breast, and awakening, looked, and it being bright moonlight, did clearly see Bridget Bishop, or her likeness, sitting upon my stomach. And putting my arms off of the bed to free myself from that great oppression, she presently laid hold of my throat and almost choked me. And I had no strength or power in my hands to resist or help myself. And in this condition she held me to almost day.

     —John Londer, June 1692 (as cited in Boyer & Nissenbaum, 1993)

It happened right after my grandmother died. I slept in my parents' room that night on the floor. I started hearing loud noises, like Times Square. I opened my eyes, and then I didn't see anything, but just heard noise and I couldn't move. Then I felt a pressure on me, and something was around my neck, strangling me. I started praying to get out of it. It seemed to help.

     —Female student interviewed by first author, October 2012

SLEEP PARALYSIS IN FOLKLORE

Though separated by 320 years, these two vignettes display some of the more consistent and paradigmatic aspects of sleep paralysis. They are particularly good examples of what has been termed the "Nightmare" (e.g., Jones, 1949) or, more recently, the "incubus" subtype of the phenomenon (Cheyne, Rueffer, & Newby-Clark, 1999). The overwhelming senses of fear, vulnerability, and powerlessness are clearly apparent in both. Further, the vividness of these descriptions, especially the first, make it easy to understand how sleep paralysis hallucinations could be misinterpreted as "real-world" nocturnal assaults if neurological and psychological explanations are not kept in mind. However, as described in the following pages, interpretations of sleep paralysis have not been limited to attacks by *human* agents. In fact, the paranormal and/or supernatural attributions of this phenomenon appear to be much more prevalent throughout recorded history, and these interpretations are also what attract attention from the lay public (e.g., Zakin & Grant, 2012; MacKinnon, 2013).

The true scope of sleep paralysis can be seen in appendix A. Here, we have collected 118 terms from around the world and from numerous languages and cultures. Very few come from the scientific literatures; instead, the majority was derived from collections of "folk" understandings and narratives. These terms range widely in age, from ancient Greece to the contemporary West.

Several patterns in the appendix are noteworthy. In general, we were struck by the strong convergence of the descriptions across time and place. This likely speaks to some degree of cultural invariance for sleep paralysis phenomena. For instance (and in line with both vignettes), the sense of fear/dread evinced by the events is fairly universal, and none of the terms listed in the appendix is associated with pleasant feelings. However, a number do indeed appear to be influenced by culture-specific content. Many also denote a sense of pressure or crushing on the body. The particular "crusher," however, varies widely (e.g., from China's "ghost oppression" to Roman Italy's incubus/succubus). Some cultures see the "oppressors" as common animals from their environment (e.g., black sheep, birds, dogs), whereas others envision shape-shifting humans, incorporeal spirits, malevolent demons, and other supernatural entities. As discussed at length in chapter 6, the sensed (or sometimes actually seen and felt) presence appears to be a key sleep paralysis hallucination with at least some neurological substrata. This does not mean, however, that biological explanations alone are sufficient to exhaust the full range of sleep paralysis phenomena.

Indeed, for much of history most cultures lacked what might be termed a *scientific* understanding of sleep and sleep disorders. As a result, they not surprisingly relied upon other available explanatory categories (i.e., paranormal/supernatural/godlike, or otherwise) and folk psychology. The very fact that these experiences were named and written down speaks to the cultural and personal importance that they held regardless of time and locale.

The geographic, temporal, and cultural gulf between the sources of these indigenous terms (i.e., ranging from Iceland to Laos) appears to argue against mere cultural transmission as an explanation for sleep paralysis's pervasiveness. From our perspective, a more likely conceptualization would be that the common root experiences found in sleep paralysis episodes are universally human. Though prevalence rates do vary somewhat according to group, we are not aware of any evidence that sleep paralysis is not universal. Further, although these root experiences have at least a partially biological basis, the causality of sleep paralysis *as an experience* appears to be complex. For instance, did sleep paralysis create these cultural narratives, eventually leading to subsequent cultural "embellishments" for the basic experience, or did pre-existing cultural narratives instead serve to make sleep paralysis more likely to occur, or to occur in a particular (and culturally understandable) way? These questions have yet to be sufficiently answered.

Thus, there appear to be three distinct, yet interacting contributions to the experience of sleep paralysis. First, there is a root neurological basis in terms of the paralysis itself and the tendency toward vivid hallucinations. By themselves, both of these roots may be fairly ambiguous, and therefore allow for varied interpretations and understandings, be they catastrophic or otherwise. Second, the person experiencing the sleep paralysis is situated in a particular time, place, and context. They can therefore avail themselves of the predominant social narratives and cultural constructs. For example, is the sensed presence more likely to be a technologically advanced extraterrestrial, a black and hairy bat from an unknown part of the jungle, or a malevolent demon bent upon physical and spiritual corruption? In other words, what particular flavor of the scary and unknown was bequeathed to you by virtue of birth and chance? Third, personal contributions are also important. These would consist of such things as idiosyncratic appraisals, personal beliefs at variance with society, and possibly recent and meaningful real-life experiences (i.e., what was termed the day's "residue" by Freud [1953]; see also Cipolli, Bolzani, Tuozzi, & Fagioli, 2001). We would argue that a full understanding of the experience of sleep paralysis for any particular individual requires understanding at all three of these levels.

However, understanding sleep paralysis at the second level (viz., time, place, and context/culture) is even more challenging. As mentioned, the causality is difficult, if not impossible, to discern. Are sleep paralysis hallucinations *the cause* of the predominant beliefs of a particular group of people, or do the pre-existing beliefs actually influence the particular manifestation of the hallucinations? In all likelihood a to-and-fro movement between sleep paralysis experience as a *part*, and the culture as *whole* (what could be termed a "hermeneutic circle" as in Gadamer, 1975) occurred and served to mutually influence one another.

As demonstrated in what follows, there are a number of relevant supernatural beliefs that appear to arise in particular societal contexts. Along with the already mentioned difficulties of causality, fully tracing out the connections between sleep paralysis and supernatural beliefs is likely impossible given the paucity of source material and other difficulties inherent in the historical analysis of ancient phenomena. However, we should preface the next section with another important caveat. Namely, we are not claiming that sleep paralysis is, in effect, the proto-cause of all of the various mythological beliefs we are about to describe. This would be going well beyond the bounds of available historical evidence and a gross oversimplification of a clearly multi-determinant process. We hope to make the much smaller claim that sleep paralysis likely played an important part in the genesis, maintenance, and/or elaboration of these beliefs. This is particularly the case with the hallucinatory content of sleep paralysis and the effects of these experiences on the pre-scientific mind.

SLEEP PARALYSIS AND THE "NIGHTMARE"

When reading literature relevant to the history of sleep paralysis, the terminology can become confusing. For although the term "sleep paralysis" was coined almost two centuries ago, a perusal of appendix A demonstrates that the experience of sleep paralysis is far older (e.g., ancient Greece's *ephialtes*), and predates its formal medical naming. Further adding to this complexity is the fact that the most common term, "the Nightmare," carries a definition quite different from colloquial English. Whereas a "nightmare" typically denotes a scary or disturbing dream, a "Nightmare" is much more specific (Sharpless, 2014). As eloquently described by Macnish (1834):

> They are a thousand times more frightful than the visions conjured up by necromancy or diablerie; and far transcend everything in history or romance, from the fable of the writhing and asp-encircled Laocoon to Dante's appalling picture of Ugolino and his famished offspring, or the hidden tortures of the Spanish Inquisition. The whole mind, during the paroxysm, is wrought up to a pitch of unutterable despair; a spell is laid upon the faculties, which freezes them into inaction; and the wretched victim feels as if pent alive in his coffin, or overpowered by resistless and unmitigable pressure .... Everything horrible, disgusting or terrific in the physical or moral world, is brought before him in fearful array; he is hissed at by serpents, tortured by demons, stunned by the hollow voices and cold touch of apparitions .... (pp. 122–123)

Clearly, this is not merely a scary dream.

In Jones' sustained discussion of the Nightmare (from a primarily psychoanalytic perspective), he derived its three cardinal features from cases found in the historical record (Jones, 1949). First, he noted the sense of overwhelming *angst* experienced by the sufferer. Our English term "anxiety" inadequately conveys the intensity and sense of dread found in the German term. *Angst* more accurately implies a more direct threat of non-being than our colloquial sense of "anxiety" or "anxious apprehension." Second, Nightmares always include the sensation of weight or some other form of pressure on the sufferer's chest. This sense of physical oppression is also associated with difficulties breathing and smothering feelings. Third, Nightmares include the sensation of paralysis. Given the fact that most Nightmares occur when a person is in the supine position (and also given the fact that people are rarely as vulnerable as when they are sleeping), this paralysis engenders feelings of profound helplessness. Haga (1989) notes that the risk of *mara* (i.e., a ghost that rides humans and animals) increases when one sleeps in a supine position. As discussed in the next chapter, only the third of these features is necessary for a sleep paralysis diagnosis. Thus, the Nightmare in Jones' sense of the term could best be considered a vivid and particularly frightening subtype.

Golther (1895, as cited in Jones, 1949, p. 74) proposed that the Nightmare was an originator of beliefs in a soul. He states that "the belief in the soul rests in great part on the conception of torturing and oppressive spirits. Only as a gradual extension of this did the belief arise in spirits that displayed other activities than torturing and oppressing. In the first place, however, the belief in spirits took its origin in the Nightmare." The Nightmare in this sense was an independently existing "night-fiend" with malicious intent that was physically responsible for these terrible ordeals. As time went on, the original meaning of the term became lost, and Nightmares became synonymous with the "dreams" themselves (i.e., nightmares) rather than being viewed as the causal agents of the experiences (Jones, 1949).

One may wonder about the links, if any, between Nightmares and actual horses. The famous painting by Fuseli (1781) clearly connects the two, but the parallels seem loose at best. Although it is beyond the scope of this chapter to go into too much etymological detail (the interested reader is directed to Davies, 2003 and Jones, 1949), mention should be made of this interesting issue on at least three different fronts. First, there is the term "*mare*" itself. It is believed to be of Indo-European origin, but scholars disagree on its original meaning (Davies, 2003). Nightmare has been linked to the German terms *nacht* for night and *mara* for incubus/ crusher. But what is the connection between *mara* and mare? Of course, the similarity in sound and appearance of the terms is apparent. However, Jones (1949) noted a number of myths that link the two more directly. For instance, numerous classical tales involve humans/gods metamorphosing into horses and tormenting others. There is also an idea contained in the Nightmare of being "ridden" by a spirit/witch/demon. This experience of oppression has been likened to having horse hooves on the chest. More generally, the logic of mythology appears to be fluid with regard to *riding* and *being ridden*. This inversion of meaning could easily lead to such a connection.

Second, there previously existed a belief that horses manifesting odd behaviors (e.g., sweating, anxiety attacks) were themselves likely visited by a Nightmare in the form of a horse, human being, or spirit. Thus, they were not only potentially Nightmares themselves, but could be *victims* of them as well. It was also thought that horses could be exhausted just like humans, or could even be ridden to death by one of these spiritual entities.

Finally, according to Jones (1949), it was widely believed that a horse's head could actually *prevent* a Nightmare's attack. Thus, putting these links together, horses could be Nightmares themselves, victims of Nightmares, or used to protect people from Nightmares. Given humans' dependence on the horse for much of human history (especially in the Old World), these links become easier to understand. One also must wonder if the real physical danger from a horse stumbling/falling could have been an early, and very literal, simile for the fear and oppression so characteristic of the experience of Nightmare. As demonstrated in the following, the Nightmare has not only been associated with horses, but also has more specific supernatural connotations.

THE DEVIL

Graf (1893, as cited in Jones, 1949) noted that the presence of the Devil usually elicits feelings of dread, paralysis, coldness, and an inability to speak and act. The Devil is generally associated with darkness, the unknown, and the mysterious; his powers were also held to be most formidable at night. Thus, it is no great stretch for sleep paralysis to be interpreted as having Luciferian origins. Although our common conceptions of Satan derive from the Middle Ages, there are earlier and more topic-relevant historical linkages. For instance, the Devil and the Greek god Pan have always maintained a close association for mythologists. Pan was the personification of nature, was also very libidinal, had animal features, and could cause humans to go into a "panic" or even die. The Greek term for Nightmare, *ephialtes*, often had *pan* added as a prefix (Cheyne et al., 1999). Thus, we note here what is likely the earliest association found between sleep paralysis and panic attacks which we have not seen elsewhere described. Further, Pan was later described by Christian theologians as the "Prince of the Incubi."

The Devil's ability to assault humans could occur in two ways. First, he could attack from without, and this was properly termed "obsession." Second, he could influence a person from within through the more commonly known process of "possession." We surmise that most people's beliefs in a satanic origin of sleep paralysis would be characterized by the former rather than the latter.

INCUBI, SUCCUBI, AND OTHER MINOR DEMONS

Most cases of sleep paralysis were believed to be caused by much lesser beings than the Devil. Depending upon time and place, this could include general demonic entities or the more specific *incubi* (male) and *succubi* (female). The latter two were believed to be nocturnally assaulting demons that not only tormented and obsessed people, but often sexually attacked them as well. The results of such attacks could be pregnancy, physical harm, and high levels of sexual enervation leading to exhaustion or even death. *Succubi* in particular were believed to be responsible for male nocturnal emissions and general distress. Davies also noted the possibility that widespread belief in demonic attacks could have been used to excuse away evidence of masturbation or illicit affairs (Davies, 2003). One also wonders if incest, a crime happening at much higher rates than was believed in earlier times, may have been covered up and/or the experience distorted into a putative demonic assault?

Etymologically, the Latin term *incubus* derives from *incubare* (to lie down upon), as in (Davies, 2003; Mack, 1989), so it is easy to see how the common feelings of pressure found in sleep paralysis could be conceptually linked to these entities. Indeed, as early as 1900 Höfler concluded that the belief in demons was caused by Nightmares (Jones, 1949).

It is probably difficult for the contemporary reader to comprehend the degree of seriousness that beliefs in demons held for the general population during these earlier times. This unwavering conviction was not just found in peasants and the uneducated, but was found in the ranks of the learned as well. For instance, the *Malleus Maleficarum* (Kramer & Sprenger, 1971), sometimes translated as "Hammer of Witches" or "Women who commit *Maleficia*" (i.e., evil acts against others, as noted in Kors & Peters,

2001) was a 15th century manual for the detection, diagnosis, and "purification" of witches. This book took the existence of demons completely for granted. Within this work (written in response to a 1484 papal bull) serious discussions took place on such topics as whether or not incubi could legitimately impregnate human women and also the many ways in which demons could disturb sleepers (see also the 1608 *Compendium Maleficarum* by Guazzo, 2004). The authors noted that:

> *Theologians have ascribed to them certain qualities . . . there is in them a natural con-cupiscence, a wanton fancy, as is seen from their spiritual sins of pride, envy, and wraith. For this reason they are the enemies of the human race: rational in mind, but reasoning without words; subtle in wickedness, eager to do hurt; ever fertile in fresh deceptions, they change the perceptions and befoul the emotions of men, they confound the watchful and in dreams disturb the sleeping . . . they seek to get a mastery over the good, and molest them to the most of their power . . . . (p. 23)*

The purported behaviors of demons were even discussed by luminaries such as Saints Thomas Aquinas and Augustine. The latter noted in his *City of God* that:

> *There is, too, a very general rumor, which many have verified by their own experience, or which trustworthy persons who have heard the experience of others corroborate, that sylvan and fauns, who are commonly called 'incubi', had often made wicked assaults upon women, and satisfied their lusts upon them; and that certain devils called Duses by the Gauls, are constantly attempting and effecting this impurity is so generally affirmed, that it were impudent to deny it. (Augustine, 1952, p. 416)*

Therefore, at least in the European world, a pervasive *non-belief* in demons is a relatively recent historical development.

Returning to the relationships between sleep paralysis and demons, one can find a number of intriguing similarities. Along with the aforementioned feelings of pressure, sensed presence, and nocturnal assault (which are all fairly paradigmatic sleep paralysis hallucinations), there is also a connection with cold. This sensation is found in a fairly high percentage of sleep paralysis patients (e.g., Sharpless et al., 2010). Montague Summers' work on witchcraft described the unnatural coldness attributed to demons' bodies by witches, as well as the belief that ectoplasm is itself cold to the touch (Summers, 1987). Davies noted additional descriptions of demonic sex organs being similarly cold (it is also curious that one current meaning of incubation is to provide *warmth* so that eggs may hatch—this may be another instance of mythological meaning inversion). Linkages can also be found with the enervating aspects of *incubi/succubi*. As shown in subsequent chapters, sleep paralysis is more likely to occur when sleep is disrupted, and the episodes themselves can result in feelings of tiredness and a subsequent avoidance of sleep. Thus, sufferers of sleep paralysis (who may simultaneously experience hallucinations, as noted) often feel a great deal of lassitude, and could attribute their weakness to supernatural origins. In addition, there is the interesting belief that demons must depart, and magical enchantments must fail, upon cock's crow (Summers, 1987). As sleep paralysis episodes are much more likely to occur upon awakening than when going to sleep, one can see how the external stimulation of a loud rooster could be associated with cessation of sleep and/or sleep paralysis hallucinations. Finally, demons, nocturnal emissions, and sexual assaults were all linked with Lilith. Lilith was an important mythological figure originating in Jewish, Babylonian, and Sumerian mythologies (but possibly having earlier roots). There are many depictions of Lilith in the historical record. Summers reported that the purpose of an ancient Babylonian cylinder seal depicting Lilith was to stave off the frightening nocturnal visits of her and her sisters, as Lilith was held to be queen of the *succubi* (Summers, 1991). Lilith has also been discussed as the first vampire, and we now turn our attention to this creature and its relation to sleep paralysis.

THE VAMPIRE

Very few mythological beings have captured the attention of the contemporary lay public as much as the vampire. From Bram Stoker's popularization of the Eastern European version of this particular revenant (i.e., a being that returns after death) to current films and television shows, the vampire has been an important part of our culture. Prior to this, vampire myths were found in Assyria, China, Mexico, Greece, and many other locales (Summers, 1991).

The origin of the term "vampire" can be traced to a southern Slav word that came into use in the 18th century, but the concept is much older. The classic European vampire was elegantly described by John Heinrick Zopfius in 1733 (cited in Summers, 1991). Zopfius states that:

> Vampires issue forth from their graves in the night, attack people sleeping quietly in their beds, suck out all their blood from their bodies and destroy them.

They beset men, women and children alike, sparing neither age nor sex. Those who are under the fatal malignity of their influence complain of suffocation and a total deficiency of their spirits, after which they soon expire. Some who, when at the point of death, have been asked if they can tell what is causing their disease, reply that such and such person, lately dead, have arisen from the tomb to torment and torture them. (pp. 1–2)

This ubiquity of the revenant, and the similarities found across time and place (esp. in terms of nocturnal attacks, some form of "draining," etc.), raises a number of important issues and questions about how people came to believe in vampires. As shown in the following, sleep paralysis is likely a small part of this complex story. Before discussing sleep paralysis, however, mention should be made of the richness of the myth itself. In our limited review of the vampire literature, we see origins of vampirism as a multideterminant process involving certain naturalistic processes in combination with humans' general conceptions of death and possibilities for an afterlife.

At a fundamental level, the belief that the dead are not merely reduced to non-existence, but in some way can survive the demise of their body, appears to be a fairly universal human idea. This belief may originate in religion, a wish to *not* be eternally separated from deceased loved ones, survivor guilt, fear of one's own finitude, and so on. One need only look to the prevalence of mediums and other psychics to see how strong these wishes for reconnection can be as well as the lengths people will go to reconnect. Regardless, a post-death existence allows not only for the possibility to visit loved ones (in dreams or in person), but also allows for the possibility of some form of torment *from the deceased*. As noted by Jones (1949), such visitations often occurred at night. Presumably, this observation holds irrespective of the emotional valence of the visit (i.e., fear or joy), and examples of both can be found in any number of literatures.

Along with general discomfort over death, a number of other naturalistic explanations for vampirism have been proposed. For instance, porphyria is an enzymatic disorder that results in such things as photosensitivity, necrosis of the gums and skin, and various forms of mental disturbance. Given the relative infrequency of this condition, however, its contribution to the vampire mythos is likely minimal. A much more likely candidate would be the misunderstood natural decay processes of the human body (e.g., occasional lack of blood coagulation, collection of gases leading to distention and noise when the body is disinterred) catalogued by Barber (1988). Prior to systematic observational studies of the effects of different environmental conditions on human decay, variations in a corpse's disposition would have likely been seen as quite remarkable, especially for a non-scientifically educated population. Similarly, the symptoms of tuberculosis (previously called "consumption") could have played a larger role. In this contagious disease caused by the *mycrobacterium tuberulae*, sufferers become pale and slowly waste away. Fluid and blood may collect in the lungs if they sleep in a supine position and, when advanced, patients may awaken to the sight of visible blood on their bed linens. Thus, Bell hypothesized that the symptoms of tuberculosis could be misconstrued as nocturnal vampire attacks (Bell, 2001). Finally, premature burials (due to any number of reasons and fairly common before modern embalming techniques and autopsies) also likely played a role in the vampire mythos. When such a corpse was disinterred, onlookers would witness a contorted body, damaged coffin (e.g., scratch marks), and other signs of recent (i.e., post-mortem) animation. Such burials were not uncommon, as evidenced by the fact that in 1874 the city of Vienna made plans for a temporary morgue that included bells attached to each body that rang at the slightest movement (Editors of Time-Life Books, 1988, p. 93). Considering these many naturalistic possibilities together, there appears to have been no lack of interpretable "evidence" for the existence of revenants in general, and vampires in particular.

So how might the experience of sleep paralysis contribute to and/or influence vampire beliefs and mythologies? We propose that there are at least four main ways. First, the most obvious connection between the two is that vampire attacks are held to typically occur at night while the victim is in bed. In the prototypical example, an intruder, usually malevolent, is sensed, felt, or seen in the room. This figure (if seen) is often known to the victim, and may even be a recently deceased relative. Though not as common in modern film adaptations, the manifestations of vampire beliefs in real-world American and European history often began with a single death in a small village. This death was followed shortly thereafter by nocturnal visits by the deceased person to one or more relatives or neighbors (e.g., the 1892 Mercy Brown case in Exeter, Rhode Island described in Bell, 2001). Given that sleep paralysis often includes hallucinations of recently deceased relatives and others known to the victim (Sharpless & Grom, 2013), one can see how these nocturnal experiences could easily become blended with vampire lore (see also Roscher, 2007, p. 107). The dead often weigh heavily on a conscious mind, and it is only natural that they would become part of our REM activity.

Taken further, the sensations of pressure/oppression and difficulties breathing may give the illusion of being lain upon or throttled by this figure and, as seen with *incubi/succubi* experiences, sleep paralysis often has a sexual cast. Part of the popular allure of vampires is their unnatural, unhinged, and dangerous sexuality (e.g., Florescu & McNally, 1994). They need not necessarily even use force to achieve their libidinal or hematophagic aims, as hypnotic powers are also often ascribed to them (i.e., their ability to "charm" or "glamour" humans, which is an ability they share with fairies, which are also mythological beings who attack humans at night [Briggs, 1978]). Summers (1991) noted that, "The vampire is... generally believed to embrace his victim who has been thrown into a trance-like sleep... (p. 184)." They can therefore leave their victims paralyzed and immobile without necessarily having to use any physical force.

A third possible connection between vampire attacks and sleep paralysis would be the exhaustion that is a common consequence to both. As the Zopfius quote illustrates, visits by vampires are often followed by lassitude. This is found in the vampire myths of other cultures, too. For instance, natives of Grenada who experience tiredness upon awakening often blame this on a visit from the *longaroo* (a corruption of *loup garou*; Summers, 1991). This creature shares a number of similarities to the classic European vampire, as it must leave by morning (cock's crow), and attacks can be foiled by scattering grains of rice or sand. Vampires, for some reason, are apparently afflicted with arithmomania, and must obsessively count small objects even if it means losing their prey (see also chapter 14).

Regardless, in sleep paralysis, exhaustion and disrupted sleep patterns appear to be both a cause and consequence of the phenomenon (see chapter 6). As one example, Davies reported that strenuous exercise was a proximal cause of purported visits by a revenant in late 16th century Breslau (Davies, 2003). He contended that such experiences may have been more common in earlier time periods due to more intensive physical labor and much longer work days. It also appears likely that the lack of clean drinking water during time periods such as the Middle Ages, and the corresponding greater intake of alcoholic beverages such as low alcohol beer (even by children) may have also made sleep paralysis more likely to occur (Hornsey, 2003). This is because alcohol (and certain other substances) can actually suppress REM activity and cause a rebound effect to occur later in the night.

We also surmise that the symptoms of tuberculosis (esp., the corresponding sleep disturbances) could make sleep paralysis more likely to occur as well. Should bloody sputum suddenly appear on bedclothes following the nocturnal visit of a malevolent (hallucinated) "intruder," one can easily see how real experiences could become intermingled with pre-existing beliefs. The resulting mixture would serve to lend further credence to vampirism.

In ending this section on the vampire, it is noteworthy that several of the "preventative measures" and "treatments" for vampires are also shared with folk remedies for sleep paralysis. These are primarily discussed in chapter 14, but we provide one interesting "vampire detection" technique here. Summers reported that a virginal boy would be placed upon a similarly untouched (and coal-black) young stallion. The pair was then led to-and-fro over cemetery plots until the vampire was ultimately revealed through the stallion refusing to cross over the revenant's daytime resting place (Summers, 1991, p. 200). The connections to our earlier discussion of the Nightmare's equine elements are striking, and also foreshadow our discussion of Henri Fuseli's classic (1781) painting in chapter 4.

THE WEREWOLF

Links between sleep paralysis and werewolf beliefs are less extensive than with the other supernatural beings described, but some connections are apparent. As with the vampire, most readers are familiar with the basic mythology of the Western conception of this particular shape-shifter, so no extensive background details are provided here.

Shape-shifting is pervasive in many mythologies (e.g., from Native American "skin walkers" to ancient Greek tale of Zeus and Lycaon and Ovid's *Metamorphoses*). These physical transformations can be traced back to the very dawn of humanity, and cave paintings at *Lascaux* and *les Trois Freres* caves in France reportedly display vivid depictions of these supernatural metamorphoses (Editors of Time-Life Books, 1989). Throughout much of mythology, there appears to be a fluidity and lack of a sharp disjuncture between humans and animals and the respective traits of each (e.g., intelligence, brutality). This fluidity is likely difficult to fully appreciate from our contemporary vantage points.

It has also been proposed that werewolf mythology, and lycanthropy in general, may have partially arisen as a means to explain the acts of those we would now term serial killers/lust murders (e.g., Peter Stubbe's 1589 German case and Gilles Garnier in 1573 France as described in Masters & Lea, 1963). The bestial yet meticulous (i.e., indicative of a human-like intelligence) and episodic attacks would have led many to interpret these events as due neither to human nor animal, but something in between that partook of both characteristics. Other, less likely explanations included the fairly rare conditions of hypertrichosis and porphyria, but these are not further discussed.

Several aspects of these myths have relevance for sleep paralysis. At the level of phenomenology, werewolves were supposed to only roam at night (at least European werewolves) and, along with waylaying travelers, would attack people in the safety of their own beds (e.g., Baring-Gould, 1973; Summers, 1966). Although night-hags typically entered houses through keyholes, werewolves entered through water vents (Jones, 1949). Characteristic werewolf noises (e.g., growling, scraping, guttural sounds) are also not uncommon auditory hallucinations experienced during sleep paralysis. Similar to vampires, a sensed presence or actual perception of a large being in the room, possibly fuzzy/indistinct/hairy, and with a malicious intent, may be perceived as oppressing/attacking a person under sleep paralysis. As seen in appendix A, a number of animals are perceived during sleep paralysis, so blends of human and animal could easily become part of REM activity. Interestingly, we have heard from several native French speakers that, as children, they were told not to misbehave or the *loup garou* (meaning "wolf" and "man who changes into an animal") would get them at night. Such children's tales of "bogeymen" may not only plant the seed for experiencing frightening sleep paralysis episodes, but may also be reflective of scary experiences that occurred while sleeping.

It is also important to note the many historical similarities between the werewolf and the nightmare/night-hag. For instance, seventh sons were believed to turn into werewolves, whereas seventh daughters turned into night-hags (Davies, 2003). As another example, werewolves and hags can be identified through the presence of a unibrow (Jones, 1949). More connections between the two can be found in Woodward's work, as he noted that Scandinavian werewolves were typically old women with claws who could *paralyze* people and animals with their gaze (Woodward, 1979). Thus, depending upon time and place, connections with sleep paralysis and lycanthropy can be identified.

GHOSTS

Disembodied spirits who possess the capacity to be seen by and interact with humans can be found in most (if not all) cultures. These beliefs are likely also tied to fundamental human death anxieties and fears of the unknown that were discussed in the vampire section of this chapter. As can be seen in appendix A, many translations of sleep paralysis terms directly relate to ghosts. Indeed, even a cursory review of the extensive folklore on hauntings and ghosts reveals many similarities with sleep paralysis. Specters are usually viewed at night, and they are often perceived as shadowy, indistinct, or otherwise lacking in "full" corporeal human form (e.g., missing legs or shrouded in mist). Most sightings are terrifying ordeals, especially if there is also a corresponding paralysis. Ghosts are also often associated with feelings of coldness (as are demons and undead vampires). Popular press narratives of ghostly encounters often discuss rapid reductions in air temperature, which serve as a prelude to ghosts making themselves known (e.g., Editors of Time-Life Books, 1988; see also Sharpless et al., 2010 for empirical frequencies of cold sensations during isolated sleep paralysis).

There also appear to be connections between certain ghosts and psychopathology/stress. For instance, *poltergeists* (i.e., "noisy spirits") have typically been associated with individuals experiencing high levels of emotional tension (e.g., Fodor, 1964). Classic examples often center the *poltergeist* on an emotionally troubled adolescent who is touched/attacked, witnesses the movement of inanimate objects, hears anomalous sounds (e.g., banging, scraping, and knocking), and feels as if he or she is being moved against his or her will. As shown in chapter 9, sleep paralysis is more likely to occur in individuals who suffer from certain forms of psychopathology (however, we are not aware of data associating it more specifically with adolescent tumult). Therefore, the presence of these fairly typical sleep paralysis hallucinations in the sleeping life of emotionally troubled individuals is not particularly surprising.

Appendix A displays a predominance of Asian countries that experience sleep paralysis as a ghostly visitation (e.g., Cambodia, China, Sri Lanka, Thailand), but this appears to be less common in the West. At present, the reasons for this are not known. It is possible that this may be due to such culturally sanctioned beliefs as ancestor worship, animism, particular conceptions of the afterlife (e.g., Shinto's beliefs in a world in between earth and eternity where spirits can interact), or other factors not yet identified.

WITCHES

Sleep paralysis is probably most associated with witchcraft, and a number of the terms in appendix A are indeed witch-related (e.g., *hexendrücken*, *hagge*, hag, *boszorkany-nyomas*, *Madzikirira*). Along with beliefs in demonic *incubi* and *succubi*, many of the learned elite and the uneducated alike truly believed in the mortal threat of witches (especially during the Renaissance and, ironically, the Enlightenment). This sometimes reached conspiratorial levels. However, we should note again that belief in witches was often variable and, even in some true believers, was tempered with some degree of skepticism. For example, the Reverend Montague Summers, who took many of the phenomena described in this section with deadly seriousness, believed that experiences of "witchcraft" were often due to non-supernatural factors (e.g., hallucinations, hysteria, or disease, as in Summers, 1987). Similarly, the famous "witch-hunter/witch-pricker" John Stearne (Davies, 2003) and the 12th century John of Salisbury also expressed qualifying statements. The latter noted a possible origin of witch beliefs in dream experiences (Jones, 1949). A notable proponent of the more skeptical view of witchcraft would be Reginald Scott (Kors & Peters, 2001).

In spite of these qualifications, many witches were arrested, questioned, tortured, tried, convicted, and executed/immolated. Whereas estimates vary widely in terms of the total number of deaths attributed to the witch persecutions in Europe (e.g., 12,000 to 9 million), most historians are uncomfortable going beyond 50,000 deaths between the 15th and 18th centuries (Kors & Peters, 2001). Given the high costs in terms of time, expense, and human life, it is clear that witchcraft was imbued with a high degree of cultural importance. It is also clear that the historical and sociological literatures devoted to the witch craze are much too wide and nuanced to adequately deal with in this context, so only a thumbnail sketch is provided in order to set the stage for sleep paralysis' role in this multi-determined phenomenon.

The idea that a segment of the population possessed knowledge, power, or abilities that ordinary people did not was common. You can see this in shamans, medicine men, magi, and other social roles that maintain and/or withhold "esoteric" knowledge. This privileged position could be very provocative, however, as those with esoteric knowledge often aroused suspicion. The pervasiveness of certain conspiracy theories involving government agencies, secret knowledge, and financial elites may be a contemporary reinterpretation of these older perspectives, as those seen as having more power/influence are often simultaneously envied and maligned. This went for the witch as well.

While certainly powerful (e.g., abilities to fly, manipulate weather patterns, and influence people/objects), many unsavory attributes were attributed to the witch regardless of gender (e.g., pacts with the devil, sexual debauchery, infanticide). In most countries except France the majority of victims were women (Kors & Peters, 2001), and many have interpreted this fact as indicative of misogyny and discomfort with female sexuality.

Giving misogyny too much explanatory power would be a mistake, however, and as noted by Christina Larner, "witchcraft was not sex-specific, but it was sex related" (Larner, 1981, p. 91). Indeed, descriptions of trials and methods used to extract testimony are replete with sexual accusations and personal violations. For example, witches were often publicly examined in the nude for "devil's marks" and other signs of satanic influence, and it is hard to overlook the obviously prurient nature of these acts in the midst of the prevailing religious beliefs and sexual mores.

Extensive documentation is available for a number of witch trials, and source material includes archival documents of actual testimony and proceedings. Many are translated and collected in *Witchcraft in Europe: 400-1700* (Kors & Peters, 2001). Witch trials were not only localized to the old world, however. America was home to one of the more infamous trials that also yielded extensive historical documentation. David Hufford (1982) may have been the first to suggest that sleep paralysis was experienced by one or more persons involved in the Salem village witch trials, and if one looks at the actual trial documents, this appears plausible, and indeed probable. For instance, the opening quote to this chapter by John Londer is taken from his actual trial testimony used against Bridget Bishop (Boyer & Nissenbaum, 1993). Examples of testimony provided by other individuals involved in the trial are also consistent with sleep paralysis (e.g., Richard Coman's testimony in Boyer & Nissenbaum, 1993).

Modern psychological and psychiatric interest in the connection between sleep paralysis and witches appears to have been primarily stimulated by Ness' work on the "old hag experience" in Newfoundland, Canada (Ness, 1978) and Hufford's much more extensive book-length work (Hufford, 1982). Numerous first-hand accounts of sleep paralysis episodes were collected and analyzed under this folkloric conception of being "hagged." The "old hag" and the act of being "hagged" were the colloquial phrases used for Nightmares in Newfoundland. In these interviews, various beliefs in the ability to "hag" others (i.e., cause oppressive episodes of paralysis) as well as means to prevent being "hagged" were commonly discussed in these communities (e.g., Hufford, 1982, p. 18). Therefore, in these first-hand accounts of the old hag, one finds a contemporary analogue to prior notions of witchcraft, at least in certain important respects. Moreover, there is much less possibility for a "presentist" distortion of these experiences. This is clearly not as easy when interpreting material that is more temporally and culturally remote.

Keeping these caveats in mind, one can reasonably infer that sleep paralysis did indeed play at least some role in both the genesis and maintenance

of witchcraft beliefs and also in the actual testimony used against purported witches. In archival trial records, this was only really possible due
to the allowance of what was termed "spectral evidence." Spectral evidence is testimony based upon the content of visions and dreams. During
the Salem witch trials, chief justice William Stoughton allowed this testimony to be admitted into evidence. Ignoring the legal dilemmas that are
apparent in this evidence, we again find in these actions further evidence
of the importance of anomalous nocturnal experiences.

So what are the experiential consistencies found between witchcraft
and Nightmares/sleep paralysis? Again, one finds the typical sensed presence, chest pressure, stifled breath, and fearful paralysis. More unique
facets may be related to the purported movement of "witches." Witches
have historically had the power to travel great distances through various
means of conveyance (e.g., via broomsticks). This was thought necessary
so that they could gather in groups for sabbaths and other diabolical rites
(Summers, 1987). Thus, they had the ability to both hover above a sleeper
and descend from above. Along with flying abilities, witches were reputed
to be able to move inanimate objects and other people (viz., telekinesis).
The common sleep paralysis experiences of being levitated, turned, or otherwise moved without one's own volition is in keeping with traditional
witch powers (Kramer & Sprenger, 1971). As seen in chapter 6, these hallucinations constitute the vestibular-motor subtype of sleep paralysis
(Cheyne et al., 1999). Other hallucinations are potentially relevant. In
Wales, for instance, the *gwrach-y-rhibyn* ("dribbling hag" or "hag of the
mist") was not only frightening and repulsive, but also made scraping
noises and inarticulate moans (Editors of Time-Life Books, 1988, p. 42).

One also finds pronounced sexual components in both witchcraft
beliefs and sleep paralysis. This is especially the case when one reads the
actual trial documents (see also Davies, 2003) and witchcraft "manuals"
(e.g., *The Compendium Maleficarum*, Guazzo, 2004). What remains unclear,
however, is whether or not the sexual components accurately reflected
the nocturnal experiences themselves or were partially artifacts of the
type of testimony that was likely to titillate a courtroom. Regardless, the
ideas that witches "ride" (i.e., sexually assault) people and spend their free
time copulating with the devil or lesser demons was a popular belief (e.g.,
Kramer & Sprenger, 1971). This can be seen in certain colloquial phrases
as well. For instance, the German term *es reiten ihn Hexen* (the witch
rides him) and *dich hat geriten der Mar* (the night fiend has ridden you)
were synonymous with what we would today term nocturnal emissions
or "wet dreams" (Jones, 1949). Ness reported that some contemporary
Newfoundlanders would complain of genital soreness upon awakening

due to the belief that they were sexually manipulated by the old hag (Ness, 1978). Witches could also remove or otherwise negatively affect genitals through shrinking or various other means (e.g., Kramer & Sprenger, 1971, question IX). This can be seen today in mass hysteria and "witch killings" that have taken place recently in West Africa (e.g., Radford, 2013). Though this particular belief is more likely due to the experience of *koro* than sleep paralysis, it helps to instantiate the fact that witchcraft and malevolent sexual magic have long been linked and, at least in some parts of the world, this link continues.

Witchcraft has also been more generally connected with the bedroom and sleeping habits, and this is additional, albeit indirect evidence for a partial origin in sleep paralysis. For instance, Kramer and Sprenger (1971, p. 184) advised those individuals who felt they were bewitched to thoroughly search all corners of their bed and mattresses for any tools of witchcraft. Presumably this was due to the fact that "witches" often attacked at night when one was most helpless and vulnerable. They also reputedly possessed the power to induce sleep and/or paralyze limbs through the use of soporific potions, spells, or "strange lights" (Guazzo, 2004, pp. 83–88).

Of all the supernatural phenomena documented in this chapter, the fever pitch of hysteria brought on by witchcraft caused the highest body count and had the most societal impact. This appears to be quite different in scale from that brought on by demons, vampires, and ghosts. It is hard for the contemporary reader to situate him- or herself in a time period when anxiety about witchcraft was so pronounced. Given that anxiety in general appears to be a proximal cause of sleep paralysis episodes, it is interesting to speculate on the reciprocal nature of anxiety over witchcraft, subsequent sleep paralysis, and increased anxiety due to vivid and scary experiences. The testimony of Salem Village would appear to be consistent with this hypothesis.

ALIEN ABDUCTIONS

Whereas many of the supernatural entities described thus far have few believers in the West (with the exception of the devil and ghosts), the belief in extraterrestrials is somewhat different. There has been serious speculation about life on other planets since at least the ancient Greek philosophers (e.g., Democritus; McKirahan, 1994, pp. 326–327), and this continues to the present. Several polls indicate that many people take the possibility of alien life very seriously. A 2002 nationally representative

Roper poll of 1021 individuals in the United States explored this topic (Roper ASW, 2002). The poll indicated that no less than 67% of Americans believe in other forms of intelligent life in the universe. A total of 48% believe that UFOs have visited the earth, 12% reported that they or someone they know have seen a UFO at close range, and 3% reported seeing a UFO effect some sort of physical change on objects, animals, or humans. A 2012 survey of 1359 adults in the United Kingdom conducted by *Opinion Matters* found fairly similar results (as cited in Kumar, 2012). Almost 10% saw a UFO, and 52% believed that UFO evidence has been covered up by government agencies.

So how many individuals believe they were abducted by aliens? This is difficult to assess. The Roper poll reports a figure of 1.4%. This would be a staggering number because, assuming there are 320,217,750 individuals in the United States (census.gov/popclock), 4,483,049 of these would believe they were abducted. This is roughly the entire population of the state of Kentucky. However, if one looks closer at the poll, the 1.4% did not endorse abduction directly, but endorsed at least four of five dubious "signs" of abduction, and many of these are consistent with sleep paralysis phenomena (e.g., "feeling that you left your body"). This approach has been used in other surveys of "abduction" as well (as reviewed in French & Stone, 2013).

There have been a number of theories put forth to explain the belief in alien abductions. Though some of these may appear convincing to a greater or lesser degree, the heterogeneity of abduction narratives makes it unlikely for any one explanation to take precedence. Prior to this review, it is important to note that few empirical differences have been found between "abductees" and non-abductees, and some of these are quite subtle. Whereas there is a prevalent conception that you can dismiss abductees as psychotic or more generally "crazy," there are scant data to support this. In fact, studies that have measured abductees' level of psychopathology have revealed that they do not appear to grossly differ from non-abductees (e.g., Holden & French, 2002; McNally & Clancy, 2005).

Certain specific characteristics do appear to differentiate abductees and non-abductees, however. Abductees were found to more likely display memory distortions and false memory creation in certain laboratory paradigms than non-abductees (e.g., Clancy, McNally, Schacter, Lenzenweger, & Pitman, 2002); these same authors found that hypnotic suggestibility was related to these memory task results as well. However, one study did not replicate the false memory findings using the same Deese/Roediger-McDermott task, and the researchers hypothesized that sample differences may have been at least partially responsible (French, Santomauro, Hamilton, Fox, & Thalbourne, 2008).

Abductees in several studies were also found to have higher levels of schizotypy than controls (e.g., Spanos, Cross, Dickson, & DuBreuil, 1993). Schizotypy is a personality characteristic that may manifest through such things as unusual beliefs, perceptual aberrations, social anhedonia, and magical ideation. Closely related to schizotypy, abductees are also more prone to fantasy than non-abductees (e.g., Bartholomew, Basterfield, & Howard, 1991; French et al., 2008). Individuals high in fantasy-proneness have active and vivid fantasy lives, and may sometimes experience difficulties differentiating fantasy from reality. This may also be related to general capacities for creativity.

Forrest (2008) provided a medical hypothesis for alien abduction experiences. He noted the similarities between paradigmatic alien abduction beliefs (e.g., seeing "grays" examinations/surgeries on helpless victims) and dimly recalled childhood surgeries. Forrest proposed that certain altered states of consciousness described by abductees resemble anesthesia. Presumably this may trigger state-dependent memories. Forrest claimed that the pronounced eyes of "gray" aliens and their greenish/gray appearance correspond to viewing physicians in scrubs and surgical masks. He also contended that the bright lights of the surgical room and the nature of the surgery itself (i.e., invasive procedures conducted on a helpless person in a supine position) bear more than a passing resemblance to many alien abduction scenarios. However, as of yet we are not aware of empirical evidence demonstrating that abductees are more likely to have undergone childhood surgeries than non-abductees. Interestingly, an earlier study linked anesthesiology with sleep paralysis (Spector & Bourke, 1977).

Along with endogenous personality traits and possible childhood experiences, abductees have been known to seek out certain therapeutic techniques that may increase the risk of memory creation and distortion. For example, Clancy reviewed literature on the use of clinical hypnosis to refresh memories, and noted that abductees have often sought out hypnotic inductions for this very purpose (Clancy, 2007). Hypnosis, especially when used improperly or carelessly, can lead to false memory creation (e.g., Spanos, Cross, Dickson, & DuBreuil, 1993) and may lend real-life vividness to illusory situations (e.g., an abductee seeing his or her human/alien hybrid children). Of note, even when awake, abductees experienced sympathetic arousal when listening to recordings of their abductions that were at least equivalent to, if not greater than, the reactions of combat veterans and rape victims who listened to their own traumatic narratives (McNally et al., 2004). It is possible that this may be related to higher dissociative capacities to become absorbed in experiences. Regardless, hypnosis, particularly in individuals prone to vivid fantasy, may serve to distort or create memories that unfortunately possess high levels of subjective veracity.

More specifically, sleep paralysis potentially provides a non-extraterrestrial explanation for bedroom abduction scenarios. Hufford (2005) noted the pervasiveness of bedroom abductions in the early abduction literature. Seeing non-human beings with distorted features approach you while simultaneously uttering inarticulate (alien?) speech would be scary and memorable experiences for anyone to have. This is especially the case if a person in also paralyzed and feels that he or she is being levitated (tractor beam?), feels sensations of pain or cold (invasive surgeries, metallic operating tables, and alien medical instruments?), or experiences genital stimulation (sperm/egg extraction?). In this framework, it is fairly easy to see how these otherwise anomalous experiences could be interpreted as an "abduction" if one is primed with pre-existing beliefs and cultural narratives about aliens. This has led some to claim that alien abductions may be our most current supernatural attribution to sleep paralysis hallucinations (e.g., Susan Clancy and Richard McNally). Whereas prior epochs with powerful church influences may have presumed demonic or satanic influences in these events, 21st century Westerners may find technologically advanced extraterrestrials to be more palatable and compelling causal agents of malevolence. Abductions only began to be discussed by the media in 1962 (Clancy, 2007). At least in the West, this is a time period riddled with new technologies and scientific achievements. It is also the publication date of the first edition of Thomas Kuhn's *The Structure of Scientific Revolutions* (Kuhn, 1996), a groundbreaking work that proposed a theretofore unconsidered worldview.

Related to the preceding, Susan Clancy aptly notes that an entire worldview/paradigm is engendered through a belief in aliens that she argued was similar to a religion in many regards (Clancy, 2007). The nature of the universe is made more parsimonious, predictions of events are possible, and experiences are able to be more easily explained. There may also be prospects for a better life than the one a person currently has, which may now be imbued with meaning, order, and even the possibility of various means of escape. Wishes have long been known to have a powerful capacity to organize human experiences.

In ending this section, two other comments may be noteworthy. First, many otherwise normal and psychologically healthy individuals may have strange beliefs or a "pocket" of beliefs that lack empirical support, but are fervently believed nonetheless. For instance, we have clinically worked with several individuals reporting to possess "psychic" abilities. There are also a number of people today who believe they have seen and/ or interacted with fantastic creatures such as "the Jersey Devil" from the Pine Barrens of southern New Jersey (McCloy & Miller, 2002) or the more famous "Nessie" of Loch Ness, Scotland. Are these individuals "crazy?" We would contend that they are not, but that they clearly have beliefs or perceptual experiences that deviate from the norm. Further, we contend that they are doing their best to explain a sometimes mysterious world in which standard scientific explanations may not seem compelling, or in which science does not appear to possess adequate explanatory power for their perceptions.

Second, several academicians have come out on the non-skeptical side of alien abductions. For instance, Harvard psychiatrist, psychoanalyst, and Pulitzer prize–winning author John Mack (2007) created perturbations throughout the academic world when his *Abduction: Human Encounters with Aliens* was first published in 1994. He described interviews with more than 200 abductees, and noted the unexplained nature of many of their reports. Mack is quite possibly the most prominent intellectual figure to address the subject, and he is often cited as an intellectual resource by abductees. In an interview shortly before his death (Hind, 2005), he stated his ultimate position as, "I would never say, yes, there are aliens taking people. [But] I would say there is a compelling powerful phenomenon here that I can't account for in any other way, that's mysterious. Yet I can't know what it is but it seems to me that it invites a deeper, further inquiry." Thus, Mack appears to be open to the possibilities of abduction and is simultaneously sensitive to the beliefs of abductees. Other scholars have made stronger claims. For instance, David Jacobs, emeritus professor of history at Temple University and author of *The Threat: Revealing the Secret Alien Agenda* (Jacobs, 1999) describes a fairly nefarious alien conspiracy involving inter-species breeding of human/alien hybrids using both fetal implantation procedures and forced mating. This breeding program is supposedly oriented toward infiltrating human society and supplanting existing power structures.

SHADOW PEOPLE

This last phenomenon, "shadow people," has only recently received popular attention (as evidenced by several films such as *Shadow People*) (Ohoven & Arnold, 2013). Some claim that it is far older and found all over the world. Unfortunately, we were unable to locate scholarly articles on this subject in psychology or psychiatry. As a result, much of the information that follows was derived from blogs and popular writings (e.g., Offutt, 2009, 2013). Shadow people are indistinct humanoid shapes that flicker and move quickly. These silhouettes are purported to be apparent primarily in one's *peripheral* vision, and are often seen at night when one is resting in bed. Appearances can range from hooded figures to shadows with glowing red eyes.

No consensus about their origin or intentions has yet solidified. Some believe them to be ghosts. Others believe that, much like shades of Hades described in the *Odyssey* (Homer, 1963), they were formerly human, but the process of death removed aspects of their personality, essentially leaving them as psychologically impoverished shells of their former selves. Some believe they are visual representations of astral projection. Finally, others claim that they are inter-dimensional beings (or time travelers), technologically advanced or otherwise.

In one Internet poll of 504 individuals (cited in Offutt, 2009, 2013), the majority of experiencers who responded (viz., 47%) believed them to be beings from different dimensions. This was followed (in descending order) by belief that they are demons (21%), ghosts (16%), manifestations of psychological disorders (13%), omens of impending doom (1%), and extraterrestrials (1%). Regarding their intentions, some claim they are helpful, others malevolent, and others believe their intentions are as varied as the individuals from whom they ultimately derive. In many of the narratives of purported encounters, the shadow people are not usually oblivious to those they visit, and behaved in frightening, sometimes assaultive, manners.

A number of descriptions of encounters with these shadow people correspond well to sleep paralysis. First, meetings often occur at night and in bedrooms. Shadow people are seen as indistinct human forms that elicit fear and dread, and many people report being unable to move. Much like alien abduction scenarios, this is consistent with the "intruder" subtype of sleep paralysis hallucinations (e.g., Cheyne et al., 1999). In the future, it will be interesting to see if the frequency of these visitations increases over time as this idea of shadow people becomes more well-known. As with extraterrestrials, these shadow people, if considered in the interdimensional/time traveler perspective, possess markedly advanced technology. This may resonate with our contemporary, technology-obsessed society more than spiritual and demonic explanations. The latter likely appear anachronistic to 21st century Westerners.

CONCLUSIONS

In this chapter we have surveyed many legends that appear to have been influenced by the experience of sleep paralysis. These myths ranged across time and place, and we noted two contemporary examples of these trends (i.e., alien abductions and shadow people). All of these beings, for whatever reason, often visit their victims in the bedroom. Perhaps this is due to primal fears of the dark and the uncertainty that arises when we attempt to sleep. In a real way, people are never as vulnerable as when they are sleeping. In sleep we are usually reclining, lack typical conscious awareness, and are not able to be vigilant when faced with potential threats.

The overlap among these many creatures/beings is striking, and it almost appears that they are really variations on two basic themes (i.e., disembodied spirits on the one hand, such as ghosts and shadow people, and supernaturally powered corporeal humans/demons on the other). Regardless, all of them exude a malevolent presence that the victim is ill-equipped to deal with and powerless to combat. They also evoke a corresponding sense of mortal terror. As discussed more thoroughly in chapter 14, a theme of desperation in the aftermath of sleep paralysis is also apparent. As a result, certain safeguards were taken and treatment recommendations were solicited by putative "experts." Whereas some sought spiritual counsel and support, modern experiencers of sleep paralysis are likely more prone to seek out hypnotists and other, more secular sources of assistance. Now that the many intersections between folklore and sleep paralysis have been elaborated, we now turn to artistic representations of this provocative phenomenon.

REFERENCES

Augustine. (1952). City of god. In R. M. Hutchins (Ed.), *Great books of the western world volume 18: Augustine* (M. Dods, trans., pp. 129–618). Chicago: Encyclopedia Britannica.

Barber, P. (1988). *Vampires, burial, and death: Folklore and reality*. New Haven, CT: Yale University Press.

Baring-Gould, S. (1973). *Book of were-wolves*. London: Forgotten Books.

Bartholomew, R. E., Basterfield, K., & Howard, G. S. (1991). UFO abductees and contactees: Psychopathology or fantasy proneness? *Professional Psychology: Research and Practice, 22*(3), 215.

Bell, M. E. (2001). *Food for the dead: On the trail of New England's vampires*. Middletown, CT: Wesleyen University Press.

Boyer, P., & Nissenbaum, S. (Eds.). (1993). *Salem-village witchcraft: A documentary record of local conflict in colonial New England*. Boston: Northeastern.

Briggs, K. M. (1978). *An encyclopedia of fairies: Hobgoblins, brownies, bogies, and other supernatural creaturs*. New York: Pantheon Books.

Cheyne, J. A., Rueffer, S. D., & Newby-Clark, I. R. (1999). Hypnagogic and hypnopompic hallucinations during sleep paralysis: Neurological and cultural construction of the night-mare. *Consciousness and Cognition: An International Journal*, 8(3), 319–337. doi: 10.1006/ccog.1999.0404

Cipolli, C., Bolzani, R., Tuozzi, G., & Fagioli, I. (2001). Active processing of declarative knowledge during REM dreaming. *Journal of Sleep Research, 10*, 277, 284.

Clancy, S. A. (2007). *Abducted: How people come to believe they were kidnapped by aliens*. Cambridge, MA: First Harvard University Press.

Clancy, S. A., McNally, R. J., Schacter, D. L., Lenzenweger, M. F., & Pitman, R. K. (2002). Memory distortion in people reporting abduction by aliens. *Journal of Abnormal Psychology, 111*(3), 455–461. doi: 10.1037//0021-843X.111.3.455

Davies, O. (2003). The nightmare experience, sleep paralysis and witchcraft accusations. *Folklore, 114*(2), 181.

Editors of Time-Life Books (Ed.). (1988). *Mysteries of the unknown: Phantom encounters*. Alexandria, VA: Time-Life Books.

Editors of Time-Life Books (Ed.). (1989). *Mysteries of the unknown: Transformations*. Alexandria, VA: Time-Life Books.

Florescu, R., & McNally, R. T. (1994). *In search of Dracula: The history of Dracula and vampires* (rev. sub. ed.). Wilmington, MA: Mariner Books.

Fodor, N. (1964). *Between two worlds*. West Nyack, NY: Parker Publishing.

Forrest, D. (2008). Alien abduction: A medical hypothesis. *Journal of the American Academy of Psychoanalysis and Dynamic Psychiatry, 36*(3), 431.

French, C. C., Santomauro, J., Hamilton, V., Fox, R., & Thalbourne, M. A. (2008). Psychological aspects of the alien contact experience. *Cortex; A Journal Devoted to the Study of the Nervous System and Behavior, 44*(10), 1387–1395. doi: 10.1016/j.cortex.2007.11.011

Freud, S. (1953). In Strachey J. (Ed.), *Volume IV: The interpretation of dreams (first part)* [Die Traumdeutung] (J. Strachey trans.). The Standard Edition of the Complete Psychological Works of Sigmund Freud. London: Hogarth Press.

Fuseli, H. (1781). *The nightmare*. London: Royal Academy of London.

Gadamer, H. (1975). *Truth and method* [Wahrheit und Methode] (J. Wiensheimer, D. Marshall, trans., 2nd ed.). New York: Continuum.

Guazzo, F. M. (2004). *Compendium Maleficarum: The Montague Summers edition* (E. A. Ashwin, trans.). Minneola, NY: Dover.

Haga, E. (1989). The nightmare—A riding ghost with sexual connotations. *Nordisk Psykiatrisk Tidsskrift. Nordic Journal of Psychiatry, 43*(6), 515–520.

Hind, A. (2005). Alien thinking. Retrieved from http://news.bbc.co.uk/2/hi/uk_news/magazine/4071124.stm

Holden, K. J., & French, C. C. (2002). Alien abduction experiences: Some clues from neuropsychology and neuropsychiatry. *Cognitive Neuropsychiatry, 7*(3), 163–178.

Homer. (1963). *The odyssey* (R. Fitzgerald, trans.). Garden City, NY: Doubleday.

Hornsey, I. S. (2003). *A history of beer and brewing*. Cambridge, UK: The Royal Society of Chemistry.

Hufford, D. J. (2005). Sleep paralysis as spiritual experience. *Transcultural Psychiatry, 42*(1), 11–45. doi: 10.1177/1363461505050709

Hufford, D. (1982). *The terror that comes in the night: An experience-centered study of supernatural assault traditions*. Philadelphia: University of Pennsylvania Press.

Jacobs, D. (1999). *The threat: Revealing the secret alien agenda*. New York: Simon & Schuster.

Jones, E. (1949). *On the nightmare* (2nd ed.). London: Hogarth Press and the Institute of Psycho-analysis.

Kors, A. C., & Peters, E. (Eds.). (2001). *Witchcraft in Europe 400-1700: A documentary history* (2nd ed.). Philadelphia: University of Pennsylvania Press.

Kramer, H., & Sprenger, J. (1971). In Summers M. (Ed.), *The Malleus Maleficarum* (N. Summers, trans.). Mineola, NY: Dover.

Kuhn, T. S. (1996). *The structure of scientific revolutions* (3rd ed.). Chicago: The University of Chicago Press.

Kumar, A. (2012). More Brits believe in aliens than god, survey claims. *The Christian Post*, October 1, 2014.

Larner, C. (1981). *Enemies of god: The witch hunt in Scotland*. London: Johns Hopkins University Press.

Mack, J. E. (1989). *Nightmares and human conflict*. New York: Columbia University Press.

Mack, J. E. (2007). *Abduction: Human encounters with aliens*. New York: Charles Scribner's Sons.

MacKinnon, C. (Producer), & MacKinnon, C. (Director). (2013). *Devil in the room*. [motion picture]. London: Rich Pickings.

Macnish, R. (1834). *The philosophy of sleep* (1st American ed.). New York: D. Appleton and Company.

Masters, R. E. L., & Lea, E. (1963). *Sex crimes in history: Evolving concepts of sadism, lust-murder, and necrophilia from ancient to modern times*. New York: The Julian Press.

McCloy, J. F., & Miller, R. J. (2002). *The 13th child: Legend of the Jersey devil volume I*. Moorestown, NJ: Middle Atlantic Press.

McKirahan, R. D. (1994). *Philosophy before Socrates: An introduction with texts and commentary*. Indianapolis: Hackett.

McNally, R. J., & Clancy, S. A. (2005). Sleep paralysis, sexual abuse, and space alien abduction. *Transcultural Psychiatry*, 42(1), 113–122. doi: 10.1177/1363461505050715

McNally, R. J., Lasko, N. B., Clancy, S. A., Macklin, M. L., Pitman, R. K., & Orr, S. P. (2004). Psychophysiological responding during script-driven imagery in people reporting abduction by space aliens. *Psychological Science*, 15(7), 493–497.

Ness, R. C. (1978). The old hag phenomenon as sleep paralysis: A biocultural interpretation. *Cultural, Medicine and Psychiatry*, 2, 15.

Offutt, J. (2009). *Darkness walks*. San Antonio: Anomalist Books.

Offutt, J. (2013). From the shadows. Retrieved from from-the-shadows.blogspot.com/

Ohoven, M. (Producer), & Arnold, M. (Director). (2013). *Shadow people*. [motion picture] Beverly Hills, CA: Anchor Bay Films.

Radford, B. (2013). Penis-snatching panics resurface in Africa. Retrieved from http://www.livescience.com/28015-penis-snatching-panics-koro.html

Roper A. S. W. (2002). *UFOs & extraterrestrial life: Americans' beliefs and personal experiences*. (No. C205-008232).

Roscher, W. H. (2007). *Ephialtes: A pathological-mythological treatis on the nightmare in classical antiquity*. [Ephialtes] (A. V. O'Brien, trans., rev ed., pp. 96–159). Putnam, CT: Spring.

Sharpless, B. A. (2014). Changing conceptions of the nightmare in medicine. *Hektoen International: A Journal of Medical Humanities (Moments in History Section)*.

Sharpless, B.A., & Grom, J.L. (2013). *Isolated sleep paralysis: Prevention, disruption, and hallucinations of others (poster)*. American Psychological Association Annual *Conference*, Honolulu, Hawaii.

Sharpless, B. A., McCarthy, K. S., Chambless, D. L., Milrod, B. L., Khalsa, S. R., & Barber, J. P. (2010). Isolated sleep paralysis and fearful isolated sleep paralysis in outpatients with panic attacks. *Journal of Clinical Psychology, 66*(12), 1292–1306. doi: 10.1002/jclp.20724; 10.1002/jclp.20724

Spanos, N. P., Cross, P. A., Dickson, K., & DuBreuil, S. C. (1993). Close encounters: An examination of UFO experiences. *Journal of Abnormal Psychology, 102*(4), 624–632.

Spector, M., & Bourke, D. L. (1977). Anesthesia, sleep paralysis, and physostigmine. *Anesthesiology, 46*(4), 296–297.

Summers, M. (1987). *The history of witchcraft* (1st Thus ed.). New York: Dorset Press.

Summers, M. (1991). *The vampire*. New York: Dorset Press.

Summers, M. (1966). *The werewolf*. New Hyde Park, NY: University Books.

Woodward, I. (1979). *The werewolf delusion*. New York: Paddington Press.

Zakin, R. (Producer), & Grant, E. (Director). (2012). *Secret history of UFOs*. [video/ DVD]. National Geographic Television.

CHAPTER 4
Sleep Paralysis in Art and Literature

Descriptions of sleep paralysis are also found in great works of art and literature. Our brief survey will range from classics of the Western literary canon to the visual arts. Before delving into specific works, it should be noted that a number of well-known artists and authors have experienced sleep paralysis in their personal lives (e.g., Vladamir Nabakov, Emanuel Swendeborg). However, relatively few have directly depicted sleep paralysis in their creations, and these are detailed in what follows. Needless to say, the depictions of these experiences by classic writers convey a depth and vividness to the experience that is often missing from many clinical and experimental descriptions. We describe these works and present excerpts of them in chronological order. This is certainly not an exhaustive catalogue, but covers many of the more well-known literary examples of sleep paralysis. As will be seen, there is a great deal of overlap (e.g., the sensed/seen presence is found in all written descriptions and the majority evidence fear, suffocation, a feeling of something sitting on the chest, and being touched in some way), so we concentrate on the unique features that each reveals.

SLEEP PARALYSIS IN THE WRITING OF ERASMUS DARWIN (1731 TO 1802)

Erasmus Darwin, Grandfather of Charles Darwin and a well-known natural philosopher and poet in his own right, described what appears to be sleep paralysis in the second part of his *Botanic Garden* (Darwin, 2012). Apart from the clear literary skill of this poem, many facets of sleep paralysis are presented. Noteworthy are the mentions of Henri Fuseli and the corresponding fiend/demon Ape/incubus imagery. An earlier version of Darwin's poem was actually exhibited on a plaque with Fuseli's *The Nightmare* painting. Also noteworthy in this excerpt is the inability to cry out in response to the harrowing paralytic ordeal.

> *So on his Nightmare through the evening fog*
> *Flits the squab Fiend o'er fen, and lake, and bog;*
> *Seeks some love-wildered maid with sleep oppressed,*
> *Alights, and grinning sits upon her breast.*
> *—Such as of late amid the murky sky*
> *Was marked by Fuseli's poetic eye,*
> *Whose daring tints, with Shakespeare's happiest grace,*
> *Gave to the airy phantom form and place.—*
> *Back o'er her pillow sinks her blushing head,*
> *Her snow-white limbs hang helpless from the bed,*
> *While with quick sighs, and suffocative breath,*
> *Her interrupted heart-pulse swims in death.*
> *—Then shrieks of captured towns, and widows' tears,*
> *Pale lovers stretched upon their blood-stained biers,*
> *The headlong precipice that thwarts her flight,*
> *The trackless desert, the cold starless night,*
> *And stern-eyed murderer with his knife behind,*
> *In dread succession agonize her mind.*
> *O'er her fair limbs convulsive tremors fleet,*
> *Start in her hands, and struggle in her feet;*
> *In vain to scream with quivering lips she tries,*
> *And strains in palsied lids her tremulous eyes;*
> *In vain she wills to run, fly, swim, walk, creep;*
> *The will presides not in the bower of Sleep.*
> *—On her fair bosom sits the Demon-Ape*
> *Erect, and balances his bloated shape;*
> *Rolls in their marble orbs his Gorgon-eyes,*
> *And drinks with leathern ears her tender cries.*
> (Darwin, 2012)

SLEEP PARALYSIS IN THE WRITING OF HERMAN MELVILLE (1819 TO 1891)

Sleep paralysis can also be found in the classic American novel, *Moby Dick* (Melville, 1952), which was originally published in 1851. Along with many of the paradigmatic features of sleep paralysis (e.g., fear, distress, and the feeling of being touched by an alien presence), Melville aptly captures in Ishmael's childhood narrative both the post-episode confusion and apprehension that patients often report (Sharpless et al., 2010). It is perhaps not surprising that many patients do not disclose their concerns to others for fear of embarrassment, and instead worry over anomalous events in private. A subsequent author, Joseph Herman, noted that a number of predisposing factors to sleep paralysis, such as stress and some degree of physical discomfort, were present in *Moby Dick* as well (Herman, 1997).

At last I must have fallen into a troubled nightmare of a doze; and slowly waking from it—half steeped in dreams—I opened my eyes and the before sunlit room was now wrapped in outer darkness. Instantly I felt a shock running through all my frame; nothing was to be seen and nothing was to be heard; but a supernatural hand seemed placed in mine. My arm hung over the counterpane, and the nameless, unimaginable silent form or phantom, to which the hand belonged, seemed closely seated by my bedside. For what seemed ages piled on ages, I lay there, frozen with the most awful fears, not daring to drag away my hand; yet ever thinking that if I could but stir it one single inch, the horrid spell would be broken. I knew not how this consciousness at last glided away from me; but waking in the morning, I shudderingly remembered it all, and for days and weeks and months afterwards I lost myself in confounding attempts to explain the mystery. Nay, to this very hour, I often puzzle myself with it. (Melville, 1952)

SLEEP PARALYSIS IN THE WRITING OF GUY DE MAUPASSANT (1850 TO 1893)

One of the more frightening depictions of sleep paralysis can be found in French writer Guy de Maupassant's *Le Horla* (Maupassant, 1945), originally published in 1887. Maupassant had a sophisticated understanding of psychology and neurology, attended lectures of Jean-Martin Charcot at the Salpetriere (Alvaro, 2005), and later earned the admiration of no less a philosophical psychologist than Friedrich Nietzsche. In his autobiography, *Ecce Homo*, Nietzsche stated that, "I do not see from what century of the past one could dredge up such inquisitive and at the same time delicate psychologists as in contemporary Paris...to single out one of the strong race, a genuine Latin to whom I am especially well-disposed, Guy de Maupassant" (Nietzsche, 1967, pp. 243–244).

Like Nietzsche, Maupassant also struggled with a number of psychological issues likely exacerbated by syphilis contracted when he was young. Maupassant was quite disposed to paranoia as well, at times experienced hallucinations, and made at least one suicide attempt (i.e., cutting his own throat) which resulted in hospitalization until his relatively early death (e.g., see Ignotus, 1968).

His writings clearly draw from his intellectual and experiential knowledge of these matters, and are quite rich in psychological insights beyond sleep paralysis. With regard to sleep paralysis specifically, Maupassant may have been the first writer to note the anticipatory anxiety and dread of sleep that some individuals report in clinical settings. Especially in individuals who have frequent episodes, a conditioned anxiety response to bedroom settings and avoidance behaviors may occur. Maupassant also vividly noted the many symptoms of sympathetic nervous system activation that occur during these events. Finally, he noted the feelings of strangulation common in sleep paralysis, along with the sense that some malevolent entity is the causal agent.

As the evening comes on, an incomprehensible feeling of disquietude seizes me .... I dine quickly, and then try to read, but I do not understand the words, and can scarcely distinguish the letters. Then I walk up and down my drawing-room, oppressed by a feeling of confused and irresistible fear, a fear of sleep and a fear of my bed. Then, I go to bed, and I wait for sleep as a man might wait for the executioner. I wait for its coming with dread, and my heart beats and my legs tremble, while my whole body shivers beneath the warmth of the bedclothes, until the moment when I suddenly fall asleep, as a man throws himself into a pool of stagnant water in order to drown. I do not feel this perfidious sleep coming over me as I used to, but a sleep which is close to me and watching me, which is going to seize me by the head, to close my eyes and annihilate me.

I sleep—a long time—2 or 3 hours perhaps—then a dream—no—a nightmare lays hold of me. I feel that I am in bed and asleep—I feel it and I know it—and I feel also that somebody is coming close to me, is looking at me, touching me, is getting onto my bed, is kneeling on my chest, is taking my neck between his hands and squeezing it—squeezing it with all his might in order to strangle me.

And then suddenly I wake up, shaken and bathed in perspiration; I light a candle and find that I am alone, and after that crisis, which occurs every night, I at length fall asleep and slumber tranquilly until morning. (Maupassant, 1945, pp. 44–45)

SLEEP PARALYSIS IN THE WRITING OF
THOMAS HARDY (1840 TO 1928)

The English author and Victorian realist, Thomas Hardy, also published an account of sleep paralysis (1999). In *The Withered Arm* (originally published in 1888), Hardy documented a case of sleep paralysis that occurred after a hard day's work (as is similarly described in chapter 3) and also evidenced hallucinations that contained a day's residue of the character's recent concerns. Specifically, the bride from a recent wedding (whom the character clearly recognized) sat on her chest and mocked her. Interestingly, Hardy called the oppressing bride an "incubus," whereas "succubus" would seemingly have been more sex-appropriate. The episode ceases with an act of movement, and the character is left in a state of confusion and fear.

> One night, two or three weeks after the bridal return... Rhoda sat a long time over the turf ashes that she had raked out in front of her to extinguish them. She contemplated so intently the new wife... that she forgot the lapse of time. At last, wearied by her day's work, she too retired.
>
> But the figure which had occupied her so much during this and the previous days was not to be banished at night. For the first time Gertrude Lodge visited the supplanted woman in her dreams. Rhoda Brook dreamed—since her assertion that she really saw, before falling asleep, was not to be believed—that the young wife... was sitting upon her chest as she lay. The pressure of Mrs Lodge's person grew heavier... and then the figure thrust forward its left hand mockingly, so as to make the wedding-ring it wore glitter in Rhoda's eyes. Maddened mentally, and nearly suffocated by pressure, the sleeper struggled; the incubus, still regarding her, withdrew to the foot of the bed, only, however, to come forward by degrees, resume her seat, and flash her left hand as before.
>
> Gasping for breath, Rhoda, in a last desperate effort, swung out her right hand, seized the confronting spectre by its obtrusive left arm, and whirled it backward to the floor, starting up herself as she did so with a low cry.
>
> 'O, merciful heaven!' she cried, sitting on the edge of the bed in a cold sweat; 'that was not a dream—she was here!'
>
> She could feel her antagonist's arm within her grasp even now—the very flesh and hone of it, as it seemed. She looked on the floor whither she had whirled the spectre, but there was nothing to be seen. (Hardy, 1999, pp. 335–336)

Francis Scott Key Fitzgerald also vividly described an episode of sleep paralysis in his novel, *The Beautiful and the Damned* (Fitzgerald, 1950), originally published in 1922. Interestingly, Fitzgerald may have himself experienced sleep paralysis, but the historical evidence is far from conclusive (e.g., Schneck, 1971). As he did, however, definitely suffer from chronic alcoholism (and likely also tuberculosis), his body was certainly primed for these episodes to occur. Regardless of his personal experience or lack thereof, he aptly portrays the peculiar state of consciousness as well as the acute awareness of one's actual surroundings that are so characteristic of sleep paralysis episodes. Like Thomas Hardy, Fitzgerald's character also recognizes the hallucinatory figure, and the entire episode ends abruptly through a physical movement (Sharpless & Grom, in press).

She shut her eyes .... She lay there for something over two hours ... She was conscious, even aware, after a long while that the noise down-stairs had lessened .... She was in a state half-way between sleeping and waking, with neither condition predominant ... and she was harassed by a desire to rid herself of a weight pressing down upon her breast. She felt that if she could cry the weight would be lifted, and forcing the lids of her eyes together she tried to raise a lump in her throat ... to no avail ....

She became rigid. Some one had come to the door and was standing regarding her .... She could see the outline of his figure distinct against some indistinguishable light. There was no sound anywhere, only a great persuasive silence ... only this figure, swaying, swaying in the doorway, an indiscernible and subtly menacing terror, a personality filthy under its varnish, like smallpox spots under a layer of powder. Yet her tired heart, beating until it shook her breasts, made her sure that there was still life in her, desperately shaken, threatened ....

The minute or succession of minutes prolonged itself interminably, and a swimming blur began to form before her eyes, which tried with childish persistence to pierce the gloom in the direction of the door ... and then the figure in the doorway—it was Hull, she saw, Hull—turned deliberately and, still slightly swaying, moved back and off, as if absorbed into that incomprehensible light that had given him dimension.

Blood rushed back into her limbs, blood and life together. With a start of energy she sat upright, shifting her body until her feet touched the floor over the side of the bed. (Fitzgerald, 1950, pp. 242–243)

SLEEP PARALYSIS IN THE WRITING OF
ERNEST HEMINGWAY (1899 TO 1961)

In Hemingway's short story, *The Snows of Kilamanjaro* (originally published in 1938), one can find a different emphasis in the phenomenon of sleep paralysis (Hemingway, 1987). Although at first glance the details of this episode seem fairly impoverished compared to the writings of Maupassant, Hemingway's characteristically economical style actually conveys a great deal of information. It is unknown if Hemingway himself ever experienced sleep paralysis, but his notorious alcoholism would have certainly made such experiences possible.

In this story, *Death* is described as both approaching and oppressing the main character, a person who is severely ill due to an infected thorn wound. This overt connection with death in this story is interesting, and actually foreshadows some subsequent empirical findings and speculations. For instance, it is well-known that a fear of imminent death is often present *during* sleep paralysis episodes themselves (Hinton, Pich, Chhean, & Pollack, 2005; Sharpless et al., 2010). However, Liddon (1970) noted that a more general preoccupation with death was evident in both of his case studies, and other researchers found a significant (yet fairly small) correlation between sleep paralysis and the measure of death anxiety (Arikawa, Templer, Brown, Cannon, & Thomas-Dodson, 1999). These findings are especially intriguing in light of the connections between dead relatives and sleep paralysis documented in chapter 3. Further, as demonstrated in chapter 10, intrapsychic conflicts over both death and sexuality are core components of early psychoanalytic theories of sleep paralysis as well.

> It moved up closer to him still and now he could not speak to it, and when it saw he could not speak it came a little closer, and now he tried to send it away without speaking, but it moved in on him so its weight was all upon his chest, and while it crouched there and he could not move or speak, he heard the woman say, "Bwana is asleep now. Take the cot up very gently and carry it into the tent."
>
> He could not speak to tell her to make it go away and it crouched now, heavier, so he could not breathe. And then, while they lifted the cot, suddenly it was all right and the weight went from his chest. (Hemingway, 1987, pp. 54–55)

SLEEP PARALYSIS IN THE PAINTINGS OF HENRI FUSELLI
(1741 TO 1825)

In all likelihood, Fuseli's (1781) painting *The Nightmare* is the most famous visual representation of sleep paralysis. This almost archetypal image has graced the covers of several books on the subject (e.g., Adler, 2011; Hufford, 1982) and the frontispiece of an earlier edition of Jones' work on the Nightmare (Jones, 1949). It also served as inspiration for the poem by Erasmus Darwin (Darwin, 2012).

In this oil painting, a voluptuous woman dressed in sheer white night-clothes is shown lying in a supine position with her head and arms hanging from the bed. On her chest sits a diminutive, pointy-eared brown being looking directly at the viewer. A chiaroscuro effect is pronounced, and there are many textural elements found in the room as well (e.g., velvet curtains). In the upper left corner of the painting, a black horse's head with eyes bereft of pupils is shown just penetrating the folds of the curtain.

Along with a good deal of overt sexual imagery, this painting adroitly captures many sleep paralysis elements. This is especially the case for the incubus subtype of hallucinations. Namely, there is a palpable and pronounced feeling of helplessness. The female figure is utterly defenseless and at the mercy of the malevolent-looking imp sitting upon her. As she is supine with her limbs splayed out in a lifeless fashion, she can resist neither the imp nor the mare. This powerlessness is consistent with many sleep paralysis narratives (e.g., Hufford, 1982). There is also a strong sense of fear, found not so much on the face of the woman, but in the reactions of viewers to this work. *The Nightmare* conveys a sense that something bad is going to happen, and far sooner than later. Fuseli also clearly pays homage to earlier folkloric beliefs described in chapter 3 through his inclusion of both the mare and the demonic-looking imp/incubus (see also some of the malevolent stories of fairies in Briggs, 1978). Fuseli played with this imagery in several other works, with variations in placement for the main figures and differing degrees of malevolence shown upon the face of the oppressive demon. However, it is our opinion that this particular version was never surpassed.

CONCLUSIONS

In ending this survey of sleep paralysis as found in the literary and visual arts, one can see vivid depictions of sleep paralysis predating the phenomenon's formal medical naming. This is the case for at least one well-known text in the Western literary canon (e.g., *Moby Dick*). In at least one other case, content from one artistic medium served as subsequent inspiration for another (i.e., Fuseli's influence on Darwin). As we have now described sleep paralysis in folklore, legend, and art, we now turn to medical history.

REFERENCES

Adler, S. (2011). *Sleep paralysis: Night-mares, nocebos, and the mind-body connection.* Newark, NJ: Rutgers University Press.

Alvaro, L. (2005). Hallucinations and pathological visual perceptions in Maupassant's fantastical short stories—A neurological approach. *Journal of the History of the Neurosciences, 14,* 100–115.

Arikawa, H., Templer, D. I., Brown, R., Cannon, W. G., & Thomas-Dodson, S. (1999). The structure and correlates of kanshibari. *The Journal of Psychology, 133*(4), 369–375.

Briggs, K. M. (1978). *An encyclopedia of fairies: Hobgoblins, brownies, bogies, and other supernatural creatures.* NY: Pantheon Books.

Darwin, E. (2012). *The botanic garden.* part II. containing the loves of the plants. A poem with philosophical notes. [kindle version]. Retrieved from www.amazon.com

Fitzgerald, F. S. (1950). *The beautiful and the damned.* New York: C. Scribner's Sons.

French, C. C., & Stone, A. (2013). *Anomalistic psychology: Exploring paranormal belief and experience.* London: Palgrave Macmillan.

Fuseli, H. (1781). *The nightmare.* London: Royal Academy of London.

Hardy, T. (1999). In Brady K. (Ed.), *The withered arm and other stories.* New York: Penguin Books.

Hemingway, E. (1987). The snows of Kilimananjaro. *The complete short stories of Ernest Hemingway* (Finca Vigia edition ed., pp. 39–56). New York: Scribner.

Herman, J. (1997). Literature and sleep an instance of sleep paralysis in moby-dick. *Sleep, 20*(7), 577–579.

Hinton, D. E., Pich, V., Chhean, D., & Pollack, M. H. (2005). The ghost pushes you down: Sleep paralysis-type panic attacks in a Khmer refugee population. *Transcultural Psychiatry, 42*(1), 46–77. doi: 10.1177/1363461505050710

Hufford, D. (1982). *The terror that comes in the night: An experience-centered study of supernatural assault traditions.* Philadelphia: University of Pennsylvania Press.

Ignotus, P. (1968). *The paradox of Maupassant.* New York: Funk and Wagnalls.

Jones, E. (1949). *On the nightmare* (2nd Impression ed.). London: Hogarth Press and the Institute of Psycho-analysis.

Liddon, S. C. (1970). Sleep paralysis, psychosis, and death. *The American Journal of Psychiatry, 126*(7), 1027–1031.

Maupassant, G. d. (1945). In Commins S. (Ed.), *The best stories of Guy de Maupassant.* New York: Modern Library.

Melville, H. (1952). In Hutchins R. M. (Ed.), *Great books of the western world volume 48: Melville.* Chicago: Encyclopedia Britannica.

Nietzsche, F. (1967). Ecce homo. In W. Kaufmann (Ed.), *On the geneology of morals and ecce homo* (W. Kaufmann, trans., pp. 217–335). New York: Vintage Books.

Schneck, J. M. (1971). Sleep paralysis in F. Scott Fitzgerald's the beautiful and the damned. *New York State Journal of Medicine, 71*, 378–379.

Sharpless, B. A., & Grom, J. L. (in press). Isolated sleep paralysis: Fear, prevention, and disruption. *Behavioral Sleep Medicine.*

Sharpless, B. A., McCarthy, K. S., Chambless, D. L., Milrod, B. L., Khalsa, S. R., & Barber, J. P. (2010). Isolated sleep paralysis and fearful isolated sleep paralysis in outpatients with panic attacks. *Journal of Clinical Psychology, 66*(12), 1292–1306. doi: 10.1002/jclp.20724

CHAPTER 5

Early Medicine and the "Nightmare"

He who wishes to know what Night-Mare is, let him eat chestnuts before going to sleep, and drink after them feculent wine.
      —Franz Hildesheim, 1612

Although the formal christening of the term "sleep paralysis" didn't occur until the 1920s (Wilson, 1928), speculation about the etiology and treatment of this phenomenon can be found in earlier medical literatures. We have attempted to be wide ranging in this survey, and sampled physicians from the ancient world to modernity. In order to concentrate more fully on several interesting historical and medical themes that go beyond any one individual theorist, a timeline of important dates in the history of sleep paralysis can be found in Figure 5.1.

Several trends in this brief survey will be apparent. First, sleep paralysis, whether termed "ephialtes, incubus, Nightmare, cataplexy of the waking state," or otherwise, was carefully described and taken quite seriously as a disease by early physicians. In making a shift from a supernatural and "external" view of sleep paralysis (i.e., someone/something is doing this "to me") to the scientific view with endogenous natural causes, there was an increased emphasis on physiological explanations for these scary paroxysms. Perhaps not surprisingly, relatively little attention was paid to *psychological* factors related to sleep paralysis, but those we were indeed able to locate (or reasonably infer) are mentioned. It is also noteworthy that sleep paralysis was usually viewed as potentially dangerous, either because it was seen as a prelude to more serious conditions (e.g., apoplexy and the "sacred disease" of epilepsy) or because it could lead to death on its own. Although this may sound

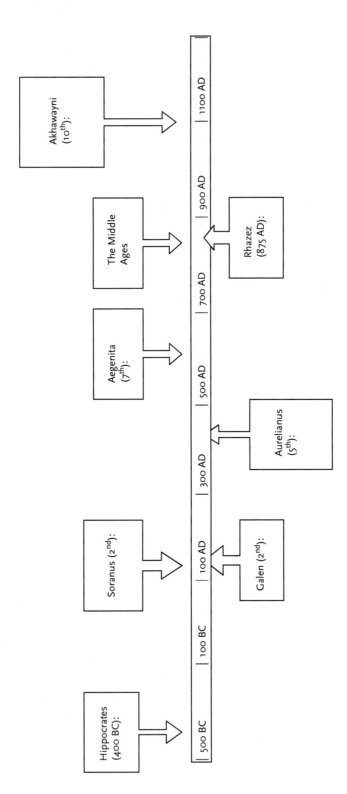

Figure 5.1:
Timeline of important dates in the history of sleep paralysis.

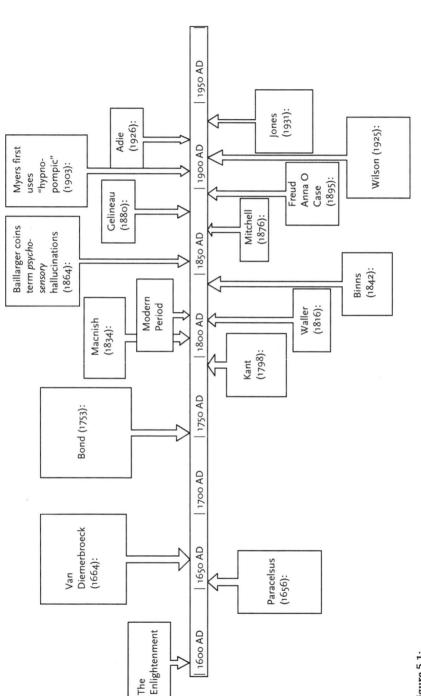

Figure 5.1:
Continued.

strange to contemporary readers, a belief in the terminal nature of sleep paralysis was widespread, and appears to have originated in ancient Rome. Finally, it may be somewhat surprising to see how little treatment approaches changed over the 1500 years we surveyed. Many of the treatments conducted in ancient Rome would have been recognizable to doctors of the 18th and 19th centuries.

Not surprisingly, these physicians' theories were intimately colored by their time and place. Thus, they are not so different from us and the conceptual limits we all experience when using the (limited) explanatory categories available to us at any point in human history. Interestingly, however, we also found more *personal experiences* influencing theory, as several of those who wrote most voluminously on sleep paralysis were themselves chronic sufferers. This intimate, first-hand knowledge, when coupled with a physician's careful eye for detail, led to some sophisticated theoretical speculations and clinical descriptions.

Throughout this chapter we use the term "Nightmare" in most cases. The use of one consistent term instead of varying terminology by author (e.g., "incubus, ephialtes") will hopefully reduce reader confusion. In general, we consider Nightmare to be a subtype of sleep paralysis/isolated sleep paralysis. Namely, Nightmares consist of paralysis characterized by feelings of weight/oppression on the chest and an inability to cry out for help. These are often but not always accompanied by frightful hallucinations and other symptoms (Sharpless, 2014).

WHO WAS THE FIRST PHYSICIAN/SCIENTIST TO DESCRIBE SLEEP PARALYSIS?

When discussing any phenomenon from a historical standpoint it is common to discuss the person who first "discovered" or described it. However, in reviewing the secondary literature on sleep paralysis and isolated sleep paralysis, there appears to be a lack of consensus over whose description of the phenomenon actually takes historical precedence. Four physicians have been repeatedly discussed; some have claimed it was Edward Binns in 1842 (e.g., Bell et al., 1984), and others have claimed Robert Macnish in 1834 or Isbrand van Diemerbroeck in 1689.

However, one of the most common citations for the first descriptions of sleep paralysis is Weir Silas Mitchell in 1876 (e.g., Awadalla et al., 2004). In reading Mitchell's original article, however, he appears to be discussing another phenomenon entirely. The female patient in the case that he presented (p. 778) was reported to have only experienced a partial paralysis during sleep in the exact place where she previously experienced palsy (i.e., on only one side of her body). This is clearly inconsistent with sleep paralysis proper.

So who was the first to present an authentic case of sleep paralysis? We would agree with previous authors that Binns, Macnish, and van Diemerbroeck (among others in the early modern period) all published vivid cases. In reviewing other works of medicine, however, we found many earlier descriptions, and some were actually cited by the authors just mentioned. For instance, Caelius Aurelianus's (5th century A.D.) translation of the medical works of Soranus of Ephesus (2nd century A.D.) from Greek to Latin contains some interesting passages. Aurelianus, a younger contemporary of Galen, wrote, "there is a feeling of heaviness and oppression and a sort of choking. They imagine that someone has suddenly attacked them and stunned their senses, exhausting them and preventing outcry (Aurelianus, 1950, p. 475)." He then stated that sufferers often jump up and cry out, but it is unclear whether or not this was a response to the incubus or an associated symptom during the attack. Although it is probably the former, it is certainly not definitive.

A likelier candidate for primacy would be Paulus Aeginita, a 7th century Byzantine Greek physician (Aegineta, 1844). He wrote in his section titled *On Incubus, or Nightmare*:

> It attacks persons after a surfeit, and who are laboring under protracted indigestion. Persons suffering an attack experience incapability of motion, a torpid sensation in their sleep, a sense of suffocation, and oppression, as if from one pressing them down, with inability to cry out, or they utter inarticulate sounds. Some imagine often that they even hear the person who is going to press them down, that he offers lustful violence to them, but flies when they attempt to grasp him with their fingers. (p. 388)

Thus, Aegineta described a paralytic state clearly differentiated from normal sleep that also contained many of the prototypical, common elements of sleep paralysis (an inability to cry out; hypnopompic hallucinations that disappear when paralysis ends). Roscher (2007) claimed that Themison of Laodicea (died 43 B.C.E.) was the first to write on the topic of *pgnalion* (i.e., "throttle"), but all that exists is the term being used in several letters, not actual descriptions (p. 110).

EARLY MEDICAL VIEWS ON THE ETIOLOGY OF NIGHTMARE

Along with descriptions of individual cases, many early physicians proposed etiological hypotheses for the Nightmare, and several suffered themselves from chronic and sometimes lifelong attacks (e.g., Bond, 1753; Waller, 1816). Their thoughts may be particularly illuminating. As will be apparent, though, theories were wide ranging, and this fact makes simple classification difficult. Jones, (1949) preferred to dichotomize into 1) theories of peripheral irritation (e.g., indigestible foods) and 2) various mechanical sources (e.g., sleeping posture), whereas Dahlitz and Parkes (1993) broke them down by organ system (e.g., alimentary, respiratory, circulatory, nervous). We have found it most useful to discuss these various causes in terms of gastric disturbances, environmental impingements, congestion, psychological predispositions, and moral theories.

Several gastric disturbances purportedly led to Nightmare. For instance, eating foods that were difficult to digest (such as the chestnuts described in the epigraph) was thought to be a proximal cause. Almonds, certain cheeses, cucumbers, and "alligator pears" (viz., avocados), have all been implicated in Nightmare (e.g., Macnish, 1834; Waller, 1816), as has indigestion in general. Relatedly, a theory of a pH balance was proposed by Waller (1816) such that an overabundance of acidity was the problem. We can see how certain attempts to "cure" the Nightmare logically followed from these theories in Table 5.1. Waller himself reported success with the regular ingestion of a drink containing ammonia (i.e., an alkaline substance).

Similar to discussions in chapter 3 on the difference between obsession and possession in demonology, some early physicians discussed causes of Nightmare that also derived from forces external to the body. For instance, Splittgerber proposed that certain phases of the moon could elicit Nightmare, and Binz believed carbon dioxide poisoning of the brain was a cause (as cited in Jones, 1949). Waller, himself a sailor, believed this class of workers to be particularly prone, and he often experienced Nightmare at sea (Waller, 1816). He did not elaborate on the cause, but we speculate that the long hours required of sailors as well as the constant rocking so characteristic of sea travel could easily lead to disturbed sleep and anomalous sensations in a slumbering body.

Various congestion theories (derived from a humoral understanding of disease) have, perhaps not surprisingly, been used to explicate Nightmares. We will do our best to avoid too much discussion of antediluvian theories of animal spirits and rising vapors of various thicknesses, but it is clear that congestion of organs and organ systems was widely held to be at the root of Nightmare for pre-19th century medicine. For example, the medieval Persian physician Akhawayni held that vapors from the stomach would rise to the brain, resulting in feelings of suffocation for the sleeper (Golzari et al., 2012). Baillarger (as cited in Jones, 1949) held

Table 5.1. EARLY MEDICAL TREATMENTS FOR THE NIGHTMARE

Treatment	Source
Ammonia: Drink a solution of ammonia mixed with warm water.	Waller, 1816
Astringents: Iron and its derivatives Wild valerian root and a cold bath. Pitch plasters	Aurelianus, 1950; Bond, 1753

Bleeding:
Therapy includes blood-letting from the superficial vein in the
    arm, ankle, or leg.
Bond found that his own practice of 4- to 6-week bleedings
    elicited nightmares, so he reduced frequency to once a year.
Attempt to take pressure off of the pulmonary veins and inferior auricle.
	Aegineta, 1844; Bond,
	    1753; Golzari et al.,
	    2012

Dietary Changes:
Thinning of the diet (restrict and attenuate)
Avoid difficult to digest/flatulent foods (e.g., cheese, cucumbers,
    almonds).
Add vinegar to meals.
Eat an acrid diet.
Eat soft, easy to digest foods.
Avoid alcohol.
	Aurelianus, 1950;
	    Bond, 1753; Golzari
	    et al., 2012; Macnish,
	    1834; Roscher, 2007;
	    Waller, 1816

Evacuants/Purgatives:
Induce vomiting/purging using radishes.
Apply certain ointments to the head (e.g., ones that contain castor)
Sneezing and gargling
	Aegineta, 1844; Golzari
	    et al., 2012; Macnish,
	    1834; Roscher, 2007;
	    Waller, 1816

Head Shaving	Aurelianus, 1950

Herbal and Vegetable Remedies:
Black hellebore
Hiera (wild gourd)
Black pips of peony
Scammony mixed with aromatics (e.g., anise, wild carrots, Macedonian
    parsley)
	Aegineta, 1844;
	    Aurelianus, 1950;
	    Roscher, 2007

Olive Oil Treatment: Have patient lie in a moderately lit and warm room and keep mind/body at rest. Cover head and region of chest with scoured wool dipped in olive oil. Have patient wash mouth with warm water.	Aurelianus, 1950
Beaver Oil Treatment Rubbed in to prevent help prevent epilepsy	Roscher, 2007

Sleep Changes:
Not to sleep on their backs (viz., this is the position of dead bodies)
Avoid sleeping when slumped over/don't compress the body
    (e.g., head resting on a desk while sitting).
	Bond, 1753; Macnish,
	    1834; Van
	    Diemerbroeck, 1689

this view as well. Congestion in the form of a plethora of blood was also discussed as a cause of this "disease." This view is probably most associated with Aegineta (1844), but is very much in keeping with humoral theories in general. Regarding the plethora hypothesis, a quick perusal of Table 5.1 makes it once again easy to see how treatment recommendations can be readily (and logically) deduced once one has committed to an etiological model. Van Diemerbroeck (1689) believed that an excess of blood caused muscle failure, and therefore the paralysis so characteristic of Nightmare. Bond (1753) treated himself with bleeding, but reported that too much venesection actually intensified his Nightmares. Galen (reviewed in Davies, 2003) believed that a general stagnation in the blood could be the result of vapors, which caused distension of the stomach, and Waller (1816) similarly noted that Nightmare attacks may be preceded by excessive flatulence.

As time passed, personal character, habits, and other psychological factors came to be understood as having roles in the Nightmare. This appears to have become a more serious consideration in the 18th century. For instance, a general excitation during the preceding day/night was thought to be a proximal trigger. This could occur due to frightful dreams or other factors (e.g., Bond, 1753; Jones, 1949).

Those with a hypochondriacal, hysterical, or seemingly neurotic temperament were thought to be at risk (Macnish, 1834; Waller, 1816). More specifically, contemplative individuals who are prone to long study and who also tend towards solitary rumination were held to be extremely vulnerable. It is interesting to note recent associations between isolated sleep paralysis and the constructs of anxiety sensitivity, negative affect, and death anxiety (Arikawa, Templer, Brown, Cannon, & Thomas-Dodson, 1999; Ramsawh, Raffa, White, & Barlow, 2008; Sharpless et al., 2010). Jones credits Franz Splittgerber as primarily responsible for foreshadowing later psychoanalytic theories of the Nightmare when he found their origin in, "hidden tendencies of the mind and the agonies of an evil conscience (Jones, 1949, p. 36)." Thus, the Nightmare for Splittgerber had its origins in guilt, conflict, and other subterranean forces.

Mention should also be made of what one could term "moral" theories for the Nightmare. These are theories very much in keeping with particular societal values, especially those associated with a protestant work ethic and personal temperance. For instance, individuals with sedentary lifestyles who do not engage in outdoor physical activities or exercise were thought to be at risk (Macnish, 1834). Thus, hard work and physical endurance were seen as preventatives. Similarly, and somewhat presciently, Waller (1816) noted that sleep disruptions in the form of sleeping too long, too deeply, or going to bed at too late of an hour and sleeping in too late could all cause Nightmare. These scary paroxysms could also be caused by gluttony in general, heavy foods in particular (Macnish, 1834), and being a "drunkard (Bond, 1753)." It is perhaps not surprising that one would look toward deviations in lifestyles and personal habits when ferreting out answers for these otherwise anomalous experiences. We should also note here the fairly stark contrast between many of the medieval explanations discussed in chapter 3 (e.g., witches, vampires) and these Enlightenment/Early Modern theories.

In ending this section, we would also like to note that Waller (1816) made another prescient hypothesis about the origin of Nightmare. Specifically, he wrote:

> Everything connected with the phenomena of sleep, is extremely obscure; and nothing on this subject appears to be more extraordinary, than the sudden transition from the sleeping to the waking state. Whatever it is which takes place at that moment in the brain, and in the whole system, takes place only partially in the Night-Mare. Is it very absurd to suppose that a part of the system may recover the waking state, while the brain, or some other part, remains asleep, for want of sufficient stimulus to rouse them? . . . It seems that the brain continues to present a succession of images to the mind as in sleep, whilst at the same time, the body is become susceptible of external impressions, and conscious of internal ones? . . . (pp. 87–88)

Subsequent scientifically-based elaborations on this insight can be found in chapter 10.

THE NIGHTMARE AND FEMALE SEXUALITY

As may be apparent, especially from our survey of myths and supernatural creatures in chapter 3, the Nightmare has been frequently associated with sex and sexuality. It often occurs at night, in dimly lit bedrooms, and commonly involves feelings of pressure and sensations that someone (or something) is on top of a terrified victim. These narratives remain ubiquitous in contemporary sleep paralysis research and practice. Early physicians saw these connections as well, but they linked the Nightmare more closely with female sexuality than most would today. Although more women experience sleep paralysis than men, the rates are not drastically different (Sharpless & Barber, 2011). Therefore, with the observations discussed in the following, it is unclear if these physicians were either astute observers of authentic etiological factors, or whether a fascination with female sexuality and/or a predisposition to see women differently from men was a root cause of these speculations. And, of course, these possibilities need not be mutually exclusive.

Bond (1753) presented several cases of Nightmare occurring in close proximity to menstruation. In his first case of a 15-year-old girl, he reported that she had very troubled sleep for several consecutive nights. One night she experienced a Nightmare of a man coming in her room, lying on top of her, and oppressing her as she slept. The next day she experienced "a copious eruption of the Menses which, for a time, remov'd all her complaints (p. 47)." His third case described another young woman who experienced Nightmare 2 to 3 nights prior to every menstrual period. Interestingly, Bond also included a case attributed to van Diemerbroeck of a woman whose Nightmare attacks began *after* her periods.

Female sexual activity, or a lack of, also appears to be a predisposing condition. Waller (1816) claimed that women were actually *less* prone to Nightmare in general, but that virgins and pregnant women were particularly at risk. Macnish (1834) also thought pregnancy created a greater risk, and you can see this belief in non-medical, occult writings as well (e.g., Paracelsus, 1656, pp. 58–59).

So what can be made of these connections? We have found no evidence that pre-, peri-, or post-menstrual factors are directly associated with sleep paralysis. Certainly, sleep in general can be affected by menses (e.g., periodic hypersomnia preceding onset, as in D'Ambrosio & Baron, 2009), and these factors could induce sleep paralysis, but more direct links are lacking. Given that many of these early physicians believed that a *plethora* of blood was a proximal cause of Nightmare, the association makes logical sense from this particular etiological viewpoint. However, empirical support would be helpful.

Regarding pregnancy, these early physicians may be on relatively firmer empirical footing. One recent study found that, whereas parasomnias decreased overall during pregnancy, sleep paralysis actually *increased* (Hedman, Pohjasvaara, Tolonen, Salmivaara, & Myllyla, 2002). Specifically, sleep paralysis episodes declined in the first trimester, but increased in the second and third. Following birth, sleep paralysis essentially disappeared. It is possible that sleep disruptions increase during the course of pregnancy (Berndt, Diekelmann, Alexander, Pustal, & Kirschbaum, 2014) and that this, in combination with increased sensations of pressure on the torso and mounting anxiety/anxiety sensitivity, may all be proximal factors leading to sleep paralysis.

NIGHTMARE AS POTENTIALLY CONTAGIOUS?

Several medical writers also proposed that Nightmare had contagious elements, and was involved in several epidemics/public hysterias. Although we were unable to locate any recent "outbreaks," there are certainly precedents for these social elements in other manifestations of psychopathology. For instance, there have been epidemics of *Koro* (Mattelaer & Jilek, 2007). *Koro* is the delusional belief that your genitals are shrinking/receding into your body, and when they fully retract, you die. Much like isolated sleep paralysis, *koro* was initially (and possibly mistakenly) thought to be a culturally bound disorder (viz., limited to East Asian populations). However, cases in Africa, Europe, and the United States have been documented (e.g., Mattelaer & Jilek, 2007; Radford, 2013). What is particularly interesting is the fact that it often occurs as a public health phenomenon, and not just in individual cases.

The earliest description of Nightmare "contagion" that we were able to locate was described by Silimachus, a Roman follower of Hippocrates (cited in Aurelianus, 1950). However, Roscher states that "Silimachus" is a mistaken rendering of "Callimachus" (Roscher, 2007). Regardless, he reports that many of his fellow Romans were affected by Nightmare, and that it spread like a plague through the populace. Bond (1753) believed that Roman decadence may have been a proximal cause of the outbreak, noting that the Romans made supper their principle meal, were prone to excessively imbibing alcohol, and "indulged themselves in all kinds of intemperance at night (p. 67)." As we show in subsequent chapters, support exists for some of these claims.

A more recent case of "contagious" Nightmare was told by one "Dr. Laurent," a French battlefield surgeon (Millingen, 1839). Dr. Laurent reported on an entire regiment being overcome by Nightmare. Details are scant, but this event transpired after a lengthy forced march ended with the men garrisoning in the small town of Tropea. Unfortunately, they experienced little comfortable rest that night due to overcrowding in the makeshift barracks, which coincidentally was also a monastery with a local reputation for being haunted. Although the soldiers initially laughed at the ghost stories told by the townsfolk, they subsequently changed their minds. Many awoke in the middle of the night to find themselves suffocated by what they described as a large black dog. The beast disappeared suddenly and, as a result of this experience, many men left the barracks screaming. If these descriptions are accurate, it may be possible that a combination of the forced march and the uncomfortable bedroom surrounds served to dysregulate sleep patterns and encourage frequent awakenings during the night. Both of these factors make sleep paralysis more likely to occur. The interrater reliability for the putative cause of these attacks (i.e., the malevolent large black dog) is interesting. If this report is indeed true, it may be the case that a shared hallucination, analogous to the group genital retraction delusion experienced in *koro*, can arise in sleep paralysis as well, at least under certain conditions. Interestingly, Krauss (cited in Roscher, 2007) described these shared hallucinations as deriving from an *Alpmiasma*, some form of redolent "bad air," which predisposed groups of people of Nightmare

SLEEP PARALYSIS AS A PRELUDE TO SERIOUS DISEASES

Another commonly held belief throughout the early history of medicine was that Nightmare was, in effect, a "gateway" disorder. There was a fair degree of unanimity that sleep paralysis was a disease that could lead to other, more serious conditions. For example, physicians ranging from Galen (as cited in Bond, 1753 and Aurelianus, 1950) to Macnish (1834) believed that prolonged Nightmare led to the development of epilepsy. Waller (1816) noted that the ancients, in particular, believed Nightmare to be a specific form of epilepsy. The "sacred disease," like Nightmare/ sleep paralysis, has also often been associated with the supernatural. At present, some have noted phenomenological similarities between sleep paralysis and certain seizure disorders (Galimberti, Ossola, Colnaghi, & Arbasino, 2009), bur more work needs to be done.

Apoplexy has also been thought to result from longstanding Nightmare. Apoplexy is a historically ambiguous term that may refer to bleeding from the internal organs, what we would now term a stroke, or, "a sudden Privation of all the Animal functions, except the Act of Respiration" (Van Diemerbroeck, 1689, p., 185). Thus, chronic Nightmare could result in a state akin to coma. Discussions of sleep paralysis and apoplexy can be found in the works of both Van Diemerbroeck (1689) and Bond (1753).

Although epilepsy and apoplexy are the most commonly held endpoints of Nightmare, it was also thought to be the forerunner of other conditions. For instance, Bond (1753) noted that vertigo, madness in general, and melancholy in particular, can result from Nightmare. The more frequent the paroxysms, the sooner that Nightmare progresses into these more serious conditions. Macnish (1834) reported that Nightmare can lead to "hysterical afflictions...which prove extremely harassing" (p. 138).

Finally, Waller (1816) made an interesting observation about the experience of Nightmare over time. He reported that, "for the frequent repetition of the paroxysms gives greater strength to the disease, and that in proportion to the length of the duration" (p. 111). Thus, sleep paralysis was believed to, in a sense, feed off itself and intensify over time. It is also possible that habitual experiences may lead a sufferer to engage in compensatory behaviors that serve to make Nightmare episodes more frequent and amplified in severity (e.g., avoidance of sleep; catastrophic attributions to sleep paralysis). There is also some limited empirical evidence that those who have more frequent or severe episodes also make more attempts to prevent episodes from occurring, whether these attempts are successful or not (Sharpless & Grom, in press).

SLEEP PARALYSIS AS A POTENTIAL CAUSE OF DEATH?

Was sleep paralysis thought to result in death? It is clear that many early medical writers thought this to be the case (e.g., Macnish, 1834). A main (the main?) source for what could be called the "terminal Nightmare hypothesis" is Silimachus (Aurelianus, 1950). Silimachus claimed that Nightmare was responsible for the deaths of many Roman citizens, although without further details, this report should be considered with some degree of skepticism.

The mechanism through which Nightmare led to death appears to have been in dispute. According to Aurelianus (1950), Nightmare caused death from severe choking. Bond (1753) believed that Nightmare was associated with stagnation in the blood, and that this formed obstructions in the body that could eventuate in sudden death. He also thought that the common sensations of suffocation could lead to death as well, and that "drunkards" were particularly susceptible (p. 70). Finally, Binns (1842) reported on the interesting case of the death of John William Polidori. Polidori was a medical doctor who wrote his thesis on sleepwalking. He is probably most famous, however, for penning *The Vampyre*, one of the first vampire stories written in English and a watershed moment for the entire genre. Although speculation about Polidori's death from suicide abounded among his contemporaries, Bond noted that he was rumored to have died of either Nightmare or the use of laudanum in order to stave off the attacks. Regardless of the veracity of Nightmare's possible role in his death, this story implies at the very least that there was a firm belief in the seriousness of attacks.

Unfortunately, apart from individual observations and heavy (and repetitive) citations of Silimachus, there is little evidence that nightmare can be terminal. However, Bond and others strongly believed that sleep paralysis could even cause sudden death in fairly healthy individuals. Similarly, a recent book by Shelley Adler (2011) associated the Night-Mare with sudden unexpected nocturnal death syndrome.

Interestingly, at least one luminary of the Enlightenment viewed the Nightmare and its relationship to death quite differently. Although not a physician, the eminent philosopher Immanuel Kant also wrote on the Nightmare and, as with much of his overall thought, believed that it served a *teleological* function. From his perspective it was not a deadly affliction, but was actually a means of *protecting* individuals from death. Specifically, the terror of the Nightmare's paroxysms and the extreme nature of these experiences served as a warning, or stimulus to action, that the body was in mortal danger due to insufficient blood flow. Thus, Nightmare was not a cause of death, but portended (and attempted to stave off) its possibility.

EARLY MEDICAL TREATMENT OF SLEEP PARALYSIS

Table 5.1 displays many of the treatments for Nightmare that were found in the course of our historical survey. Several observations are noteworthy. The reader is probably first struck by the non-medical cast of the interventions, or at least it seems this way to our contemporary eyes. With the exception of venesection, the interventions seem more akin to herbalism and healing rituals. Readers of these histories can also find inconsistencies between treatments (e.g., one physician recommends an acidic diet whereas another wants to make the body more basic). What is perhaps most striking is the lack of significant change (progress?) in Nightmare treatments from ancient Rome to the middle of the 19th century. What seemed to change most were the proposed etiologies of the Nightmare as opposed to the actual treatments. We should note that some seem potentially useful, and have been applied by contemporary sufferers. Namely, avoiding going to sleep on one's back and attempting to reduce stress have been reported to be helpful interventions (Sharpless & Grom, in press).

CONCLUSIONS

In conclusion, we have reviewed a number of primary sources dealing with the phenomenon of the Nightmare/sleep paralysis. Debate over the Nightmare's origins, health implications, and treatments were found to have an extensive history in early medical literatures, and certain themes may warrant attention from contemporary researchers and scholars.

REFERENCES

Adler, S. (2011). *Sleep paralysis: Night-mares, nocebos, and the mind-body connection.* Newark, NJ: Rutgers University Press.

Aegineta, P. (1844). In F. Adams (Ed.), *The seven books of Paulus Aegineta.* Translated from the Greek with a commentary embracing a complete view of the knowledge possessed by the Greeks, Romans, and Arabians on all subjects connected with medicine and surgery. (F. Adams Trans.). London: Syndeham Society.

Arikawa, H., Templer, D. I., Brown, R., Cannon, W. G., & Thomas-Dodson, S. (1999). The structure and correlates of kanshibari. *The Journal of Psychology, 133*(4), 369–375.

Aurelianus, C. (1950). In I. E. Drabkin (Ed.), *On acute diseases and chronic diseases* (I. E. Drabkin Trans.). Chicago: University of Chicago Press.

Awadalla, A., Al-Fayez, G., Harville, M., Arikawa, H., Tomeo, M. E., Templer, D. I., & Underwood, R. (2004). Comparative prevalence of isolated sleep paralysis in Kuwaiti, Sudanese, and American college students. *Psychological Reports, 95*(1), 317–322. doi: 10.2466/PR0.95.5.317-322

Bell, C. C., Shakoor, B., Thompson, B., Dew, D., Hughley, E., Mays, R., & Shorter-Gooden, K. (1984). Prevalence of isolated sleep paralysis in black subjects. *Journal of the National Medical Association, 76*(5), 501–508.

Berndt, C., Diekelmann, S., Alexander, N., Pustal, A., & Kirschbaum, C. (2014). Sleep fragmentation and false memories during pregnancy and motherhood. *Behavioural Brain Research, 266,* 52–57. doi: 10.1016/j.bbr.2014.02.030

Binns, E. D. (1842). *The anatomy of sleep; or, the art of procuring sound and refreshing slumber at will.* London: John Churchill.

Bond, J. (1753). *An essay on the incubus, or night mare.* London: D. Wilson and T. Durham.

D'Ambrosio, C. M., & Baron, J. (2009). Postrtraumatic and recurrent hypersomnia. In T. L. Lee-Chiong (Ed.), *Sleep medicine essentials* (pp. 57–60). Hoboken, NJ: Wiley-Blackwell.

Davies, O. (2003). The nightmare experience, sleep paralysis and witchcraft accusations. *Folklore, 114*(2), 181.

Dahlitz, M., & Parkes, J.D. (1993). Sleep paralysis. *Lancet, 341,* 406–407.

Galimberti, C. A., Ossola, M., Colnaghi, S., & Arbasino, C. (2009). Focal epileptic seizures mimicking sleep paralysis. *Epilepsy & Behavior, 14*(3), 562–564. doi: 10.1016/j.yebeh.2008.12.018

Golzari, S. E., Khodadoust, K., Alakbarli, F., Ghabili, K., Islambulchilar, Z., Shoja, M. M., & Ansarin, K. (2012). Sleep paralysis in medieval Persia—the hidayat of Akhawayni (?-983 AD). *Neuropsychiatric Disease and Treatment, 8,* 229–234. doi: 10.2147/NDT.S28231; 10.2147/NDT.S28231

Hedman, C., Pohjasvaara, T., Tolonen, U., Salmivaara, A., & Myllyla, V. V. (2002). Parasomnias decline during pregnancy. *Acta Neurological Scandinavica, 105,* 209–214.

Jones, E. (1949). *On the nightmare* (2nd Impression ed.). London, United Kingdom: Hogarth Press and the Institute of Psycho-analysis.

Macnish, R. (1834). *The philosophy of sleep* (First American ed.). New York: D. Appleton and Company.

Mattelaer, J. J., & Jilek, W. (2007). Koro—the psychological disappearance of the penis. *The Journal of Sexual Medicine, 4*(5), 1509–1515. doi: JSM586 [pii]

Millingen, J. G. (1839). *Curiosities of medical experience* (2nd ed.). London: Richard Bentley.

Mitchell, S. W. (1876). On some of the disorders of sleep. *Virginia Medical Monthly, 2*(11), 769–781.

Paracelsus. (1656). *Of the supreme mysteries of nature.* (R. Turner Trans.). London: N. Brook and J. Harison.

Radford, B. (2013). Penis-snatching panics resurface in Africa. Retrieved from http://www.livescience.com/28015-penis-snatching-panics-koro.html

Ramsawh, H. J., Raffa, S. D., White, K. S., & Barlow, D. H. (2008). Risk factors for isolated sleep paralysis in an African American sample: A preliminary study. *Behavior Therapy, 39*(4), 386–397. doi: 10.1016/j.beth.2007.11.002

Roscher, W. H. (2007). Ephialtes: A pathological-mythological treatise on the nightmare in classical antiquity. [Ephialtes] (A. V. O'Brien Trans.). (Revised ed., pp. 96–159). Putnam, CT: Spring Publishing.

Sharpless, B. A. (2014). Changing conceptions of the nightmare in medicine. *Hektoen International: A Journal of Medical Humanities (Moments in History Section).*

Sharpless, B. A., & Grom, J. L. (in press). Isolated sleep paralysis: Fear, prevention, and disruption. *Behavioral Sleep Medicine.*

Sharpless, B. A., & Barber, J. P. (2011). Lifetime prevalence rates of sleep paralysis: A systematic review. *Sleep Medicine Reviews, 15*(5), 311–315. doi: 10.1016/j.smrv.2011.01.007

Sharpless, B. A., McCarthy, K. S., Chambless, D. L., Milrod, B. L., Khalsa, S. R., & Barber, J. P. (2010). Isolated sleep paralysis and fearful isolated sleep paralysis in outpatients with panic attacks. *Journal of Clinical Psychology, 66*(12), 1292–1306. doi: 10.1002/jclp.20724

Van Diemerbroeck, I. (1689). *The anatomy of human bodies, comprehending the most modern discoveries and curiosities in that art. To which is added a particular treatise of the small-pox and measles. Together with several practical observations and experienced cures.* (W. Salmom Trans.). London: W. Whitwood.

Waller, J. (1816). *A treatise on the incubus, or night-mare, disturbed sleep, terrific dreams, and nocturnal visions with the means of removing these distressing complaints.* London: E Cox and Son.

Wilson, S. A. K. (1928). The narcolepsies. *Brain, 51,* 63–109.

CHAPTER 6
Sleep Paralysis

Typical Symptoms and Associated Features

Each day is a little life for which our waking up is the birth and which is brought to an end by sleep as death. Thus going to sleep is a daily death and every waking up a new birth. In fact to complete the simile, we could regard the discomfort and difficulty of getting up as labour pains.
—Schopenhauer, 1974, p. 435

Sleep is a private process that one must do alone. It is presumably similar to dying in the sense that receding from one's typical conscious awareness is, almost by definition, a solo event regardless of whether or not other people are in the room. Therefore, whenever we sleep, we are alienated from others. However, when experiencing sleep paralysis, the discordance in sleep architecture that characterizes this phenomenon typically makes sleep a far from peaceful experience, and as we show, can even lead to feelings of discomfort and alienation from the sleeper's own body. For although conscious awareness is present, at least to some degree, it is almost as if the sufferer was trapped, with no ability to agentically act, or even any ability to secure help or reassurance from another.

The available literature suggests that there is a great deal of heterogeneity in sleep paralysis experiences, yet certain features seem fairly ubiquitous. In order to provide a better clinical picture of this, we present a vignette of a fairly typical (and quite graphic) episode below extracted from the *Fearful Isolated Sleep Paralysis Interview* (Appendix B). The individual is a 21-year-old, mixed-ethnicity woman with a long history of isolated sleep paralysis episodes. She reported that her first remembered episode took place at the age of six.

CASE EXAMPLE

"When it [sleep paralysis] happens, I can't breathe. I feel like someone or something is moving me. I feel like my chest is heavy. I can hear things and see things. I can see squares, silhouettes, shadows, and sometimes people. I can hear a lot of random dialogue, and sometimes it sounds like children playing in a park. A lot of times the voices are talking to me, talking about music or about how they're going to attack me or something."

"One time I saw a girl. I used to sleep on a bunk bed freshman year. It was just in the center of the room with no ladder. I physically saw a girl . . . she looked like a vampire or something. She had really long teeth and her face was really white. She had blood all over her mouth and looked very 'gothic.' It was weird because she was still talking to me while she was pulling me and she told me she was going to get back at me for helping her twin brother [note: participant did not understand this dialogue]. She was pulling my leg from the bed and I was freaking out, but obviously I couldn't move."

"Sometimes I'm at the foot of the bed and looking down at myself laying in bed. One time during the paralysis I left my body and went to Cleveland, I think. I heard my boyfriend's friends talking."

As can be seen in this case, sleep paralysis episodes demonstrate a number of interesting clinical characteristics that are not found in other disorders, at least not simultaneously. The essential and "minimal" criteria required for diagnosis of an episode are the presence of conscious awareness in conjunction with temporary atonia (American Academy of Sleep Medicine, 2005). The reader should note that the hypnagogic/hypnopompic hallucinations, arguably the most dramatic symptoms of sleep paralysis, are not required for diagnosis at present (see also chapter 11). Several other features not tied to diagnostic criteria are also apparent. For instance, some may be surprised by the *clinical consequences* of sleep paralysis (viz., significant fear and mild apprehension over the possibility of additional episodes and/or sleep). These are neither mentioned in most articles nor are they required to meet *recurrent isolated sleep paralysis* diagnostic criteria per ICSD-2 (American Academy of Sleep Medicine, 2005) guidelines (see chapter 11), but have recently been added to ICSD-3 (American Academy of Sleep Medicine, 2014). Thus, the minimal diagnostic criteria for sleep paralysis, if the sole focus of a clinician's attention, will not paint a very vivid picture of the experience, and if these other features are not inquired into, they may be missed by the interviewer entirely. The remainder of this chapter will be devoted to reviewing what we believe to be the most distinctive and clinically relevant facets of sleep paralysis and isolated sleep paralysis (viz., atonia, hallucinations, and fear). The associated features and clinical consequences will be discussed as well.

ATONIA

The paralysis component of sleep paralysis has a strong and fairly well-understood neurological basis. However, what is unusual about it is the fact that this atonia coincides with a relatively clear sensorium. During standard periods of REM sleep, skeletal muscles are immobile (at least in adults). Interestingly, EEG activity during REM appears to be very similar to that seen in wakefulness, but there are some crucial differences in the *expression* of this neural activity. Namely, in spite of their level of activation, motor neurons are *suppressed* during REM. This is presumed to be evolutionarily adaptive, as expressing motor activity during dreams would likely be dangerous to both the sleeper and anyone unfortunate enough to be sleeping next to the sleeper. So how does REM paralysis occur at a neurological level? As Marks (2009) stated, "This phenomenon appears to be dependent on the activation of a population of neurons in the caudal pontine reticular formation projecting to, and facilitating activity in, the medial medullary reticular formation that provides the inhibition to the motor neurons" (p. 9; see also chapter 10). Perhaps not surprisingly, dysfunctions, or what could be termed "miscues" in the tasks of the reticular formation have been implicated in a number of other parasomnias involving sleep–wake transitions (e.g., exploding head syndrome as reviewed in Chakravarty, 2007 and Sharpless, 2014).

More recently, Terzaghi, Ratti, Manni, and Manni (2012) reported neurophysiological data on a patient who experienced sleep paralysis in the context of narcolepsy. Their interpretation of the spectral EEG data was that the patient was actually in a transitional state between sleep and wakefulness during the episode, and not clearly in one or the other. The authors invoked Mahowald and Schenk's (2005) important theory on dissociated states of mind (i.e., that wakefulness, REM sleep, and NREM sleep are not mutually exclusive states of being) to understand their results, and this is consistent with other aspects of sleep paralysis experience. For although there is an awareness of the external world during sleep paralysis (and usually a good ability to remember events), episodes are often overlain with a patina of unreality and bizarreness (Sharpless, in press). Out-of-body experiences and more traditional dissociative phenomena may be present as well, and all of these are consistent with Terzaghi et al.'s line of speculation.

At a more strictly phenomenological level, the atonia leads to other unusual experiences for the sufferer. Although REM activity clearly involves eye movements, it is not common for most people to experience REM activity juxtaposed with wakeful awareness. The majority of individuals with sleep paralysis that we have encountered, however, have their eyes open during episodes. A very small percentage report an inability to open their eyes, which, if experienced in conjunction with the somatic or auditory hallucinations (described in the next few sections), could potentially be even more terrifying. In these cases, not even the position of the putative threat could be precisely determined, and the sufferer would simultaneously feel vulnerable, threatened, and unaware.

Respiration may also be affected—or at least *perceived* to be affected—by the atonia of sleep paralysis. Going back to some of the earliest reports of Nightmares and incubi/succubi, breathing difficulties have always been key components of sleep paralysis narratives (Aurelianus, 1950; Macnish, 1834). As shown in Table 6.1, contemporary research findings are consistent with these earlier reports. Sharpless, McCarthy, Chambless, Milrod, Khalsa, and Barber (2010) found that 57.7% of a clinical sample of patients with fearful isolated sleep paralysis reported chest pressure and/or smothering sensations during attacks. The origin of this particular symptom is somewhat unclear. A higher BMI could certainly lead to sensations of oppression, as could fear-induced sympathetic nervous system activation. It is also possible, as noted in chapter 3, that certain cultures may be predisposed to experience sleep paralysis as nocturnal smothering from a malevolent agent (e.g., the "old hag," succubus). Relatedly, individuals sometimes report having to "force" themselves to breath when experiencing exploding head syndrome, another condition likely caused by asynchrony of reticular formation activities (Sharpless, 2014).

Given that speaking requires voluntary muscle control just as much as moving one's limbs, sleep paralysis narratives often include speechlessness and an inability to cry out for help when in the grip of these scary paroxysms. Over half of the clinical sample in Table 6.1 reported this experience. The unexpected mutism contributes to additional feelings of powerlessness, as the sufferer cannot even gain the attention of the person sleeping next to them for assistance.

Table 6.1. FREQUENCY AND SEVERITY OF SLEEP PARALYSIS
HALLUCINATIONS AND EXPERIENCES

Sleep Paralysis Symptom	Study	% of Sample	0–8 Severity
Auditory Hallucinations	1, 2	11.37	1.99
	3	38.50	2.23
Bodily Sensations and Kinesthetic/			
Tactile Hallucinations			
Body pressure	1, 2	12.18	2.41
Pressure on chest/smothering	3	57.70	3.58
Try to speak or call out for help, but can't	3	61.50	4.31
Cold	3	23.10	1.08
Pain	3	19.20	0.85
Falling/flying/floating/spinning	3	34.60	1.81
Floating	1, 2	10.69	2.50
Feel like being touched	3	23.10	1.38
Feel like being strangled	3	19.20	1.04
Feel that body has moved/been moved	3	38.50	2.08
Leave or see body from the outside	3	30.80	1.69
Erotic/sexual feelings	3	19.20	0.69
The Sensed Presence	1, 2	15.00	2.05
	3	50.00	2.81
Visual Hallucinations	1, 2	8.62	1.54
	3	34.60	1.96

Notes: Adapted from Sharpless (in press) and reprinted with permission from Elsevier. 1 = Cheyne, Newby-Clark, & Rueffer, 1999 (student sample), 2 = Cheyne, Rueffer, & Newby-Clark, 1999 (student sample only included here), and 3 = Sharpless et al., 2010 (clinical sample). As not all of the categories from these three studies perfectly overlapped, we have included all of the experiences separately. As the severities in Cheyne et al.'s publications ranged from 0–7, whereas Sharpless et al.'s ranged from 0–8, all of the severities in Cheyne's studies were expanded to a 0–8 scale in order to standardize interpretation.

Although it does not appear possible to generate articulate speech during sleep paralysis, many reports of guttural moans and groans have been described (Bond, 1753; Macnish, 1834; Roscher, 2007), especially near the termination of attacks. Some sufferers have relied upon these plaintive sounds as a means to secure help. For instance, Bond (1753) reported the case of an otherwise healthy individual who was so troubled by his frequent attacks that he required his servant to sleep in bed with him. When the servant heard the master's moans, he was instructed to rouse him.

We should also note that a fixed and paralyzed body posture may lead to other sensations. For instance, Yu's recent (2012) study of dreams indicated that sensations of pressure (esp. on the face, chest, and genitals) can be converted into dream images/narratives. Given that historical documents clearly link sleep paralysis/nightmare episodes with sexuality, especially in women, this observation is quite interesting. In men specifically, there have been reports of nocturnal emissions resulting from pressure exerted upon the genitalia during sleep (e.g., Roscher, 2007). The extent to which these sensations predispose individuals to experience the typically traumatic sexual encounters of sleep paralysis are yet unknown, but the possible connections are intriguing nonetheless.

HALLUCINATIONS

The hallucinatory experiences of sleep paralysis are provocative at best, and terrifying at worst. Indeed, the vast majority of individuals with sleep paralysis do suffer from hallucinations. Estimates range from approximately three quarters in a large student sample (Cheyne, Newby-Clark, & Rueffer, 1999) to 88.5% in a clinical sample (Sharpless et al., 2010). Thus, only a relatively small minority of sufferers experience paralysis alone. Further, and as exemplified in the case example, multiple hallucinations during a single episode are the rule rather than the exception. There is also some evidence for a monotonic increase in sleep paralysis hallucinations as the frequency of episodes increases (Cheyne, 2005).

The level of elaboration found in the "story told in the hallucinations" varies, but usually involve several sensory modalities (e.g., touch, sound, and vision). Sleep paralysis hallucinations can either be hypnagogic (when going to sleep) or hypnopompic (when waking up), but we will follow convention and not differentiate between the two in this section (Mavromatis, 1988).

The range of sleep paralysis hallucinations is broad. As seen in Table 6.1, many can be found in psychotic disorders, and several are common to dissociative disorders (esp., the out-of-body experiences). Most data indicate that they are also more frightening than the contents found in a typical scary dream (e.g., Parker & Blackmore, 2002; Schredl & Doll, 1998). Whether this is due to differences in the specific content of sleep paralysis REM hallucinations or to the fact that they occur within the context of conscious awareness remains to be determined. As with other hallucinations, they can be perceived in different sensory formats, and these will be described in turn.

Auditory Hallucinations

As detailed in Table 6.1, auditory hallucinations are fairly common accompaniments to sleep paralysis, with the clinical sample experiencing them more often than students. Some of the more frequently heard sounds are various types of speech (indistinct or otherwise), footsteps, "movement" sounds (e.g., scraping, scratching), and general environmental noises. In contrast to standard dreams, where sounds are heard internally (i.e., "inside the head"), sounds in sleep paralysis are typically experienced as external to the body (e.g., Cheyne, 2001; Symons, 1995). Thus, sleep paralysis hallucinations can possess levels of real-world veracity not usually found in normal dreaming, as they occur in the context of wakefulness and concurrent paralysis. The case example demonstrates that this combination can be quite uncomfortable to experience (see also Sharpless, in press). Interestingly, auditory hallucinations in sleep paralysis are experienced as external even more than in schizophrenia (e.g., Cheyne & Girard, 2004; Nayani & David, 1996). Care must therefore be taken in differential diagnosis (chapter 13).

The hallucination of voices merits some discussion. They run the gamut from background whispers and alien-sounding "gibberish" to intelligible speech. Studies of hypnagogic/hypnopompic hallucinations in general (viz., not limited to sleep paralysis) find that speech in these states is more often unclear than clear, and that voices of known persons are more common than strangers (Jones, Fernyhough, & Laroi, 2010). When the source of the "speech" is known to the sufferer, it can be a quite disconcerting experience. For instance, we have interviewed several individuals who have heard their boyfriend utter hurtful personal comments or heard deceased relatives prophesize an unpleasant future for the paralyzed individual. These various forms of speech are often combined with visual hallucinations. In the limited literature on the subject (e.g., Sharpless & Grom's 2013 study of a college-aged sample), these "encounters" were found to be rarely pleasant, and often involved a recently deceased relative.

There also remains a question as to the *source* of the auditory hallucinations in sleep paralysis. Do they arise from within (i.e., are they endogenously generated?) or are they more often interpretations of existing exogenous stimuli that are somehow perceived by the sufferer? This question has yet to be answered. However, it is well-known that sleepers will incorporate environmental impingements into their dreams (e.g., Cipolli, Bolzani, Tuozzi, & Fagioli, 2001). For example, a sleeping man who hears the sound of a blender in the next apartment may dream that he is undergoing a cavity repair at a dentist's office. It seems reasonable to conclude that sleep paralysis hallucinations could be influenced in an analogous fashion. Further, given the human tendency to try to make sense of ambiguous perceptions, the vaguer the sound, the more ways it could be interpreted/incorporated. White noise from a clock radio now becomes the hiss of a serpent or feedback from a scary piece of extraterrestrial medical equipment; the pounding of a hammer becomes the ominous footsteps of a large intruder. One can also see how pre-existing cultural narratives about sleep, dreams, Nightmares, and demonic nocturnal attacks could be seamlessly woven into the tapestry that is the individual's efforts to disambiguate environmental noises.

Tactile and Kinesthetic Hallucinations

Tactile hallucinations are also frequently found in sleep paralysis. These can include general sensations of cold or heat on the skin/extremities, but more frequently involve a feeling of pressure or weight on the chest. Jones (1949) considered pressure to be one of the three defining characteristics of the classic Nightmare, and as will be shown, this construct corresponds well to recent factor analytic data. Along with these more "passive" tactile sensations, episodes may involve more "active contact" such as feeling as if someone (or something) is grabbing at your wrists/arms, or even throttling you. And as with auditory hallucinations, it remains unclear whether these tactile events arise endogenously or are interpretations of real external stimuli.

Sleep paralysis sufferers can also have any number of kinesthetic sensations. Although differing from the traditional (and very common) "falling" and "flying" dreams, sensations of both falling and flying can occur during wakeful paralysis. These are also some of the few sensations that are associated with positive affect (e.g., bliss and joy as in Cheyne & Girard, 2007). We have heard mixed reports of whether or not flight is experienced as under the sufferer's control, but levitation is almost always described as uncontrollable.

There are also hallucinations that convey a more profound sense of alienation from one's body. A particularly scary example is the sensation that one is moving without conscious volition, as can be seen in the "vampire girl" hallucination from the case example. During this, it is as if one's arms or legs were being manipulated by an outside force, with no ability to intervene. Some individuals with sleep paralysis are quite surprised to discover their body in its original (i.e., undisturbed) position when they awaken, as the kinesthetic sensations are so vivid and convincing.

Those with sleep paralysis also report *out-of-body experiences*. Hufford (2005) noted that, whereas many individuals hallucinate seeing or feeling spirits, some may hallucinate that they can act *like a spirit*. In effect, an aspect of their self "leaves" the body in some fashion (e.g., with some sufferers believing in soul travel or astral projection) and/or they "view" their body from the outside (viz., *autoscopy*). Along with the clear relations between these hallucinations and certain spiritual beliefs (irrespective of whether or not sleep paralysis is a cause or consequence of these beliefs), these out-of-body experiences may also be related to trauma and dissociation.

The connections between trauma and dissociation have long been known, at least going back to the time of Janet (1907), and it would not be surprising if both of these experiences impacted upon the specific manifestations and structures of sleep paralysis hallucinations (see also chapter 9). The distressing dreams and hypervigilance so often found in PTSD could easily lead to some of the scarier sleep paralysis hallucinations and/or make the sufferer more prone to subsequent misinterpretations of ambiguous stimuli (bodily or otherwise). The presence of a trauma history and flashbacks may also make differential diagnosis difficult. This is especially the case if traumatic scenes are re-experienced *during* sleep paralysis. Peritraumatic dissociative symptoms can include out-of-body experiences as well, and many of the narratives from victims of sexual assault or natural disasters describe autoscopy and general alienation from one's body, often conjoined with feelings of emotional numbness. In general, several studies have noted the connections between sleep paralysis/isolated sleep paralysis and traumatic events/post-traumatic stress disorder (Abrams, Mulligan, Carleton, & Asmundson, 2008; Friedman & Paradis, 2002; Sharpless et al., 2010). However, we should be clear that no direct *causal* links have yet been established.

In ending this section, it is worth noting that limb preference, perceptual biases in sleep paralysis hallucinations, and hypnagogic/hypnopompic hallucinations in general, may be related (Brugger, Regard, & Landis, 1996; Girard & Cheyne, 2004). In illusory movements, the actual movements appear to be most strongly associated with the "preferred" limb. As for the out-of-body-experiences, these appear to be more biased to the right side of the experient's sensory field.

Visual Hallucinations During Sleep Paralysis

Visual hallucinations account for some of the most vivid and memorable experiences of sleep paralysis. The depth and breadth of visual hallucinations can be truly staggering, and in some cases may eventuate in individuals feeling as if they are going crazy and/or under some malevolent nocturnal attack. We focus here first on the inanimate hallucinations, with the sensed presence and visual hallucinations of others discussed in the subsequent section.

Visual Hallucinations of Inanimate Objects

A number of visual hallucinations of inanimate objects can be present during sleep paralysis. Perhaps not surprisingly, these hallucinations evince less overall distress than hallucinations of animate, moving objects. The most commonly reported sightings are of shadows and indistinct forms that remain stationary throughout the episode, yet vanish upon awakening. "Blobs" of various colors, geometrical shapes (e.g., squares), and real-world objects such as desks, notebooks, and even train tracks have been reported. The extent to which these objects are meaningful parts of the overall hallucinatory narrative varies widely, and they can sometimes appear to be fairly random extraneous visual "noise," at least according to the sufferer.

Lights from various sources are found in sleep paralysis as well. These could be floating spheres of illumination similar to will-o'-the-wisps (aka, *ignis fatuus*/"foolish fire"), or other shapes with glowing centers. Intense flashes of light (similar to those reported in exploding head syndrome and near-death experiences) can occur as well. However, these appear to be relatively less common in sleep paralysis.

The Sensed Presence

One of the most disconcerting accompaniments to sleep paralysis is the "sensed presence." Although this experience can vary, it is essentially the feeling of an "otherness" that is not seen, but *felt* to be in the room. The otherness is usually perceived to have an ambiguous or malevolent intent (e.g., see *la Horla* excerpt in chapter 4). It feels "as if" something bad is likely to happen, and that personal safety is compromised. We have all had an analogous feeling of sensed presence at some point in our lives, but usually not when in the safety of our beds. For instance, feeling "watched" when alone in the woods or when walking down a dark and deserted city alleyway are phenomenologically identical events that leave us feeling similarly ill at ease. At these times, and also in sleep paralysis, there is the distinct feeling that one is not predator, but vulnerable "prey." Not surprisingly, this sensed presence, when coupled with prone paralysis, is associated with fear and dread for what might befall our bodily integrity (see also Sharpless, in press).

The sensed presence is very common in sleep paralysis (see Table 6.1), with approximately half of a clinical sample reporting it. Solomonova et al. (2008) found an even higher rate of 68.9%. So what is the nature of the particular presence that is sensed? In the one study we are aware of that addressed this question (Sharpless & Grom, 2013), it appeared that the majority felt a distinctly *non-human presence*. This is consistent with literary depictions such as Maupassant's *la Horla*, which as Cheyne (2001) notes, is likely derived from the French term *le hors-la*, or "outside there." Presumably, the sense of presence that is generated is "neutral," or at the very least ambiguous. This is where efforts at interpretation based upon personal history or available cultural narratives may come to the fore and add a more specific identity to the presence (see chapter 3 and appendix C).

The alien, threatening, and "other" nature of the sensed presence led some to speculate that it is associated with some type of "threat-activated vigilance system" found in the activity of the limbic and associated struc-tures of the brain (e.g., Cheyne, 2001). The *raison d'etre* for this system is presumed to be evolutionarily adaptive, and oriented toward survival of the organism via a close attunement to relevant environmental stimuli. The threat-activated vigilance system comes into play when some source of danger is identified, and then subsequently serves to monitor the organ-ism's surroundings for additional safety information and cues. In the case of sleep paralysis, the source material is found in REM phenomena and possibly certain environmental impingements. As will be seen, visual hal-lucinations may be the end results of these active attempts to make sense of ambiguously threatening phenomena.

Another question relates to the sensed presences themselves. Namely, are they hallucinations or delusions? Some (e.g., Simard & Nielsen, 2005) have considered them to be the former whereas others (e.g., Cheyne, 2001) have argued for the latter. This confusion is understand-able given the fact that the sensed presence is a somewhat "fuzzy" idea resting on the boundary between these two constructs. Unfortunately, a full discussion of the nature of the sensed presence from an ontolog-ical standpoint is beyond the purview of this book. From a *pragmatic* standpoint, however, the decision rests upon the particular definition of psychotic phenomena that is used. Per the most current *Diagnostic and Statistical Manual of Mental Disorders* (American Psychiatric Association,

2013), delusions are defined as, "fixed beliefs that are not amenable to change in light of conflicting evidence (p. 87)." Hallucinations, on the other hand, are "perception-like experiences that occur without an external stimulus. They are vivid and clear, with the full force and impact of normal perceptions, and not under voluntary control (p. 87)." Therefore, at least when using these specific (and some may say "imperfect") definitions, sensed presences appear to be more akin to hallucinations for at least two reasons. First, they lack the fixity of typical delusional beliefs, as the feeling of presence abates upon awakening. Granted, some individuals may continue to believe in the veracity of the presence's existence beyond this point, but the presence itself is no longer "sensed" as would appear to be the case in delusional disorders (e.g., continual CIA surveillance). Second, the sensed presence does indeed appear to be a perception, although it is a perception of a somewhat different sort from other varieties of hallucinations. It is an indistinct *perception* of another without any direct sensory input.

Visual Hallucinations of "Others"

During many sleep paralysis episodes, there is a transition from merely *sensing* a presence to actually *seeing* a presence. The limited evidence implies that the sequence occurs in that order. Cheyne and Girard (2007) conducted a mediational analysis of sleep paralysis hallucinations and fear and found that the sensed presence emerged relatively early, fear emerged soon after that, and visual hallucinations manifested later in the episode. Thus, these usually malevolent figures are sensed before they are seen. These bedroom intruders are usually human (or at least humanoid), but animal forms have been reported as well (Cheyne, 2001; Davies, 2003). Interactions with "others" are usually tinged with higher levels of aggression, sexuality (especially in female experients), and conflict than in normal dreams (Parker & Blackmore, 2002), and this is consistent with the earlier historical and medical narratives. Again, as with most of the above-mentioned hallucinations, these interactions with others often evoke intense fear and anxiety. Girard and Cheyne (2004) hypothesized that these levels of intense affect may implicate greater right than left hemispheric involvement.

So who/what are these "others?" Chapter 3 and appendix A list many of the supernatural intruders. Further, a recent sample of undergraduates with isolated sleep paralysis found that slightly more perceived non-human "beings" than humans (Sharpless & Grom, 2013). As for the former, the most commonly viewed beings were "shadow people," ghosts/ spirits, and hooded humanoid figures. Regarding those participants who hallucinated other people, strangers were perceived more often than recognized persons. Interestingly, of those who recognized the hallucinated others, 42.86% saw a recently deceased loved one. One other study (Hinton, Pich, Chhean, & Pollack, 2005), which focused on Cambodian refugees, reported isolated sleep paralysis hallucinations of others known to the victim. These researchers reported that some of their participants saw Kmer Rouge uniforms on their *intruders*.

This finding that sleep paralysis hallucinations can incorporate known others is interesting in several respects. It could imply that, much like normal dreaming, the REM components of sleep paralysis may possess a personal salience for the sufferer that is not merely random or fortuitous. In the case of the reported visions of the Kmer Rouge, they may be the most readily accessible experiential categories found when the threat-activated vigilance system attempts to disambiguate the otherwise vague threat cues. Similarly, with regard to the finding that college students with isolated sleep paralysis often saw recently deceased relatives, it is possible that a relative's hallucinated presence indicates not only that that the death was on the experient's mind, but also that the common "mixed feelings" surrounding unexpected deaths may be present as well. Regardless, we feel that the potential meanings found in hallucinations could have important clinical and research implications.

Factor Structure of Sleep Paralysis Hallucinations

As can be seen from the preceding, there are any number of individual sleep paralysis hallucinations. Do any of them "hang together" in such a way as to create paradigmatic experiences? In order to assess this, Cheyne and colleagues conducted factor analyses (Cheyne et al., 1999; Cheyne, 2005; Cheyne, Rueffer, & Newby-Clark, 1999) on a number of sleep paralysis hallucinations with a self-report measure (i.e., the *Waterloo Unusual Sleep Experiences Scale;* see chapter 12). Using several relatively large samples of undergraduates and Internet respondents, they identified three broad, consistent categories of sleep paralysis experience (viz., incubus, intruder, and vestibular-motor).

In the *intruder* category, there is a sensed presence in conjunction with visual, auditory, and tactile hallucinations (including bedding being moved). High levels of fear are usually present as well, and one can see how this factor corresponds to many folkloric and literary depictions of the Nightmare. Next, there is the *incubus*. Like its namesake and the Nightmare painting by Fuseli (1781), this consists of pressure on the chest along with corresponding smothering sensations and difficulties breathing. Pain and thoughts of imminent death also load onto this factor. Finally, the vestibular-motor category of hallucinations consists of floating/flying/falling (and other general movement sensations) and out-of-body experiences. The first two categories are moderately correlated with one another and also display high levels of fear. The vestibular-motor category is less strongly associated with fear, and can actually be perceived as pleasant by some experients (see later section). Sex differences in these three factors have been found such that females tend to experience more intense incubus episodes than men in terms of their subjective fear levels. Cheyne and colleagues (Cheyne, 2005; Cheyne & Girard, 2004) noted that this moderating effect of sex on intruder hallucinations is consistent with certain cultural beliefs about demonic sexual assaults on women (or, at least primarily on women).

In general, these factor analytic findings are intriguing for a number of reasons. First, they yield rather elegant categories that dovetail nicely with narrative reports of sleep paralysis experiences. Second, the tripartite structure was *consistently* derived across several large samples. Several questions remain, however, and imply a need for additional replication. One regards the samples utilized. It is unclear if the same simple structure would emerge in clinical samples possessing higher sleep paralysis severities. It is similarly unknown if there may be differences between self-report measures like the *Waterloo* and clinician-rated interviews. Finally, we wonder about the items that were included in the factor analyses. Several of these (e.g., death thoughts, smothering sensations) do not appear to be hallucinations, at least not in the traditional sense. Death thoughts, much like the ubiquitous fear experienced during episodes, appear to be *appraisals* of the paralysis rather than truly hallucinoid phenomena. Smothering sensations and other difficulties breathing may be similarly based on a physiological reality as opposed to created/interpreted stimuli that by definition do not really exist.

ASSOCIATED FEATURES OF SLEEP PARALYSIS

Although more empirical work is needed, several associated features of sleep paralysis and isolated sleep paralysis have been identified. First, sleep paralysis appears to have a fairly early age of onset. Most individuals have their first episode as teenagers, mainly between the ages of 14 and 17 (e.g., Fukuda, Miyasita, Inugami, & Ishihara, 1987; Gangdev, 2004; Spanos, McNulty, DuBreuil, & Pires, 1995). However, Wing & Chen's (1994) study may imply a somewhat bimodal distribution, at least in Asian samples. They found that 43% of their sample had an adolescent onset and 32.1% had an onset after age 60.

The course of sleep paralysis appears to be fairly variable, although few studies have explored this topic. Dahlitz and Parkes (1993) assessed duration in a sample of 22 individuals and found a range of 5 to 35 years. Unfortunately, we do not have more information on progression of episodes (if there is any) for this study. Certain types of hallucinations appear to become more common over time (e.g., vestibular-motor types discussed in Cheyne, 2005) and, clinically, we have observed cases of recurrent isolated sleep paralysis that do appear to increase in terms of both severity and frequency. Further, as shown in chapter 5, there has been a great deal of speculation about how sleep paralysis can even develop into more dangerous conditions (e.g., epilepsy), but data supporting these claims are lacking.

Several common sleep habits have been found to be associated with sleep paralysis. In line with early observations and first-hand accounts, sleeping on one's back makes it more likely. This has been replicated in a number of studies (e.g., Cheyne, 2002; Sharpless et al., 2010). Cheyne (2002) found that sleeping in the supine position is four times more common in sleep paralysis than in normal dreaming. Interestingly, though, sleep paralysis often emerges *from* normal dreams (Cheyne, 2003). This is consistent with some of the data on the *timing* of sleep paralysis episodes. Namely, a bimodal distribution of timing appears to be evident such that approximately 28% of episodes occurred within the first hour of bedtime and 26% of episodes occurred five or more hours after bedtime (Girard & Cheyne, 2004). However, no relationship between sleep latency and sleep paralysis has yet been found (Girard & Cheyne, 2006).

One difficult to answer question concerns the actual *duration* of sleep paralysis episodes. Reports in the literature have ranged from several seconds to two and a half hours (e.g., Davies, 2003; Rushton, 1944), with overall means of six to seven minutes found in the more recent empirical literature (e.g., Hinton et al., 2005; Sharpless et al., 2010). However, given the nature of the phenomenon (i.e., odd sensory events; dissociative symptoms) as well as the fact that self-reported durations of episodes are often the only sources of data available, these summary statistics should be taken with a grain of salt. We surmise that many reports of lengthier sleep paralysis episodes are more likely to be distortions in perception as opposed to veridical assessments of the passage of time.

FEAR/DISTRESS, IMPAIRMENT, AND OTHER CONSEQUENCES OF SLEEP PARALYSIS

In ending this chapter, we would like to briefly focus on the *consequences* of sleep paralysis, especially those which may be detrimental to individuals. This area has received surprisingly little empirical attention in spite of the repercussions described in both folklore and literature on individuals suffering from chronic cases. Clearly, the experience of fear *during* episodes is pronounced. Table 6.2 lists the levels and types of fear documented in the literature. Differences in the operationalization of "fear" (e.g., terror, distress, clinically-significant fear) make across-study comparisons difficult, but regardless, the majority of individuals with sleep paralysis find it to be a fear-laden event.

A variety of cognitive appraisals of episodes have also been identified. For instance, some individuals fear that the paralysis will be permanent (Hinton et al., 2005; Koran & Raghavan, 1993; Ramsawh, Raffa, White, & Barlow, 2008). Others feel that they are in danger of immanent death (Arikawa, Templer, Brown, Cannon, & Thomas-Dodson, 1999; Cheyne & Girard, 2007; Hinton et al., 2005; Liddon, 1970, see also folklore literatures such as Haga, 1989; Jones, 1949; and Sharpless, in press). These catastrophic misinterpretations of sleep paralysis sensations are very much in keeping with the replicated empirical finding that, much like patients suffering from panic disorder, isolated sleep paralysis experients have high levels of anxiety sensitivity (Ramsawh et al., 2008; Sharpless et al., 2010).

So beyond the peri-episode fear, what are the impacts that chronic sleep paralysis could have on an individual's functioning? There appear to be at least two broad possibilities. First, could sleep paralysis result in behavioral or emotional changes prior to sleep, and second, could it result in post-episode appraisals and changes in belief? The limited evidence supports an affirmative answer for both. Regarding pre-sleep behaviors, many early reports describe a significant level of apprehension around the various components of sleep (e.g., Alvaro, 2005; Jones, 1949). This may involve a fear of nighttime, the bedroom, or any of the various accoutrements of sleep. Some may even attempt to only sleep in chairs so as to avoid sleep paralysis (Bond, 1753). In one study, 19.23% of college students with

Table 6.2. RATES OF FEAR/DISTRESS IN SLEEP PARALYSIS

Study	% Reporting Fear/Distress	Sample/Notes
Cheyne, Rueffer, & Newby-Clark, 1999	90.00	Student sample
Cheyne et al., 1999	98.00	World Wide Web sample
dahlitz & parkes, 1993	86.36	Clinical sample of patients with SP and daytime sleepiness; % = those reporting terror
Mellman, Aigbogun, Graves, Lawson, & Alim, 2008	31.70	African American sample in primary medical care setting
Ramsawh, Raffa, White, & Barlow, 2008	89.90	African American sample; mean distress = 0.6 on 3-point scale
Sharpless et al., 2010	69.23	Clinical sample of patients with panic; % = those reporting clinically-significant fear
Sharpless & Grom, in press	75.64	Student sample; % = those reporting clinically-significant fear
Simard & Nielsen, 2005	97.78	Student sample
Spanos, McNulty, DuBreuil, & Pires, 1995	66.70	Student sample
Wing, Lee, & Chen, 1994	58.60	Chinese student sample; % = those reporting terror

isolated sleep paralysis actively made attempts to prevent future episodes (Sharpless & Grom, in press). It is unclear if older patients or those with more chronic episodes attempt to prevent episodes at higher rates.

Regarding the possible impacts on functioning as a result of sleep paralysis episodes, several have been reported. For instance, daytime sleepiness is a common sequela (e.g., Jiménez-Genchi, Ávila-Rodríguez, Sánchez-Rojas, Terrez, & Nenclares-Portocarrero, 2009; Ohayon, Zulley, Guilleminault, & Smirne, 1999; Wing et al., 1994). Many individuals with sleep paralysis, especially those who are naïve to medical explanations, have a belief that they are "crazy" or suffering from a more severe condition. They often feel shame and embarrassment in the wake of attacks (Neal, Rich, & Smucker, 1994; Otto et al., 2006). Interestingly, only a relatively small percentage seek out help (Yeung, Xu, & Chang, 2005), but it is unclear if this is due to a reticence to disclose these "embarrassing" symptoms to medical professionals or the fact that sleep paralysis is not severely distressing for the majority of individuals. Many (viz., 69.29%

of a sample of undergraduates with isolated sleep paralysis) appear to take matters into their own hands and formulate their own techniques to disrupt episodes (Sharpless & Grom, in press).

Two studies to date have assessed whether or not problematic cases of isolated sleep paralysis exist. In a clinical sample of patients with panic attacks (Sharpless et al., 2010), almost 43.58% of those with any experience of isolated sleep paralysis (N = 39) also met general DSM-5 "disorder" criteria of clinically significant distress and/or interference (American Psychiatric Association, 2013, p. 21) using recurrent fearful isolated sleep paralysis guidelines. In a large (N = 156) sample of undergraduates clinically assessed at two universities, 15.38% were found to meet recurrent fearful isolated sleep paralysis criteria using these same guidelines (Sharpless & Grom, in press). Thus, at least a certain percentage of individual do appear to experience negative impacts on their functioning as a result of episodes. More specific diagnostic criteria can be found in chapter 11 and appendix B.

CONCLUSIONS

In this chapter we reviewed literature on both the paradigmatic symptoms and the associated features of sleep paralysis. The hallucinations so common in this condition were emphasized, as were the possible *consequences* of sleep paralysis. The vast majority of individuals find episodes to be quite unpleasant and disturbing experiences, which they would rather avoid. For at least a small percentage of individuals, they experience sleep paralysis at such a frequency or overall level of severity that it causes clinically significant distress or interference in their life.

REFERENCES

Abrams, M. P., Mulligan, A. D., Carleton, R. N., & Asmundson, G. J. G. (2008). Prevalence and correlates of sleep paralysis in adults reporting childhood sexual abuse. *Journal of Anxiety Disorders*, 22(8), 1535–1541. doi: 10.1016/j.janxdis.2008.03.007

Alvaro, L. (2005). Hallucinations and pathological visual perceptions in maupassant's fantastical short stories—A neurological approach. *Journal of the History of the Neurosciences*, 14, 100–115.

American Academy of Sleep Medicine. (2005). *International classification of sleep disorders: Diagnostic coding manual* (2nd ed.). Darien, IL: American Academy of Sleep Medicine.

American Academy of Sleep Medicine. (2014). *International classification of sleep disorders: Diagnostic and coding manual* (3rd ed.). Darien, IL: American Academy of Sleep Medicine.

American Psychiatric Association. (2013). *Diagnostic and statistical manual of mental disorders* (5th ed.). Arlington, VA: American Psychiatric Association.

Arikawa, H., Templer, D. I., Brown, R., Cannon, W. G., & Thomas-Dodson, S. (1999). The structure and correlates of kanshibari. *The Journal of Psychology, 133*(4), 369–375.

Aurelianus, C. (1950). In Drabkin I. E. (Ed.), *On acute diseases and chronic diseases* (I. E. Drabkin Trans.). Chicago: University of Chicago Press.

Bond, J. (1753). *An essay on the incubus, or night mare.* London: D. Wilson and T. Durham.

Brugger, P., Regard, M., & Landis, T. (1996). Unilaterally felt 'presences': The neuropsychiatry of one's invisible doppleganger. *Neuropsychiatry, Neuropsychology, and Behavioral Neurology, 9,* 114–122.

Chakravarty, A. (2007). Exploding head syndrome: Report of two new cases. *Cephalalgia: An International Journal of Headache, 28*(4), 399–400. doi: 10.1111/j.1468-2982.2007.01522.x; 10.1111/j.1468-2982.2007.01522.x

Cheyne, J. A. (2001). The ominous numinous: Sensed presence and 'other' hallucinations. *Journal of Consciousness Studies, 8*(5-7), 133–150.

Cheyne, J. A. (2002). Situational factors affecting sleep paralysis and associated hallucinations: Position and timing effects. *Journal of Sleep Research, 11*(2), 169–177. doi: 10.1046/j.1365-2869.2002.00297.x

Cheyne, J. A. (2003). Sleep paralysis and the structure of waking-nightmare hallucinations. *Dreaming, 13*(3), 163–179. doi: 10.1023/A:1025373412722

Cheyne, J. A. (2005). Sleep paralysis episode frequency and number, types, and structure of associated hallucinations. *Journal of Sleep Research, 14*(3), 319–324. doi: 10.1111/j.1365-2869.2005.00477.x

Cheyne, J. A., & Girard, T. A. (2004). Spatial characteristics of hallucinations associated with sleep paralysis. *Cognitive Neuropsychiatry, 9*(4), 281–300. doi: 10.1080/13546800344000264

Cheyne, J. A., & Girard, T. A. (2007). Paranoid delusions and threatening hallucinations: A prospective study of sleep paralysis experiences. *Consciousness and Cognition: An International Journal, 16*(4), 959–974.

Cheyne, J. A., Newby-Clark, I. R., & Rueffer, S. D. (1999). Relations among hypnagogic and hypnopompic experiences associated with sleep paralysis. *Journal of Sleep Research, 8,* 313–317.

Cheyne, J. A., Rueffer, S. D., & Newby-Clark, I. R. (1999). Hypnagogic and hypnopompic hallucinations during sleep paralysis: Neurological and cultural construction of the night-mare. *Consciousness and Cognition: An International Journal, 8*(3), 319–337. doi: 10.1006/ccog.1999.0404

Cipolli, C., Bolzani, R., Tuozzi, G., & Fagioli, I. (2001). Active processing of declarative knowledge during REM-sleep dreaming. *Journal of Sleep Research, 10*(4), 277–284. doi: 268 [pii]

Dahlitz, M., & Parkes, J. D. (1993). Sleep paralysis. *The Lancet, 341,* 406–407.

Davies, O. (2003). The nightmare experience, sleep paralysis and witchcraft accusations. *Folklore, 114*(2), 181.

Friedman, S., & Paradis, C. (2002). Panic disorder in African Americans: Symptomatology and isolated sleep paralysis. *Culture, Medicine and Psychiatry, 26*(2), 179–198. doi: 10.1023/A:1016307515418

Fukuda, K., Miyasita, A., Inugami, M., & Ishihara, K. (1987). High prevalence of isolated sleep paralysis: Kanashibari phenomenon in japan. *Sleep: Journal of Sleep
Research & Sleep Medicine, 10*(3), 279–286.
Fuseli, H. (1781). *The nightmare.* Royal Academy of London: Detroit Institute of Arts.
Gangdev, P. (2004). Relevance of sleep paralysis and hypnic hallucinations to psy-
chiatry. *Australasian Psychiatry, 12*(1), 77–80. doi: 10.1046/j.1039-8562.2003.
02065.x
Girard, T. A., & Cheyne, J. A. (2004). Individual differences in lateralisation of hallu-
cinations associated with sleep paralysis. *Laterality:Asymmetries of Body, Brain
and Cognition, 9*(1), 93–111. doi: 10.1080/13576500244000210
Girard, T. A., & Cheyne, A. (2006). Timing of spontaneous sleep-paralysis episodes.
Journal of Sleep Research, 15(2), 222–229. doi: 10.1111/j.1365-2869.2006.005
12.x
Haga, E. (1989). The nightmare—A riding ghost with sexual connotations. *Nordisk
Psykiatrisk Tidsskrift. Nordic Journal of Psychiatry, 43*(6), 515–520.
Hinton, D. E., Pich, V., Chhean, D., & Pollack, M. H. (2005). The ghost pushes you
down: Sleep paralysis-type panic attacks in a khmer refugee population.
Transcultural Psychiatry, 42(1), 46–77. doi: 10.1177/1363461505050710
Hufford, D. J. (2005). Sleep paralysis as spiritual experience. *Transcultural Psychiatry,
42*(1), 11–45. doi: 10.1177/1363461505050709
Janet, P. (1907). *The major symptoms of hysteria: Fifteen lectures given in the medical
school of harvard university.* London, UK: The Macmillan Company.
Jiménez-Genchi, A., Ávila-Rodríguez, V. M., Sánchez-Rojas, F., Terrez, B. E. V., &
Nenclares-Portocarrero, A. (2009). Sleep paralysis in adolescents: The 'a dead
body climbed on top of me' phenomenon in mexico. *Psychiatry and Clinical
Neurosciences, 63*(4), 546–549. doi: 10.1111/j.1440-1819.2009.01984.x
Jones, E. (1949). *On the nightmare* (2nd Impression ed.). London, United
Kingdom: Hogarth Press and the Institute of Psycho-analysis.
Jones, S. R., Fernyhough, C., & Laroi, F. (2010). A phenomenological survey of
auditory verbal hallucinations in the hypnagogic and hypnopompic states.
Phenomenology and the Cognitive Sciences, 9, 213–224.
Koran, L. M., & Raghavan, S. (1993). Fluoxetine for isolated sleep paralysis.
Psychosomatics: Journal of Consultation Liaison Psychiatry, 34(2), 184–187.
doi: 10.1016/S0033-3182(93)71913-1
Liddon, S. C. (1970). Sleep paralysis, psychosis, and death. *The American Journal of
Psychiatry, 126*(7), 1027–1031.
Macnish, R. (1834). *The philosophy of sleep* (First American Edition ed.). New York: D.
Appleton and Company.
Mahowald, M. W., & Schenck, C. H. (2005). Insights from studying human sleep dis-
orders. *Nature, 437,* 1279–1285.
Marks, G. A. (2009). Neurobiology of sleep. In T. L. Lee-Chiong (Ed.), *Sleep medicine
essentials* (pp. 5–10). Hoboken, NJ: John Wiley and Sons.
Mavromatis, A. (1988). *Hypnagogia: The unique state of consciousness between wakeful-
ness and sleep.* London: Routledge and Kegan Paul.
Mellman, T. A., Aigbogun, N., Graves, R. E., Lawson, W. B., & Alim, T. N. (2008). Sleep
paralysis and trauma, psychiatric symptoms and disorders in an adult African
American population attending primary medical care. *Depression and Anxiety,
25*(5), 435–440. doi: 10.1002/da.20311
Nayani, T. H., & David, A. S. (1996). The auditory hallucination: A phenomenological
survey. *Psychological Medicine, 26,* 177–189.

Neal, A. M., Rich, L. N., & Smucker, W. D. (1994). The presence of panic disorder among African American hypertensives: A pilot study. *Journal of Black Psychology, 20*(1), 29–35.

Ohayon, M. M., Zulley, J., Guilleminault, C., & Smirne, S. (1999). Prevalence and pathologic associations of sleep paralysis in the general population. *Neurology, 52*(6), 1194–1200.

Otto, M. W., Simon, N. M., Powers, M., Hinton, D., Zalta, A. K., & Pollack, M. H. (2006). Rates of isolated sleep paralysis in outpatients with anxiety disorders. *Journal of Anxiety Disorders, 20*(5), 687–693. doi: 10.1016/j.janxdis.2005.07.002

Parker, J. D., & Blackmore, S. J. (2002). Comparing the content of sleep paralysis and dream reports. *Dreaming, 12*(1), 45–59. doi: 10.1023/A:1013894522583

Ramsawh, H. J., Raffa, S. D., White, K. S., & Barlow, D. H. (2008). Risk factors for isolated sleep paralysis in an African American sample: A preliminary study. *Behavior Therapy, 39*(4), 386–397. doi: 10.1016/j.beth.2007.11.002

Roscher, W. H. (2007). Ephialtes: A pathological-mythological treatise on the nightmare in classical antiquity. [Ephialtes] (A. V. O'Brien Trans.). (Revised ed., pp. 96–159). Putnam, CT: Spring Publishing.

Rushton, J. G. (1944). Sleep paralysis. *Medical Clinics of North America, 28,* 945–949.

Schredl, M., & Doll, E. (1998). Emotions in diary dreams. *Consciousness and Cognition, 7,* 634–646.

Schopenhauer, A. (1974). *Parerga and paralipomena Volume 1* (E.F.J. Payne, trans.). NY: Oxford University Press.

Sharpless, B. A. (in press). Isolated sleep paralysis and affect. In K. Babson, & M. Feldner (Eds.), *Sleep and affect.* NY: Elsevier.

Sharpless, B. A. (2014). Exploding head syndrome. *Sleep Medicine Reviews, 18,* 489–493.

Sharpless, B.A., & Grom, J.L. (2013). Isolated sleep paralysis: Prevention, disruption, and hallucinations of others (poster). *American Psychological Association Annual Conference,* Honolulu, HI.

Sharpless, B. A., & Grom, J. L. (in press). Isolated sleep paralysis: Fear, prevention, and disruption. *Behavioral Sleep Medicine.*

Sharpless, B. A., McCarthy, K. S., Chambless, D. L., Milrod, B. L., Khalsa, S., & Barber, J. P. (2010). Isolated sleep paralysis and fearful isolated sleep paralysis in outpatients with panic attacks. *Journal of Clinical Psychology, 66*(12), 1292–1306. doi: 10.1002/jclp.20724

Simard, V., & Nielsen, T. A. (2005). Sleep paralysis-associated sensed presence as a possible manifestation of social anxiety. *Dreaming, 15*(4), 245–260. doi: 10.1037/1053-0797.15.4.245

Solomonova, E., Nielsen, T., Stenstrom, P., Simard, V., Frantova, E., & Donderi, D. (2008). Sensed presence as a correlate of sleep paralysis distress, social anxiety and waking state social imagery. *Consciousness and Cognition: An International Journal, 17*(1), 49–63. doi: 10.1016/j.concog.2007.04.007

Spanos, N. P., McNulty, S. A., DuBreuil, S. C., & Pires, M. (1995). The frequency and correlates of sleep paralysis in a university sample. *Journal of Research in Personality, 29*(3), 285–305. doi: 10.1006/jrpe.1995.1017

Symons, D. (1995). The stuff dreams aren't made of: Wake-state and dream-state sensory experiences differ. *Cognition, 47,* 181–217.

Terzaghi, M., Ratti, P. L., Manni, F., & Manni, R. (2012). Sleep paralysis in narcolepsy: More than just a motor dissociative phenomenon? *Neurological Sciences, 33*(1), 169–172. doi: 10.1007/s10072-011-0644-y

Wing, Y., Lee, S. T., & Chen, C. (1994). Sleep paralysis in chinese: Ghost oppression phenomenon in hong kong. *Sleep: Journal of Sleep Research & Sleep Medicine, 17*(7), 609–613.

Yeung, A., Xu, Y., & Chang, D. F. (2005). Prevalence and illness beliefs of sleep paralysis among chinese psychiatric patients in china and the united states. *Transcultural Psychiatry, 42*(1), 135–143. doi: 10.1177/1363461505050725

Yu, C. K. (2012). The effect of sleep position on dream experiences. *Dreaming, 22*(3), 212–221.

CHAPTER 7

Prevalence of Sleep Paralysis

DIFFICULTIES IN DETERMINING SLEEP PARALYSIS PREVALENCE RATES

Unlike many diseases and disorders with fairly standardized diagnostic procedures (e.g., use of Multiple Sleep Latency Testing for narcolepsy; *Structured Clinical Interview for DSM-5* for major depressive disorder [SCID-5, First, Williams, Karg, & Spitzer, in press]), sleep paralysis lacks a standardized assessment procedure. This is likely due not only to the relative infrequency with which it is considered in research studies and clinical practice, but also because so few patients present with complaints of sleep paralysis in primary care settings. Thus, if patients are not disclosing, and diagnosticians are not asking, sleep paralysis can be easily overlooked.

Even in those studies that directly assess for sleep paralysis/isolated sleep paralysis, the heterogeneity of assessment procedures (see chapter 12) makes inter-study comparison difficult. This was especially the case in the earlier empirical literature where study participants were often presented with vignettes of sleep paralysis and asked if they had had similar experiences. The exclusive use of self-report measures is also potentially problematic, as certain words (e.g., "paralysis") can be understood in idiosyncratic (and sometimes blatantly incorrect) ways. In our experience, many patients confuse paralysis with excessive sluggishness and the "heavy limbs" so common when waking from sleep as opposed to paralysis in the stricter sense. This can lead to an overestimation of sleep paralysis/isolated sleep paralysis prevalence rates. Similarly, many studies of ISP do not adequately engage in differential diagnosis (see chapter 13). For instance, many do not thoroughly attempt to rule out narcolepsy and establish a diagnosis of isolated sleep paralysis over sleep paralysis, and many do not assess for substance-induced episodes or those due to hypokalemia or seizure disorders. Thus, with the exception of a few studies, rates of isolated sleep paralysis are not known. Granted, the prevalence rates of narcolepsy are fairly low (e.g., 56.3 cases per 100,000 persons, Pelayo & Lopes, 2009), but rates of sleep paralysis episodes due to other listed causes (e.g., substance-induced) are presently unknown as well.

LIFETIME SLEEP PARALYSIS PREVALENCE RATES

In order to begin the process of estimating sleep paralysis prevalence, Sharpless and Barber (2011) conducted a systematic review of lifetime rates using all available studies that used an acceptable definition of sleep paralysis and also adequately reported their assessment measures and procedures. As shown in Table 7.1, they identified a total of 35 studies (participant N = 36,533 individuals) conducted in different geographical locations with a wide array of ethnicities.

Overall Prevalence Rates

Sleep paralysis was found to be surprisingly common, especially in students and psychiatric patients (see Table 7.2). Although limitations in the existing data did not allow for analysis according to other comorbid diagnoses, individuals with panic disorder were found to have the highest overall rates. Regarding the elevated rates for students and psychiatric patients as a whole, Sharpless and Barber (2011) hypothesized that this may be due to the fact that both groups often suffer from regular sleep disturbance. Insomnia and difficulties with regular sleep (e.g., shift work, jet lag) are general risk factors for sleep paralysis (e.g., Kotorii et al., 2001).

Prevalence Rates by Ethnicity

Prevalence rates according to ethnicity can be found in Table 7.3. Although it does appear that non-Caucasians experienced sleep paralysis at higher rates than Caucasians, the differences were surprisingly

Table 7.1. PUBLISHED LIFETIME PREVALENCE RATES OF
SLEEP PARALYSIS

Citation	Date	Sample N	% SP	Assessment Modality	Sample Type	Ethnicity
Abrams et al.	2008	216	62.0	SR	G, S	Caucasian American
		5	100		G, S	African American
		21	71.7		G, S	Asian Americans
		3	66.7		G, S	Hispanic Americans
Arikawa et al.	1999	720	33.9	SR	G	Japanese
Awadalla et al.	2004	527	28.8	SR	S	Kuwaiti
		762	29.9		S	Sudanese
		649	24.5		S	American
Bell et al.	1984	36	38.9	Int	G	African American
		72	41.7		C	African American
Bell et al.	1988	31	41.9	Int	G, High BP	African American
Cheyne et al.	1999	870	29.2	SR	S	Canadian
Cheyne et al.	1999	1273	28.3	SR	S	Canadian
Dahmen et al.	2002	128	2.35	Int	G	German
Everett	1963	52	15.4	SR	S	American
Fukuda et al.	1987	635	43.0	SR	S	Japanese
Fukuda et al.	1998	149	38.9	SR	S	Japanese
		86	41.9		S	Canadian
Goode	1962	67	1.5	SR	G	American
		284	5.3		S	American
		8	12.5		C	American
Huamani et al.	2006	104	55.8	SR	S	Peruvian
Hufford	2005	254	16.5	Int	G	American
Jimenez-Genchi et al.	2009	322	27.6	SR	S	Mexican
Kotorri et al.	2001	8162	39.6	SR	G, S	Japanese
Lopez et al.	1995	1000	11.3	SR	G	Mexican
McNally & Clancy	2005	16	12.5	SR	G	American
		68	45.5		C	American
Neal et al.	1994	18	38.9	Int	C	African American
Ohaeri et al.	1989	164	26.2	SR	S	Nigerian
Ohaeri et al.	1992	95	44.2	SR	S	Nigerian
Ohayon & Shapiro	2000	1832	2.4	Int	G	Canadian
Ohayon et al.*	2002	14,008	6.2	Int	G	Spanish, German, Italian, Portuguese
Otto et al.	2006	61	19.7	SR	C	American
Paradis et al.	2009	208	25.0	SR	S	American
Penn et al.	1981	80	16.3	SR	S	American

(*continued*)

Table 7.1. CONTINUED

Citation	Date	Sample N	% SP	Assessment Modality	Sample Type	Ethnicity
Sharpless et al.	2010	23	47.8	Int	C	African American
		3	33.3		C	Asian American
		97	22.7		C	Caucasian American
		7	57.2		C	Hispanic American
Simard & Nielson	2005	434	30.4	SR	S	Canadian
Smith et al.	1999	43	48.8	Int	C	African American
		28	25.0		C	Caucasian American
Smith et al.	2008	50	40.0	SR	G	African American
Spanos et al.	1995	1798	21.5	SR	S	Canadian
Suarez	1991	30	20.0	Int	G	Spanish
		60	40.0		C	Spanish
Wing et al.	1994	603	37.0	SR	S	Chinese
Wing et al.,	1999	158	17.7	SR	G	Chinese
Yeung et al.	2005	42	26.2	Int	C	Chinese American
		150	23.3		C	Chinese

Notes: Table adapted from Sharpless & Barber (2011) and reprinted with permission from Elsevier. SP = sleep paralysis; G = general population; S = students, C = clinical psychiatric patients; SR = self-report; Int = interview; BP = blood pressure; *Data used in our gender calculations were initially reported in a previous manuscript (Ohayon et al., 1999).

small. This was somewhat unexpected, as the early literature often speculated that rates of sleep paralysis were *significantly* higher in minorities, and that isolated sleep paralysis may even be an African American variant of panic disorder. Interestingly, no general population studies reported Caucasian data, so estimates for this group are lacking.

Table 7.2. LIFETIME PREVALENCE RATES OF SLEEP PARALYSIS BY SAMPLE TYPE

Sample	Sample *N*	% with SP
All Studies	36,533	20.8
General Population	18,330	7.6
Students	9095	28.3
Psychiatric Patients	683	31.9
Patients with Panic Disorder	318	34.6

Note: Table adapted from Sharpless & Barber (2011) and reprinted with permission from Elsevier. SP = sleep paralysis; Patients with Panic Disorder is a subset of the Psychiatric Patient sample category.

Table 7.3. LIFETIME SLEEP PARALYSIS PREVALENCE
RATES BY SAMPLE TYPE AND ETHNICITY

Sample Type	Ethnicity	Sample N	% with SP
General Population	African	117	40.2
	Asian	878	31.0
	Caucasian	–	–
	Hispanic	1000	11.3
Students	African	1002	31.4
	Asian	1387	39.9
	Caucasian	613	30.8
	Hispanic	426	32.9
Psychiatric Patients	African	158	44.3
	Asian	195	24.1
	Caucasian	125	23.2
	Hispanic	*	57.1
Total	African	1282	34.1
	Asian	10,643	38.7
	Caucasian	954	36.9
	Hispanic	1436	18.0

Note: Table adapted from Sharpless & Barber (2011) and reprinted with permission from Elsevier. Total N is discrepant from previous table due to a lack of uniform reporting across samples; * = $N < 10$.

Prevalence Rates by Gender

When focusing on individual studies of sleep paralysis, the prevalence rates according to gender are fairly inconsistent (e.g., Ohaeri, Odejide, Ikuesan, & Adeyemi, 1989; Otto et al., 2006). Sharpless and Barber (2011) found a slight female (18.8%) to male (15.7%) predominance in a sample of 15,157 participants. One large study conducted in Brazil that was not included in this analysis found an even higher gender discrepancy, with a male to female ration of 1:1.2 in 1987 and 1:1.5 in 1995 (Pires et al., 2007).

RECURRENT SLEEP PARALYSIS PREVALENCE RATES

There is even less documentation on the prevalence rates for *recurrent* sleep paralysis and recurrent isolated sleep paralysis. The lack of uniform reporting and the lack of consensus on frequency thresholds required for a diagnosis makes accurate summary across articles very difficult. For instance, Pires et al. (2007) considered sleep paralysis to be habitual if it occurred at least once per month, whereas Sharpless et al. (2010) required two episodes in the past six months and Paradis, Friedman, and Hatch (1997) required four episodes per year. Given that different research questions were being asked in each protocol, this heterogeneity is not surprising. Regardless, it would appear that a relatively large percentage of individuals experience more than one episode of sleep paralysis/isolated sleep paralysis over the course of their lives (e.g., Paradis et al., 1997; Ramsawh, Raffa, White, & Barlow, 2008; Spanos, McNulty, DuBreuil, & Pires, 1995).

A minority of individuals experience sleep paralysis/isolated sleep paralysis at very high frequency rates. For instance, 2.6% of Ohaeri, Awadalla, Maknjuola, and Ohaeri's (2004), 47.0% of O'Hanlon, Murphy, and Di Blasi's (2011), and 9.3% of Ohayon, Zulley, Guilleminault, and Smirne's (1999) samples experienced *multiple isolated sleep paralysis episodes per week*. Needless to say, if the majority of these episodes are frightening and distressing, this could lead to some significant sleep and/or life disruption (see chapter 6).

CONCLUSIONS

In summary, at this early stage of research more work needs to be conducted in order to determine accurate prevalence rates. This is especially the case for recurrent isolated sleep paralysis. It is recommended that the field adopt a more systematic procedure for assessing isolated sleep paralysis in epidemiological and research studies (see chapter 12). Prior to this, empirically-based definitions and frequency thresholds for isolated sleep paralysis should be better established and, given the complexity of diagnosis, the use of clinical interviews should be prioritized over self-report measures. Accurate rates and frequencies according to ethnicity and gender should also be collected.

REFERENCES

Abrams, M. P., Mulligan, A. D., Carleton, R. N., & Asmundson, G. J. G. (2008). Prevalence and correlates of sleep paralysis in adults reporting childhood sexual abuse. *Journal of Anxiety Disorders*, 22(8), 1535–1541. doi: 10.1016/j.janxdis.2008.03.007

Arikawa, H., Templer, D. I., Brown, R., Cannon, W. G., & Thomas-Dodson, S. (1999). The structure and correlates of kanshibari. *The Journal of Psychology*, 133(4), 369–375.

Awadalla, A., Al-Fayez, G., Harville, M., Arikawa, H., Tomeo, M. E., Templer, D. I., & Underwood, R. (2004). Comparative prevalence of isolated sleep paralysis in kuwaiti, sudanese, and american college students. *Psychological Reports, 95*(1), 317–322. doi: 10.2466/PR0.95.5.317-322

Bell, C. C., Shakoor, B., Thompson, B., Dew, D., Hughley, E., Mays, R., & Shorter-Gooden, K. (1984). Prevalence of isolated sleep paralysis in black subjects. *Journal of the National Medical Association, 76*(5), 501–508.

Bell, C. C., Hildreth, C. J., Jenkins, E. J., & Carter, C. (1988). The relationship of isolated sleep paralysis and panic disorder to hypertension. *Journal of the National Medical Association, 80*(3), 289–294.

Cheyne, J. A., Newby-Clark, I. R., & Rueffer, S. D. (1999). Relations among hypnagogic and hypnopompic experiences associated with sleep paralysis. *Journal of Sleep Research, 8*, 313–317.

Cheyne, J. A., Rueffer, S. D., & Newby-Clark, I. R. (1999). Hypnagogic and hypnopompic hallucinations during sleep paralysis: Neurological and cultural construction of the night-mare. *Consciousness and Cognition: An International Journal, 8*(3), 319–337. doi: 10.1006/ccog.1999.0404

Dahmen, N., Kasten, M., Muller, M.J., & Mittag, K. (2002). Frequency and dependence on body posture of hallucinations and sleep paralysis in a community sample. *Journal of Sleep Research, 11*, 179–180.

Everett, H. C. (1963). Sleep paralysis in medical students. *Journal of Nervous and Mental Disease, 136*(6), 283–287.

First, M. B., Williams, J. B. W., Karg, R. S., & Spitzer, R. L. (in press). *Structured clinical interview for DSM-5 disorders: Patient edition.* New York: Biometrics Research Department.

Fukuda, K., Miyasita, A., Inugami, M., & Ishihara, K. (1987). High prevalence of isolated sleep paralysis: Kanashibari phenomenon in Japan. *Sleep: Journal of Sleep Research & Sleep Medicine, 10*(3), 279–286.

Fukuda, K., Ogilvie, R. D., Chilcott, L., Vendittelli, A., & Takeuchi, T. (1998). The prevalence of sleep paralysis among Canadian and Japanese college students. *Dreaming, 8*(2), 59–66. doi: 10.1023/B:DREM.0000005896.68083.ae

Goode, G. B. (1962). Sleep paralysis. *Archives of Neurology, 6*, 228–234.

Huamani, C., Martinez, A., Martinez, C., & Reyes, A. (2006). Prevalencia y presentacion de la paralisis del sueno en estudiantes de medicina humana de la UNMSM. *Anales de la Facultad de Medicina, 67*(2), 168–172.

Jimenez-Genchi, A., Avila-Rodriguez, V. M., Sanchez-Rojas, F., Terrez, B. E., & Nenclares-Portocarrero, A. (2009). Sleep paralysis in adolescents: The 'a dead body climbed on top of me' phenomenon in Mexico. *Psychiatry and Clinical Neurosciences, 63*(4), 546–549. doi: 10.1111/j.1440-1819.2009.01984.x [doi]

Kotorii, T., Kotorii, T., Uchimura, N., Hashizume, Y., Shirakawa, S., Satomura, T., et al. (2001). Questionnaire relating to sleep paralysis. *Psychiatry and Clinical Neurosciences, 55*(3), 265–266. doi: 10.1046/j.1440-1819.2001.00853.x

Lopez, A. T., Sanchez, E. G., Torres, F. G., Ramirez, P. N., & Olivares, V. S. (1995). Habitos y trasornos del dormir en residentes del metropolitana de Monterrey. *Salud Mental, 18*(1), 14–22.

McNally, R. J., & Clancy, S. A. (2005). Sleep paralysis in adults reporting repressed, recovered, or continuous memories of childhood sexual abuse. *Journal of Anxiety Disorders, 19*(5), 595–602. doi: 10.1016/j.janxdis.2004.05.003

Neal, A. M., Rich, L. N., & Smucker, W. D. (1994). The presence of panic disorder among African American hypertensives: A pilot study. *Journal of Black Psychology, 20*(1), 29–35.

Ohaeri, J. U., Adelekan, M. F., Odejide, A. O., & Ikuesan, B. A. (1992). The pattern of isolated sleep paralysis among Nigerian nursing students. *Journal of the National Medical Association, 84*(1), 67–70.

Ohaeri, J. U., Awadalla, V. A., Maknjuola, V. A., & Ohaeri, B. M. (2004). Features of isolated sleep paralysis among nigerians. *East African Medical Journal, 81*(10), 509–519.

Ohaeri, J. U., Odejide, O. A., Ikuesan, B. A., & Adeyemi, J. D. (1989). The pattern of isolated sleep paralysis among Nigerian medical students. *Journal of the National Medical Association, 81*(7), 805–808.

O'Hanlon, J., Murphy, M., & Di Blasi, Z. (2011). Experiences of sleep paralysis in a sample of irish university students. *Irish Journal of Medical Science, 180*(4), 917–919. doi: 10.1007/s11845-011-0732-2; 10.1007/s11845-011-0732-2

Ohayon, M. M., Priest, R. G., Zulley, J., Smirne, S., & Paiva, T. (2002). Prevalence of narcolepsy symptomatology and diagnosis in the general population. *Neurology, 58,* 1826–1833.

Ohayon, M. M., & Shapiro, C. M. (2000). Sleep disturbances and psychiatric disorders associated with posttraumatic stress disorder in the general population. *Comprehensive Psychiatry, 41*(6), 469–478.

Ohayon, M. M., Zulley, J., Guilleminault, C., & Smirne, S. (1999). Prevalence and pathologic associations of sleep paralysis in the general population. *Neurology, 52*(6), 1194–1200.

Otto, M. W., Simon, N. M., Powers, M., Hinton, D., Zalta, A. K., & Pollack, M. H. (2006). Rates of isolated sleep paralysis in outpatients with anxiety disorders. *Journal of Anxiety Disorders, 20*(5), 687–693. doi: 10.1016/j.janxdis.2005.07.002

Paradis, C. M., Friedman, S., & Hatch, M. (1997). Isolated sleep paralysis in African Americans with panic disorder. *Cultural Diversity and Mental Health, 3*(1), 69–76. doi: 10.1037/1099-9809.3.1.69

Paradis, C., Friedman, S., Hinton, D. E., McNally, R. J., Solomon, L. Z., & Lyons, K. A. (2009). The assessment of the phenomenology of sleep paralysis: The unusual sleep experiences questionnaire (USEQ). *CNS Neuroscience & Therapeutics, 15*(3), 220–226. doi: 10.1111/j.1755-5949.2009.00098.x

Pelayo, R., & Lopes, M. C. (2009). Narcolepsy. In T. L. Lee-Chiong (Ed.), *Sleep medicine essentials* (pp. 47–51). Hoboken, NJ: Wiley-Blackwell.

Penn, N. E., Kripke, D. F., & Scharff, J. (1981). Sleep-paralysis among medical students. *Journal of Psychology: Interdisciplinary and Applied, 107*(2), 247–252. doi: 10.1080/00223980.1981.9915230

Pires, M. L. N., Benedito-Silva, A. A., Mellow, M. T., Del Giglio, S., Pompeia, C., & Tufik, S. (2007). Sleep habits and complaints of adults in the city of Sao Paolo, Brazil, in 1987 and 1995. *Brazilian Journal of Medical and Biological Research, 40*(11), 1505–1515.

Ramsawh, H. J., Raffa, S. D., White, K. S., & Barlow, D. H. (2008). Risk factors for isolated sleep paralysis in an African American sample: A preliminary study. *Behavior Therapy, 39*(4), 386–397. doi: 10.1016/j.beth.2007.11.002

Sharpless, B. A., & Barber, J. P. (2011). Lifetime prevalence rates of sleep paralysis: A systematic review. *Sleep Medicine Reviews, 15*(5), 311–315. doi: 10.1016/j.smrv.2011.01.007

Sharpless, B. A., McCarthy, K. S., Chambless, D. L., Milrod, B. L., Khalsa, S. R., & Barber, J. P. (2010). Isolated sleep paralysis and fearful isolated sleep paralysis in outpatients with panic attacks. *Journal of Clinical Psychology, 66*(12), 1292–1306. doi: 10.1002/jclp.20724

Simard, V., & Nielsen, T. A. (2005). Sleep paralysis-associated sensed presence as a possible manifestation of social anxiety. *Dreaming, 15*(4), 245–260. doi: 10.1037/1053-0797.15.4.245

Smith, P. M., Brown, D., & Mellman, T. A. (2008). Sleep paralysis and sleep duration. *Journal of the National Medical Association, 100*(10), 1207–1208.

Spanos, N. P., McNulty, S. A., DuBreuil, S. C., & Pires, M. (1995). The frequency and correlates of sleep paralysis in a university sample. *Journal of Research in Personality, 29*(3), 285–305. doi: 10.1006/jrpe.1995.1017

Suarez, S. A. (1991). Parálisis del sueño aislada en pacientes con trastorno por crisis de angustia. *Archivos De Neurobiología, 54*(1), 21–24.

Wing, Y., Chiu, H., Leung, T., & Ng, J. (1999). Sleep paralysis in the elderly. *Journal of Sleep Research, 8*, 151–155.

Wing, Y., Lee, S. T., & Chen, C. (1994). Sleep paralysis in chinese: Ghost oppression phenomenon in hong kong. *Sleep: Journal of Sleep Research & Sleep Medicine, 17*(7), 609–613.

Yeung, A., Xu, Y., & Chang, D. F. (2005). Prevalence and illness beliefs of sleep paralysis among chinese psychiatric patients in china and the united states. *Transcultural Psychiatry, 42*(1), 135–143. doi: 10.1177/1363461505050725

CHAPTER 8

Sleep Paralysis and Medical Conditions

As demonstrated in the following, sleep paralysis bears a relation to a number of medical conditions. We discuss seven of the most important ones in this chapter (see also chapter 13 for discussions of differential diagnosis). We next evaluate the role of medication and substances in generating sleep paralysis episodes.

INSUFFICIENT SLEEP SYNDROME

Also known as "chronic sleep deprivation" or "sleep restriction," insufficient sleep syndrome (ISS) is characterized by persistently obtaining less sleep than an individual's requirements to maintain normal levels of daytime alertness (American Academy of Sleep Medicine, 2014). The hallmark complaint is that of excessive daytime sleepiness (EDS), or an exaggerated tendency to fall asleep during the daytime. This is usually associated with a feeling of lassitude or fatigue. Since sleep requirements are subject to a high level of inter-individual variability, the recommended way to properly establish the diagnosis is a trial of sleep extension for a week or more; if EDS dissipates, or is significantly reduced, the diagnosis can be made with greater confidence. Typically, sleep times are assessed with sleep logs or actigraphy to both establish the diagnosis and to monitor the effects of sleep extension. In addition, a clinical evaluation should be conducted to rule out other causes of EDS.

Although the ICSD-3 (American Academy of Sleep Medicine, 2014) discussed the potential for sleep paralysis in the context of ISS, studies into the prevalence of sleep paralysis as a function of habitual sleep times have not been conducted, nor have rates of sleep paralysis been determined in sleep-deprived populations such as shift workers. However, rebound of REM sleep has been observed on the second night of recovery sleep following total sleep deprivation (Carskadon & Dement, 1979).

NARCOLEPSY

Narcolepsy type 1 is a neurological disorder characterized by the complaint of EDS for at least 3 months along with either (1) or (2) or both of the following (American Academy of Sleep Medicine, 2014):

(1) (a) Repeated episodes of cataplexy, or brief (i.e., seconds to minutes), usually bilaterally symmetrical episodes of sudden loss of muscle control, during which consciousness is maintained. Episodes are triggered by strong emotions, usually positive ones, such as laughter or excitement. Cataplexy occurs almost exclusively in the context of narcolepsy. It is thought to represent REM-associated muscle atonia that strikes during wakefulness. It may be mild, leading to facial or limb weakness or a feeling general body weakness. Less commonly, it can lead to collapse and falls.

(2) (b) Multiple sleep latency testing (MSLT) demonstrates a mean sleep latency of less than or equal to 8 minutes and two or more sleep onset REM periods (SOREMPs). The MSLT is performed in the controlled setting of a sleep laboratory (Littner et al., 2005). Individuals are given four or five opportunities, each separated by 2 hours of wakefulness, to fall asleep during the day. The test begins shortly following patients' morning awakening time, and concludes in the afternoon or early evening. The speed of falling asleep, i.e., sleep latency, is interpreted as being inversely proportional to the level of EDS. Individuals who fall asleep rapidly during these nap tests are, therefore, considered to be highly sleepy. A SOREMP represents the occurrence of REM sleep within 15 minutes of sleep onset on any one or more nap opportunity. A SOREMP on the preceding nocturnal polysomnogram may replace one of the SOREMPs on the MSLT.

(3) Hypocretin-1 concentration of less than or equal to 110 pg/mL or less than one-third of mean values obtained in normal subjects with the same standardized assay.

The pathophysiology of narcolepsy is widely regarded as stemming from a deficiency in the hypothalamic neuropeptide hypocretin (orexin). The presence of cataplexy and an abnormal MSLT serve as surrogate markers for this condition with high specificity and sensitivity. However, the capacity to measure hypocretin levels is highly limited to a few research centers, and available for clinical purposes on a very limited basis. Therefore, from a practical, clinical, standpoint, the presence of cataplexy and abnormal MSLT findings represent the mainstay of establishing the diagnosis of narcolepsy type 1. Hypocretin deficiency is, in turn, thought to be related to an autoimmune-based hypocretin cell destruction, at least in animal models. The autoimmune basis is supported by the close link between narcolepsy type 1 and the human leukocyte antigen (HLA) subtypes DR2/DRB1*1501 and DQB1*0602. Almost all patients with cataplexy are positive for DQB1*0602, compared with 12% to 38% of the general population who have this HLA subtype. Rare cases of narcolepsy have also been identified in other disorders that affect the hypothalamus or the hypocretin system.

Narcolepsy type 2 is diagnostically similar to narcolepsy type 1, with the exception that cataplexy is absent and, if measured, CSF hypcretin-1 concentrations are above 110 pg/mL or greater than one-third of mean values obtained in normal subjects with the same standardized assay. It most likely represents a heterogenous disorder.

The prevalence of narcolepsy with cataplexy has been examined in many studies and falls between 25 and 50 per 100,000 people (Longstreth, Koepsell, Ton, Hendrickson, & van Belle, 2007). Cataplexy, which is specific to narcolepsy, is thought to represent the tendency for the occurrence of REM-related phenomena during abnormal times, that is, wakefulness. Skeletal muscle paralysis occurs normally during nocturnal REM sleep, yet its induction during wakefulness in narcoleptics results in cataplexy. Associated, yet non-specific, features of narcolepsy, include disrupted nocturnal sleep, characterized mainly by discontinuous and fragmented sleep; hypnagogic hallucinations, or vivid, dreamlike perceptual experiences occurring at the transition from wakefulness to sleep, which can encompass visual, auditory, and tactile phenomena; less commonly, hypnopompic hallucinations, which are similar but occur at sleep to wake transitions; and sleep paralysis, during which patients are cognitively awake and aware of their surroundings, but can't move their body, limbs, or even open their eyes. Sleep paralysis is one of the most distressing experiences of narcolepsy. Hypnagogic hallucinations and sleep paralysis are considered to be REM sleep dissociation phenomena (Szucs, Janszky, Hollo, Migleczi, & Halasz, 2003). Associated features are less common than cataplexy, yet their prevalence rates have not been well defined. One study noted that sleep paralysis and hypnagogic hallucination rate ranges for narcolepsy with cataplexy were 49% to 58% and 74% to 75%, and for narcolepsy without cataplexy were generally lower at 27% to 36% and 14% to 30%, respectively (Aldrich, 1996). A review of various publications by Scammel reported the rates of sleep paralysis and hypnagogic hallucinations for narcolepsy with cataplexy to be 50% to 70% and 70% to 86%, respectively, and for narcolepsy without cataplexy to be 25% to 60% and 15% to 60%, respectively (Scammell, 2003). In summary, various studies indicate that 33% to 80% of narcolepsy patients report hypnagogic hallucinations and/or sleep paralysis (American Academy of Sleep Medicine, 2014).

IDIOPATHIC HYPERSOMNIA

Like narcolepsy, idiopathic hypersomnia (IH), also referred to as idiopathic central nervous system hypersomnolence, also features the complaint of EDS for at least three months. However, cataplexy is absent, sleep onset REM periods are not evident on nocturnal polysomnography and fewer than two such phenomena are evident following MSLT testing, and either the MSLT demonstrates high levels of EDS (mean sleep latency of less than or equal to 8 minutes) or total 24-hour sleep time is greater than or equal to 660 minutes (typically 12 to 14 hours) (American Academy of Sleep Medicine, 2014). Associated features suggest a dysfunction of the autonomic nervous system, including headache, orthostatic disturbance, perception of temperature dysregulation, and peripheral vascular complaints (Raynaud-type phenomena with cold hands and feet). Sleep paralysis and hypnagogic hallucinations may also be reported, but the frequency is uncertain. Recent series (Anderson, Pilsworth, Sharples, Smith, & Shneerson, 2007) reported their frequencies to be 4% and 5%, respectively, and 10% and 4%, respectively (Ali, Auger, Slocumb, & Morgenthaler, 2009), although an earlier series reported their frequencies to be 40% and 43% (Bassetti & Aldrich, 1997).

The prevalence of IH is unknown, and its pathophysiology poorly understood. Cerebrospinal fluid (CSF) hypocretin levels are not reduced and, although CSF neurotransmitter levels have been explored, no consistent findings have been noted.

SLEEP RELATED HALLUCINATIONS

This disorder features recurrent hypnagogic or hypnopompic hallucinations, mainly visual, and not occurring in the context of narcolepsy or other disorders (American Academy of Sleep Medicine, 2014). Less commonly, auditory and tactile hallucinations occur as well. Patients with this disorder may also report experiencing episodes of sleep paralysis during the same night, or on different nights, although the extent of this association is currently unknown (Silber, Hansen, & Girish, 2005). The prevalence of this disorder is similarly unknown, although a community sample of UK residents indicated that 37% of the sample reported experiencing hypnagogic hallucinations and 12.5% reported hypnopompic hallucinations (Ohayon, Priest, Caulet, & Guilleminault, 1996). Sleep-related hallucinations are presumed to result from dream ideation of REM sleep intruding into wakefulness, but this has not been confirmed. Nevertheless, these hallucinations differ from nightmares, which are frightening dreams that awaken sufferers from sleep, are clearly identified as dreams, and which do not persist into wakefulness.

OBSTRUCTIVE SLEEP APNEA

Obstructive sleep apnea (OSA), whose main presenting symptoms include EDS and loud snoring, is characterized by repetitive episodes of complete (apnea) or partial (hypopnea) upper airway obstruction during sleep. Airflow cessations or reductions produce arousals, fragmented sleep, reductions in blood oxyhemoglobin saturation, and fluctuations in blood pressure and heart rate. The severity of the condition is primarily assessed by the average number of apneas and hypopneas per hour of sleep, or the apnea/hypopnea index (AHI). Obstructive sleep apnea is diagnosed if the AHI is greater than or equal to 5 in the presence of symptoms such as sleepiness, fatigue, inattention) or signs of disturbed sleep (restless sleep, and respiratory pauses), or an AHI greater than or equal to 15 in an otherwise asymptomatic patient (American Academy of Sleep Medicine, 2014). The prevalence of the condition is estimated to be 2% in women and 4% in men.

Obstruction of airway during sleep occurs due to anatomical as well as physiological factors. Anatomical factors include large neck size, micrognathia, crowded pharynx, tonsillar/adenoidal hypertrophy, and nasal obstruction, among others. Physiological factors contributing to upper airway collapsibility are less well understood, and are thought to be due to impaired pharyngeal muscle dilator sensitivity and diminished neural output to the upper airway muscles during sleep. Apneas occur when the respiratory drive is less than the threshold for inspiratory muscle strength needed for maintaining upper airway patency during sleep. As apnea progresses, respiratory drive increases until that inspiratory threshold is passed and inspiration can then occur. The arousal response plays a critical role in apnea termination. Sleep fragmentation and hypoxia, hypercapnia, and acidosis are thought to lead to EDS and other consequences, including hypertension, coronary artery disease and myocardial infarction, congestive heart failure, stroke, cognitive impairment resulting in motor vehicle and industrial accidents, diabetes, and major depression. The disorder also results in a decreased quality of life and decreased life expectancy (Mulgrew et al., 2008; Ohayon, Lemoine, Arnaud-Briant, & Dreyfus, 2002; Peppard, Szklo-Coxe, Hla, & Young, 2006; Young, Skatrud, & Peppard, 2004; Young et al., 1993, 2002).

Although sleep paralysis is not one of the commonly reported symptoms of the disorder, a recent study noted that 41 of 107 OSA patients (38.3%) met ICSD-2 diagnostic criteria for isolated sleep paralysis (Hsieh, Lai, Liu, Lan, & Hsu, 2010; International classification of sleep disorders, 2005). Sixty-three point four percent experienced sleep paralysis less than once a month but at least once in recent 6 months, and 22.0% experienced sleep paralysis more than once a month, 9.7% more than once a week, and 4.9% every night; 90.2% of those who suffered from isolated sleep paralysis also experienced hypnagogic or hypnopompic hallucinations. It was also an independent predictor of EDS, impairment in nocturnal sleep quality, and impairment in health-related quality of life, as assessed by the *Epworth Sleepiness Scale* (Johns, 1991), the *Pittsburgh Sleep Quality Index* (PSQI) (Buysse, Reynolds, Monk, Berman, & Kupfer, 1989), and the *Short-Form 36* (SF-36) (Leger, Scheuermaier, Philip, Paillard, & Guilleminault, 2001). Notably, the study was performed in an Asian population, and the degree to which this information applies to other cultures is unclear, especially in light of the cultural variations in rates of sleep paralysis (see chapter 7). A non-OSA control group may have assisted in clarifying this point. In addition, the study excluded narcolepsy patients from the population on the basis of clinical symptoms alone, and did not utilize the MSLT for this purpose (see the preceding), raising the possibility that some of these patients may have suffered from narcolepsy.

If the association between OSA and sleep paralysis is confirmed by other studies, what might be the mechanism? Obstructive sleep apnea may increase vulnerability for sleep paralysis through a selective or predominant fragmentation of REM sleep. The withdrawal of excitatory noradrenergic and serotonergic inputs to upper airway motor neurons during REM sleep is thought to exaggerate the reduction in pharyngeal muscle activity that accompanies sleep and substantially increase the propensity for upper airway collapse. Thus, REM sleep in patients with OSA is typically associated with increased frequency of obstructive events that are often prolonged and accompanied with severe oxyhemoglobin desaturation. In addition, 10% to 36% of OSA patients experience apneas primarily during REM sleep (Mokhlesi & Punjabi, 2012). Alternatively, OSA treatment with continuous positive airway pressure (CPAP) may produce a REM rebound, resulting in the experience of vivid dreaming and sleep paralysis (Hsieh et al., 2010).

HYPERTENSION

A study of 31 black patients with a history of hypertension noted that 41.9% reported at least one episode of isolated sleep paralysis, and 30.8% reported having sleep paralysis disorder (i.e., at least one episode of sleep paralysis a month as described in Bell, Hildreth, Jenkins, & Carter, 1988). However, the study lacked a control group and contained at least some subjects who met diagnostic criteria for panic disorder. Although no conclusive relationship can be drawn between hypertension and sleep paralysis based on this pilot study, the authors hypothesize that adrenergic dysfunction may predispose individuals to both hypertension and sleep paralysis.

WILSON'S DISEASE

Wilson's disease, or hepatolenticular degeneration, is an inherited, autosomal recessive disorder of copper metabolism. It results from mutations in the ATP7B gene, which encodes a copper transporter protein, resulting in reduced excretion of copper into the bile and its accumulation in the liver, brain, cornea, and other organs, causing damage to these organs. The prevalence of the disorder is 20 to 30 per million (Portala, Westermark, Ekselius, & Broman, 2002). Many of the systemic manifestations of the condition are related to hepatic impairment, including portal hypertension and esophageal varices, splenomegaly, cirrhosis, and even acute liver failure. However, a host of neuropsychiatric symptoms are also seen in half of all patients, including parkinsonian symptoms, tremor, frontal lobe signs, subcortical dementia, depression, anxiety, and psychosis (Ropper & Samuels, 2014). An abnormal metabolism of neurotransmitters, probably due to increased activity of copper-containing enzymes like dopamine b-hydroxylase with increased noradrenaline in the striatum, has been reported (Kish, Shannak, Rajput, Deck, & Hornykiewicz, 1992).

In a recent study, 24 patients with Wilson's disease with a mean age of 35.1 years and disease duration of 17.7 years were compared with those from a random sample of 72 individuals using a standardized sleep questionnaire (i.e., 87 questions concerning sleep habits, sleeping difficulties, and other variables). Patients were specifically asked regarding sleep paralysis in the pre-sleep period, sleep paralysis at awakening, and cataplexy. The frequencies of these symptoms in the Wilson's disease versus reference group were 20.8% versus 2.8%, 25.0% versus 8.3%, and 29.2% versus 19.4%, respectively. Objective, polysomnographic, testing was not performed to understand to what extent the sample suffered from sleep apnea, narcolepsy, or other sleep disorders. Nevertheless, if the association between WD and these manifestations of REM sleep fragmentation are confirmed, they indicate the potential role of brainstem impairment in WD, which, in turn, impair REM-off monoaminergic neurons, resulting in REM fragmentation. They may also indicate suprachiasmatic nucleus impairment, leading to circadian disturbances, which are often associated with REM sleep abnormalities.

MEDICATIONS AND SUBSTANCES

Alcohol

The first known reference to the association between alcohol consumption and sleep paralysis was made by Rhazes (865 to 925 A.D.), the Persian polymath, who noted "...and Kabus (sleep paralysis) could occur in individuals following alcohol consumption" (reference and translation from Arabic in Golzari & Ghabili, 2013). A recent cross-sectional sampling survey of Japanese adolescents (Munezawa, Kaneita, Yokoyama, Suzuki, & Ohida, 2009) noted that the prevalence of nightmares and sleep paralysis was 35.2% and 8.3%, respectively. Multiple logistic analyses revealed that female sex, drinking alcohol, poor mental health, difficulty initiating sleep, low subjective sleep assessment, presence of excessive daytime sleepiness, and presence of sleep paralysis had higher odds ratios than others for nightmares. Male sex, poor mental health, drinking alcohol (extent unclear), taking a long daytime nap, early or late bedtime, difficulty initiating sleep, low subjective sleep assessment, presence of excessive daytime sleepiness, and presence of nightmares had higher odds ratios than other factors for experiencing an episode of sleep paralysis over the prior month.

The basis for the presumed association between alcohol consumption and sleep paralysis is unclear. Alcohol is associated with shallow and interrupted sleep (Johnson & Breslau, 2001) and increases the frequency of sleep-disordered breathing, factors promoting REM fragmentation. Rapid eye movement rebound also occurs in the context of alcohol withdrawal, which, in turn, is associated with enhanced REM-related phenomena such as hypnogogic hallucinations and sleep paralysis. Nevertheless, it is possible that individuals who suffer from sleep paralysis and nightmares are more prone to alcohol consumption as a mechanism of diminishing anxiety associated with both of these phenomena.

Other Medications and Substances

Cholinergic mechanisms have long been implicated in the generation of REM sleep. In animal studies, injection of the cholinergic agonist carbachol into the dorsomedial pons produces a REM sleep-like state with muscle atonia and cortical activation, both of which are cardinal features of REM sleep (Weng et al., 2014). The sublaterodorsal nucleus (SLD), which is located within this region of the pons, is regarded to be both necessary and sufficient for generating REM sleep muscle atonia. Acetylcholine produces synergistic, excitatory pre- and postsynaptic responses on SLD neurons that, in turn, probably serve to promote muscle atonia during REM sleep. Infusion of physostigmine into human subjects induces the onset of REM sleep. However, there are no data regarding potential effects of similar medications on sleep paralysis. A sample of European community residents indicated that no associations between the severity of sleep paralysis and use of antidepressants and hypnotic medications (Ohayon, Zulley, Guilleminault, & Smirne, 1999). Similarly, the consumption of coffee and alcohol during the day or at bedtime did not differ. However, a significantly greater proportion of subjects in both the severe and moderate sleep paralysis groups reported taking anxiolytic medication, compared with the no-sleep paralysis group (severe SP, 10.6%; moderate SP, 12.2%; mild SP, 3.8%;

no SP, 3.0%; chi-square $p < .0001$). Clearly, further studies are needed in this area.

REFERENCES

Aldrich, M. S. (1996). The clinical spectrum of narcolepsy and idiopathic hypersomnia. *Neurology, 46*(2), 393–401.

Ali, M., Auger, R. R., Slocumb, N. L., & Morgenthaler, T. I. (2009). Idiopathic hypersomnia: Clinical features and response to treatment. *Journal of Clinical Sleep Medicine: JCSM: Official Publication of the American Academy of Sleep Medicine, 5*(6), 562–568.

American Academy of Sleep Medicine. (2014). *International classification of sleep disorders: Diagnostic and coding manual* (3rd ed.). Darien, IL: American Academy of Sleep Medicine.

Anderson, K. N., Pilsworth, S., Sharples, L. D., Smith, I. E., & Shneerson, J. M. (2007). Idiopathic hypersomnia: A study of 77 cases. *Sleep, 30*(10), 1274–1281.

Bassetti, C., & Aldrich, M. S. (1997). Idiopathic hypersomnia. A series of 42 patients. *Brain: A Journal of Neurology, 120*(Pt 8), 1423–1435.

Bell, C. C., Hildreth, C. J., Jenkins, E. J., & Carter, C. (1988). The relationship of isolated sleep paralysis and panic disorder to hypertension. *Journal of the National Medical Association, 80*(3), 289–294.

Buysse, D. J., Reynolds, C. F. 3rd, Monk, T. H., Berman, S. R., & Kupfer, D. J. (1989). The pittsburgh sleep quality index: A new instrument for psychiatric practice and research. *Psychiatry Research, 28*(2), 193–213. doi: 0165-1781(89)90047-4 [pii]

Carskadon, M. A., & Dement, W. C. (1979). Effects of total sleep loss on sleep tendency. *Perceptual and Motor Skills, 48*(2), 495–506.

Golzari, S. E., & Ghabili, K. (2013). Alcohol-mediated sleep paralysis: The earliest known description. *Sleep Medicine, 14*(3), 298. doi: 10.1016/j.sleep.2012.09.014; 10.1016/j.sleep.2012.09.014

Hsieh, S., Lai, C., Liu, C., Lan, S., & Hsu, C. (2010). Isolated sleep paralysis linked to impaired nocturnal sleep quality and health-related quality of life in chinese-taiwanese patients with obstructive sleep apnea. *Quality of Life Research: An International Journal of Quality of Life Aspects of Treatment, Care & Rehabilitation, 19*(9), 1265–1272. doi: 10.1007/s11136-010-9695-4

Johns, M. W. (1991). A new method for measuring daytime sleepiness: The Epworth sleepiness scale. *Sleep, 14*(6), 540–545.

Johnson, E. O., & Breslau, N. (2001). Sleep problems and substance use in adolescence. *Drug and Alcohol Dependence, 64*(1), 1–7. doi: S0376-8716(00)00222-2 [pii]

Kish, S. J., Shannak, K., Rajput, A., Deck, J. H., & Hornykiewicz, O. (1992). Aging produces a specific pattern of striatal dopamine loss: Implications for the etiology of idiopathic parkinson's disease. *Journal of Neurochemistry, 58*(2), 642–648.

Leger, D., Scheuermaier, K., Philip, P., Paillard, M., & Guilleminault, C. (2001). SF-36: Evaluation of quality of life in severe and mild insomniacs compared with good sleepers. *Psychosomatic Medicine, 63*(1), 49–55.

Littner, M. R., Kushida, C., Wise, M., Davila, D. G., Morgenthaler, T., Lee-Chiong, T.,...Standards of Practice Committee of the American Academy of Sleep Medicine. (2005). Practice parameters for clinical use of the multiple sleep latency test and the maintenance of wakefulness test. *Sleep, 28*(1), 113–121.

Longstreth, W. T. Jr., Koepsell, T. D., Ton, T. G., Hendrickson, A. F., & van Belle, G. (2007). The epidemiology of narcolepsy. *Sleep, 30*(1), 13–26.

Mokhlesi, B., & Punjabi, N. M. (2012). "REM-related" obstructive sleep apnea: An epiphenomenon or a clinically important entity? *Sleep, 35*(1), 5–7. doi: 10.5665/sleep.1570 [doi]

Mulgrew, A. T., Nasvadi, G., Butt, A., Cheema, R., Fox, N., Fleetham, J. A.,...Ayas, N. T. (2008). Risk and severity of motor vehicle crashes in patients with obstructive sleep apnoea/hypopnoea. *Thorax, 63*(6), 536–541. doi: 10.1136/thx.2007.085464; 10.1136/thx.2007.085464

Munezawa, T., Kaneita, Y., Yokoyama, E., Suzuki, H., & Ohida, T. (2009). Epidemiological study of nightmare and sleep paralysis among japanese adolescents. *Sleep and Biological Rhythms, 7*(3), 201–210. doi: 10.1111/j.1479-842 5.2009.00404.x

Ohayon, M. M., Lemoine, P., Arnaud-Briant, V., & Dreyfus, M. (2002). Prevalence and consequences of sleep disorders in a shift worker population. *Journal of Psychosomatic Research, 53*(1), 577–583.

Ohayon, M. M., Priest, R. G., Caulet, M., & Guilleminault, C. (1996). Hypnagogic and hypnopompic hallucinations: Pathological phenomena? *The British Journal of Psychiatry, 169*(4), 459–467.

Ohayon, M. M., Zulley, J., Guilleminault, C., & Smirne, S. (1999). Prevalence and pathologic associations of sleep paralysis in the general population. *Neurology, 52*(6), 1194–1200.

Peppard, P. E., Szklo-Coxe, M., Hla, K. M., & Young, T. (2006). Longitudinal association of sleep-related breathing disorder and depression. *Archives of Internal Medicine, 166*(16), 1709–1715. doi: 10.1001/archinte.166.16.1709

Portala, K., Westermark, K., Ekselius, L., & Broman, J. (2002). Sleep in patients with treated Wilson's disease: A questionnaire study. *Nordic Journal of Psychiatry, 56*(4), 291–297.

Ropper, A. H., & Samuels, M. A. (2014). *Adams and victor's principles of neurology* (10th ed.). New York: McGraw-Hill.

Scammell, T. E. (2003). The neurobiology, diagnosis, and treatment of narcolepsy. *Annals of Neurology, 53*(2), 154–166. doi: 10.1002/ana.10444 [doi]

Silber, M. H., Hansen, M. R., & Girish, M. (2005). Complex nocturnal visual hallucinations. *Sleep Medicine, 6*(4), 363–366. doi: S1389-9457(05)00064-X [pii]

Szucs, A., Janszky, J., Hollo, A., Migleczi, G., & Halasz, P. (2003). Misleading hallucinations in unrecognized narcolepsy. *Acta Psychiatrica Scandinavica, 108*, 314–317.

Weng, F. J., Williams, R. H., Hawryluk, J. M., Lu, J., Scammell, T. E., Saper, C. B., & Arrigoni, E. (2014). Carbachol excites sublaterodorsal nucleus neurons projecting to the spinal cord. *The Journal of Physiology, 592*(Pt 7), 1601–1617. doi: 10.1113/jphysiol.2013.261800 [doi]

Young, T., Skatrud, J., & Peppard, P. E. (2004). Risk factors for obstructive sleep apnea in adults. *JAMA: The Journal of the American Medical Association, 291*(16), 2013–2016.

Young, T., Palta, M., Dempsey, J., Skatrud, J., Weber, S., & Badr, S. (1993). The occurrence of sleep-disordered breathing among middle-aged adults.

The New England Journal of Medicine, 328(17), 1230–1235. doi: 10.1056/NEJM199304293281704

Young, T., Shahar, E., Nieto, F. J., Redline, S., Newman, A. B., Gottlieb, D. J., ... Sleep Heart Health Study Research Group. (2002). Predictors of sleep-disordered breathing in community-dwelling adults: The sleep heart health study. *Archives of Internal Medicine, 162*(8), 893–900.

CHAPTER 9

Sleep Paralysis and Psychopathology

Sleep paralysis, especially when seen in more chronic forms, possesses clear associations with many medical and neurological conditions (see chapter 8). Other proximal medical events (e.g., acute alcohol intoxication or excessive caffeine use) may also make episodes more likely. However, none of these relatively well-understood biological correlates of sleep paralysis/isolated sleep paralysis remove the possibility that psychological factors may also possess etiological relevance. In fact, evidence is accruing that sleep paralysis does in fact occur at greater than chance levels with certain psychological states and specific forms of psychopathology. Whether sleep paralysis episodes are *directly* caused by psychopathological processes or are instead indirectly mediated though associated *consequences of psychopathology* is currently open to debate. The most likely candidate for the latter view would be that most psychological disorders can result in sleep deprivation, sleep–wake disruptions, and/or insomnia; these disrupted sleep patterns, in turn, increase the risk for sleep paralysis. After first discussing comorbidity in general, we consider sleep paralysis within the context of more specific psychiatric conditions (e.g., panic disorder) and broader psychological constructs (e.g., anxiety sensitivity, death distress). We focus most of our attention on the complex relationships between trauma/post-traumatic stress disorder (PTSD) and isolated sleep paralysis.

PSYCHIATRIC COMORBIDITY

Before discussing specific symptoms and syndromes, we consider psychiatric comorbidity more generally. Data are consistent with the view that sleep paralysis is more likely to occur in individuals with multiple disorders. For instance, patients with anxiety disorders are more likely to have isolated sleep paralysis than those without (e.g., Ohayon, Zulley, Guilleminault, & Smirne, 1999). This was also found in Michael Otto's 2006 study, but depressive disorders did not bear a relationship with higher rates of isolated sleep paralysis. Others reviewing the available literature believe that the presence of either the anxiety and depressive disorders conveys an increased risk for sleep paralysis (Plante & Winkelman, 2006), and one study found that the occurrence of isolated sleep paralysis, regardless of the definition used (i.e., ICSD-2 or fearful isolated sleep paralysis [ISP] criteria), was linearly associated with the number of non-psychotic mood and anxiety disorder diagnoses that a patient had (Sharpless, McCarthy, Chambless, Milrod, Khalsa, & Barber, 2010).

PSYCHOTIC DISORDERS AND PSYCHOTIC SYMPTOMS

Psychosis has also been discussed in the context of sleep paralysis. We are not aware of any findings indicating that psychosis serves as a risk factor for sleep paralysis. However, Plante and Winkleman (2008) noted that psychosis may, in general, be associated with higher rates of hypnagogic and hypnopompic hallucinations.

We have experience with many patients with comorbid schizophrenia and sleep paralysis, and these can be clinically challenging. For example, a patient of the first author suffered from both isolated sleep paralysis and paranoid schizophrenia. The presence of realistic sleep paralysis hallucinations made this patient's attempts at reality-testing even more difficult. Unfortunately, the paralysis also interacted with his delusional beliefs and hallucinations, and he incorporated the atonia into his psychosis.

Moreover, as discussed in chapters 2 and 13, it may occasionally be challenging to differentiate psychosis from sleep paralysis if hypnagogic/hypnopompic hallucinations are present and acutely distressing. This is a crucial matter, however, as the conceptualization and treatment of these two disorders is quite different.

MOOD DISORDERS

Sleep difficulties are common symptoms in both unipolar and bipolar mood disorders. Hyposomnia is very common during manic episodes, and both hypo- and hypersomnia are common correlates of major depressive episodes. Rapid eye movement (REM) sleep disinhibition has been proposed as one of the possible mechanisms through which sleep disruption occurs in mood disorders (e.g., Casement, Arendt, & Armitage, 2009). In this theory, an imbalance in cholinergic/aminergic neurotransmission leads to an early onset of REM and an overall increase in REM activity. Given some of the basic science findings about sleep paralysis and its relation to disruptions in sleep architecture, one could surmise that rates may be elevated in patients with mood disorders.

In fact, there is some evidence that this may indeed be the case, but it is not unambiguous. Regarding depression, those with sleep paralysis/isolated sleep paralysis typically have higher scores on self-report measures (e.g., McNally & Clancy, 2005a; Szklo-Coxe, Young, Finn, & Mignot, 2007). Sharpless et al. (2010) administered a clinician-administered instrument (*Hamilton Rating Scale for Depression*) and found no signification relationship when utilizing standard sleep paralysis definitions; instead, a significant correlation only emerged when using more specific recurrent fearful isolated sleep paralysis criteria. Finally, one study found no association between a diagnosis of major depression and isolated sleep paralysis (Otto et al., 2006).

As for bipolar disorder, even fewer data are available. In one of the earliest empirical studies of sleep paralysis, elevated hypomania on the *Millon Clinical Multi-Axial Inventory* was associated with sleep paralysis (Bell et al., 1984). Similarly, a large epidemiological study found elevated rates of bipolar disorder in individuals with sleep paralysis (Ohayon et al., 1999). In summary, there is some limited evidence that mood disorders may be associated with sleep paralysis/isolated sleep paralysis. More specific statistical modeling is needed in order to determine whether there are any more direct relationships beyond the mood disorders' characteristic sleep disturbances and the subsequent development of sleep paralysis episodes.

POST-TRAUMATIC STRESS DISORDER/TRAUMA

Trauma is unfortunately a fairly ubiquitous human experience, and has been associated with a number of symptoms and syndromes. It has also been studied in the context of sleep paralysis. We believe that, of the many psychological syndromes, post-traumatic stress disorder (PTSD) has been looked at most thoroughly, and possesses the strongest evidence base in terms of a putative relationship with sleep paralysis. As shown in the following, however, this relationship may be quite complex.

To meet current criteria for PTSD, the DSM-5 (American Psychiatric Association, 2013) requires a "qualifying" traumatic event. These can be any of four types: the traumas can be directly experienced (e.g., a personal assault), directly witnessed (seeing someone you care about assaulted), learned of after the fact (hearing that something terrible happened to a loved one), or be repeatedly heard about from multiple sources (e.g., vicarious traumatization in a therapist who works heavily with trauma victims).

Along with a qualifying event, diagnosis of PTSD requires a combination of four other symptom clusters, such as the avoidance of trauma-related stimuli, negative alterations in cognition or mood associated with trauma, intrusive symptoms (e.g., distressing dreams or flashbacks), and alterations of arousal and reactivity (e.g., hypervigilance, exaggerated startle response, and sleep disturbances). The qualifying traumatic event and these last two symptom sets are the most directly relevant for our discussion of sleep paralysis. As demonstrated in the next section, there are a number of relevant connections.

Traumatic Events

Specific traumatic events may be linked to sleep paralysis in several ways. Parasomnias are often experienced in the wake of trauma. This is the case for sleep paralysis as well (e.g., Ohayon & Shapiro, 2000). What is particularly interesting is the way in which traumatic events and traumatic content appear to impact upon the hallucinations of sleep paralysis. For instance, Hinton, Pich, Chhean, and Pollack's (2005) study of Cambodian refugees found that sufferers of ISP occasionally experienced "intruders" that were dressed in Kmer Rouge uniforms. These hallucinations sometimes evoked additional traumatic memories and, in some cases, survival guilt (p. 48). Hudson, Manoach, Sabo, and Sternbach (1991) also reported a case in which a woman who was abducted, raped, and tortured for several days had sleep paralysis episodes with similar trauma-related hallucinatory content. Similarly, Sharpless and Grom (2013) found that a number of college students experienced their first isolated sleep paralysis episode after a close relative died, and that the deceased individual was perceived in their hallucinations. This topic has yet to receive extensive empirical attention. However, it appears to be quite reasonable that, much in same way that waking events manifest in dreams, the horrific images of trauma would come out in the REM activity of sleep paralysis. Trauma, with its tendency to shatter assumptions that the world is a safe, predictable, and stable place, possesses the power to infiltrate both our waking and dreaming minds (e.g., Sharpless & Barber, 2011).

It is also worth noting that sleep paralysis has also been conceptualized as a traumatic event in and of itself. If this is true, there may be a circularity inherent to trauma and sleep paralysis such that one could conceivably impact upon the other and even have a catalytic effect. But, this very real possibility aside, several researches have speculated that sleep paralysis, even without a pre-existing trauma history, could lead to personal impacts that are similar to "actual" traumas. For instance, Hinton et al. (2005) speculated that sleep paralysis phenomena can be terrifying enough to constitute a unique traumatic event. Looking at the characteristic hallucinations described in chapter 6, it is easy to see how a sufferer could experience episodes as "actual" assaults and threats to bodily integrity. This would be even more likely if the hallucinations were not seen as hallucinations, but as real-world happenings. In a very interesting psychophysiological study of individuals who believed themselves to be abducted by aliens (and who all experienced at least one episode of sleep paralysis/isolated sleep paralysis), further evidence of the power of improbable experiences was found. McNally et al. (2004) found that physiological reactivity and self-reported distress in response to audio recordings of abduction narratives was as high in a group of putative alien abductees as the level of reactivity found in individuals who suffered actual and verifiable traumas. These researchers did not believe that either group was feigning distress during the recordings, and instead emphasized the potential psychological (and physiological) power of these experiences for those who believed themselves to be victims of alien abduction.

Alterations of Arousal and Reactivity

Both sleep paralysis and PTSD engender heightened levels of arousal. Although a small number of individuals with sleep paralysis may experience chronic levels of activation as a result of their episodes, this activation is most frequently experienced only *during* episodes. This is clearly not the case with PTSD where a fairly high percentage of sufferers have persistent hyperarousal (e.g., Barlow, 2002; Foa, Keane, Terence, Friedman, & Cohen, 2008). These symptoms serve a protective, yet often maladaptive and non–context-relevant function for individuals with PTSD, and they often manifest hyperalertness or hypervigilance toward real and imagined threats (e.g., trauma-related stimuli that are not inherently threatening when outside the context of the original trauma). Thus, individuals with PTSD are constantly "on guard" in order to stave off potential threats. A related symptom of this is an exaggerated startle response such that many surprising, but not scary perceptions (e.g., a glass breaking) elicit increased heart-rates, eye blinks, and other acute fear responses. Needless to say, these manifestations of hyperarousal lead to tiredness and physical exhaustion (e.g., Foa et al., 2008).

Unfortunately for PTSD sufferers, hyperarousal does not end with sleep, as waking hypervigilance appears to cause both REM disruptions and insomnia. Thus, hypervigilance, startle responses, and other relevant symptoms can be proximal causes of any number of sleep problems, including sleep paralysis (e.g., Abrams, Mulligan, Carleton, & Asmundson, 2008; Hudson et al., 1991; Krakow et al., 2001). Sleep studies are consistent with this, as patients with PTSD display lighter and more fragmented sleep states, suggesting that hyperarousal occurs *during* sleep (Krakow et al., 2001). These recurrent sleep difficulties can make disruptions of REM sleep architecture more likely, thus leading to sleep paralysis (Abrams et al., 2008). In keeping with these data, a recent large review found that sexual abuse victims experienced more sleep problems (e.g., nightmares, isolated sleep paralysis, poor sleep onset) than those without comparable trauma histories (Steine et al., 2012) and, as noted, isolated sleep paralysis is found in higher rates in those with a diagnosis of PTSD (e.g., Sharpless et al., 2010).

Intrusive Symptoms

The intrusive symptoms of PTSD may also be related to sleep paralysis. It is well known that trauma patients experience not only flashbacks, but (REM-based) nightmares as well. There are likely many different causes for these intrusive symptoms, but activation and stress lead to increases in adrenaline. In fact, certain treatments for PTSD nightmares (e.g., Prazosin), inhibit adrenaline. Regardless, the content of the traumas can indeed work themselves into REM sleep mentation (e.g., Hinton et al., 2005). These nightmares can result in frequent awakenings and nocturnal distress (Abrams et al., 2008), both of which are factors that may make sleep paralysis more likely to occur.

The content of sleep paralysis hallucinations can be considered to be *an expression* of the trauma or, put differently, could be another intrusive symptom (viz., similar to a trauma-related nightmare). This was clearly the case with Hinton's Cambodian refugees, and from a REM standpoint, it makes quite a bit of sense.

Peri-traumatic Tonic Immobility

Finally, there appears to be a parallel between certain traumatic reactions and the paralysis found in sleep paralysis. Namely, immobility is a common experience during trauma. Again, this is presumably intended to serve a defensive function when confronted with life-threatening events, and has a precedent in animal behavior as well (however, we should note that tonic immobility is different from *thanatosis* or the act of playing dead/"playing possum"). Peri-traumatic tonic immobility is also a predictor of subsequent PTSD (e.g., Rocha-Rego et al., 2009) and has also been linked with higher levels of PTSD severity and peri-traumatic dissociation (e.g., Abrams et al., 2008). It may be worth mentioning that a number of childhood sexual abuse victims report tonic immobility during assaults, and this appears to be an involuntary response to these horrific events (Abrams et al., 2008). So it appears that both the paralysis in sleep paralysis and the tonic immobility found during traumatic experiences may not be under conscious control, but this does not necessarily imply similar etiological mechanisms. Interestingly, patients with sleep paralysis will sometimes report being "scared stiff" by the hallucinations, and believe the paralysis to be a secondary *consequence* of the hallucinations. This appears to be unlikely given what we know of REM-based paralysis and the sequence of hallucinations (Cheyne & Girard, 2007). Regardless, the parallel between trauma-related immobility and sleep paralysis, especially in those with pre-existing trauma histories, is intriguing. One could speculate on whether or not the paralysis in sleep paralysis could be a re-experiencing symptom of PTSD, at least partially.

DISSOCIATION

One of the more common attendant consequences of trauma is dissociation, a psychological construct that encompasses a broad range of experiences (Michelson & Ray, 1996). These range from the common and fairly ubiquitous (e.g., "zoning out" while driving a long stretch of highway) to the rare and the unusual (e.g., entering a confused "fugue state" during which you wander aimlessly and have amnesia about your own identity). Dissociative phenomena are all characterized by a lack of normal integration of such things as emotion, identity, consciousness, and so on. This discontinuity of subjective experience appears to also bear a relationship to unusual sleep phenomena such as sleep paralysis.

Considering sleep experiences more broadly than just sleep paralysis, David Watson (2001) found that dissociation and unusual sleep experiences were indeed connected. He proposed that they, in effect, constituted a "cross-state continuity" such that these unusual perceptions/experiences occurred during both the day and the night. Similarly, van der Kloet, Giesbrecht, Lynn, Merckelbach, and de Zutter (2011) built upon these data and further linked dissociation and labile sleep–wake cycles with hypnagogic/hypnopompic hallucinations, waking dreams, and nightmares. Another study found associations between chronic nightmares and dissociative phenomena such as out-of-body experiences (Agargun et al., 2003).

Other research conducted by Richard McNally and Susan Clancy looked at dissociation and isolated sleep paralysis more specifically, but these involved relatively smaller and more homogenous samples. For instance, McNally and Clancy (2005b) assessed individuals who reported being the victims of alien abductions (and who also reported at least one episode of sleep paralysis) and a control group. They found that those with isolated sleep paralysis reported higher levels of dissociation than those without isolated sleep paralysis. In a second study looking at individuals who reported repressed, recovered, or continuous memories of sexual abuse when they were children (McNally & Clancy, 2005a), those with isolated sleep paralysis also had higher levels of dissociation and absorption (a subtype of dissociation). These latter results were subsequently replicated (Abrams et al., 2008; French, Santomauro, Hamilton, Fox, & Thalbourne, 2008).

PANIC DISORDER

Panic disorder has long been associated with sleep paralysis. Even from historical and mythological perspectives, the Greek god Pan was not only prone to causing "panic," but was also sometimes considered to be the prince of the incubi. Apart from these earlier connections, the 20th century saw some theorists speculating whether or not isolated sleep paralysis may in fact be an African American variant of panic disorder. Contemporary data do not appear to bear out this claim (e.g., Mellman, Aigbogun, Graves, Lawson, & Alim, 2008).

However, one can also see certain phenomenological parallels between panic attacks and sleep paralysis episodes. Both are associated with intense, acute fear. When considered from a cognitive therapy perspective, they also both involve a catastrophic misinterpretation of physical sensations that are not objectively dangerous in and of themselves (see appendix C). Finally, some patients experience *immobilization panic*, and this clearly encompasses both sets of symptoms, even if the etiology for them may be different. Cortese and Uhde (2006) found that 18% of patients with panic disorder are always immobilized, and that 71% have experienced immobilization at least once.

Several studies identified relationships between panic symptomatology and sleep paralysis, but data are somewhat mixed. For example, three studies found higher rates in those with panic (Neal-Barnett & Crowther, 2000; Ramsawh, Raffa, White, & Barlow, 2008; Yeung, Xu, & Chang, 2005), and two did not (Ohayon et al., 1999; Otto et al., 2006). Given discrepancies in sample compositions (e.g., all three studies that found a difference were fairly heterogeneous studies of minority samples) and sample sizes, the precise relationship between panic and sleep paralysis is somewhat cloudy. It may be the case that panic disorder, post-traumatic stress disorder, and many other anxious and depressive symptoms may be fairly non-specific predictors of sleep paralysis. In ending this chapter, we now discuss two non–disorder-specific constructs that may bear relevance for sleep paralysis and potentially cut across multiple disorder domains.

ANXIETY SENSITIVITY

Anxiety sensitivity refers to a fear of sensations and/or behaviors that are associated with anxiety. People who manifest high levels of anxiety sensitivity believe that their anxious symptoms will have harmful or even potentially deadly consequences. For example, someone with pronounced anxiety sensitivity would interpret acute tachycardia as indicative of an impending cardiac event, whereas an individual with low levels of this construct would experience it as puzzling, annoying or, at worst, mildly uncomfortable. There has been some debate over the extent to which anxiety sensitivity is distinct from global trait anxiety/neuroticism (e.g., Rapee, 1996), but it is a useful construct regardless. The most common measurement is the *Anxiety Sensitivity Index* (ASI, Peterson & Reiss, 1987), a brief self-report measure.

Two studies to date have assessed individuals with isolated sleep paralysis using the ASI (Ramsawh et al., 2008; Sharpless et al., 2010), and both found significant correlations. In their sample of African Americans, Ramsawh et al. found higher ASI scores in those with isolated sleep paralysis (M = 21.1) than those without (M = 16.7). This was consistent with patient reports, as nearly two-thirds of the sample reported a fear that something was wrong with their bodies during episodes, and half of these feared that they might experience permanent paralysis as a result. Needless to say, these reports are consistent with high levels of anxiety sensitivity, and it is clear to see how these bodily sensations—dramatic though they may be—can be perceived in a catastrophic fashion. A subsequent regression indicated that the ASI contributed unique variance to predicting the cognitive symptoms of isolated sleep paralysis. Ramsawh et al. further speculated that anxiety sensitivity may also be a vulnerability factor shared with panic disorder, another disorder strongly linked with anxiety sensitivity.

In their sample of patients who all endorsed panic attacks, Sharpless et al. (2010), found similar results. However, the point-biserial correlation between isolated sleep paralysis (0 = no, 1 = yes) and the total score for the ASI (r = .17) did not reach significance when using standard diagnostic criteria, but only when using fearful isolated sleep paralysis criteria (r = .35). Given the nature of the sample and the fact that anxiety sensitivity is already elevated in patients with panic attacks, it is perhaps not surprising that the correlation only reached significance when using these more specific and clinically focused criteria. In summary, available data indicate a relationship between isolated sleep paralysis and anxiety sensitivity, even in patients with already-heightened levels of anxiety sensitivity. Additional work using larger samples would help to better understand the exact nature of this relationship.

DEATH DISTRESS

As noted in chapter 5, death and sleep paralysis seem to have always had a close relationship. Fear of immanent death has been a constant accompaniment to sleep paralysis episodes. Several learned physicians speculated that sleep paralysis could either cause death on its own or serve as a first step toward more serious and ostensibly deadly conditions (e.g., Aurelianus, 1950). Macnish even speculated that preoccupation with somber topics (or being too prone to melancholic reflection in general) was associated with the occurrence of these episodes (Macnish, 1834).

Common to all of the preceding is death distress. Death distress is a complex construct with a lack of consensus about how best to operationalize it. Essentially, though, it is concerned with negative attitudes and emotions toward death and includes subcategories such as death anxiety, death depression, and death obsession (Abdel-Khalek, 2011–2012). There has been relatively little empirical work on this topic. Cheyne and Girard (2007) noted that death thoughts were generally common in sleep paralysis. Feeling as if one might die during sleep paralysis episodes is also common (Sharpless et al., 2010). As for death anxiety more specifically, Arikawa et al. found a significant, but relatively small (i.e., $r = .14$) correlation (Arikawa, Templer, Brown, Cannon, & Thomas-Dodson, 1999). More work on this topic is needed, as it is possible that death distress could be one of the many risk factors for chronic and severe sleep paralysis.

CONCLUSIONS

In conclusion, sleep paralysis/isolated sleep paralysis appears to be related to an array of psychopathological symptoms and syndromes in a fairly non-specific way. The available evidence does not point toward any one specific risk factor, but trauma and traumatic sequelae likely play large roles. There is also no way at present to determine whether or not general sleep disturbances or a more specific psychopathological contribution explains the relation between sleep paralysis and the mentioned symptoms/disorders. A good first step for future research may be to utilize large samples of well-assessed patients and look for "points of rarity" between isolated sleep paralysis and specific disorders and symptoms. Large samples would also allow for a better statistical modeling of the relative contributions of broad psychological constructs (e.g., anxiety sensitivity, dissociation, death distress) to the occurrence and intensity of sleep paralysis and associated symptoms.

REFERENCES

Abdel-Khalek, A. M. (2011–2012). The death distress construct and scale. *Omega*, 64(2), 171–184.
Abrams, M. P., Mulligan, A. D., Carleton, R. N., & Asmundson, G. J. G. (2008). Prevalence and correlates of sleep paralysis in adults reporting childhood sexual abuse. *Journal of Anxiety Disorders*, 22(8), 1535–1541. doi: 10.1016/j. janxdis.2008.03.007
Agargun, M. Y., Kara, H., Ozer, O. A., Selvi, Y., Kiran, U., & Ozer, B. (2003). Clinical importance of nightmare disorder in patients with dissociative disorders. *Psychiatry and Clinical Neurosciences*, 57(6), 575–579. doi: 1169 [pii]

American Psychiatric Association. (2013). *Diagnostic and statistical manual of mental disorders* (5th ed.). Arlington, VA: American Psychiatric Association.

Arikawa, H., Templer, D. I., Brown, R., Cannon, W. G., & Thomas-Dodson, S. (1999). The structure and correlates of kanshibari. *The Journal of Psychology, 133*(4), 369–375.

Aurelianus, C. (1950). In Drabkin I. E. (Ed.), *On acute diseases and chronic diseases* (I. E. Drabkin, trans.). Chicago: University of Chicago Press.

Barlow, D. H. (2002). *Anxiety and its disorders: The nature and treatment of anxiety and panic* (2nd ed.). New York: Guilford Press.

Bell, C. C., Shakoor, B., Thompson, B., Dew, D., Hughley, E., Mays, R., & Shorter-Gooden, K. (1984). Prevalence of isolated sleep paralysis in black subjects. *Journal of the National Medical Association, 76*(5), 501–508.

Casement, M. D., Arendt, J. T., & Armitage, R. (2009). Mood disorders. In T. L. Lee-Chiong (Ed.), *Sleep medicine essentials* (pp. 249–252). New York: Wiley-Blackwell.

Cheyne, J. A., & Girard, T. A. (2007). Paranoid delusions and threatening hallucinations: A prospective study of sleep paralysis experiences. *Consciousness and Cognition: An International Journal, 16*(4), 959–974.

Cortese, B. M., & Uhde, T. W. (2006). Immobilization panic. *American Journal of Psychiatry, 163*(8), 1453–1454.

Foa, E. B., Keane, T. M., Terence, M., Friedman, M. J., & Cohen, J. A. (2008). *Effective treatments for PTSD: Practice guidelines from the international society for traumatic stress studies* (2nd ed.). New York: Guilford Press.

French, C. C., Santomauro, J., Hamilton, V., Fox, R., & Thalbourne, M. A. (2008). Psychological aspects of the alien contact experience. *Cortex; a Journal Devoted to the Study of the Nervous System and Behavior, 44*(10), 1387–1395. doi: 10.1016/j.cortex.2007.11.011 [doi]

Hinton, D. E., Pich, V., Chhean, D., & Pollack, M. H. (2005). The ghost pushes you down: Sleep paralysis-type panic attacks in a Khmer refugee population. *Transcultural Psychiatry, 42*(1), 46–77. doi: 10.1177/1363461505050710

Hudson, J. I., Manoach, D. S., Sabo, A. N., & Sternbach, S. E. (1991). Recurrent nightmares in posttraumatic stress disorder: Association with sleep paralysis, hypnopompic hallucinations, and REM sleep. *Journal of Nervous and Mental Disease, 179*(9), 572–573. doi: 10.1097/00005053-199109000-00010

Krakow, B., Germain, A., Warner, T. D., Schrader, R., Koss, M., Hollifield, M., … Johnston, L. (2001). The relationship of sleep quality and posttraumatic stress to potential sleep disorders in sexual assault survivors with nightmares, insomnia, and PTSD. *Journal of Traumatic Stress, 14*(4), 647–665.

Macnish, R. (1834). *The philosophy of sleep* (1st American ed.). New York: D. Appleton and Company.

McNally, R. J., & Clancy, S. A. (2005a). Sleep paralysis in adults reporting repressed, recovered, or continuous memories of childhood sexual abuse. *Journal of Anxiety Disorders, 19*(5), 595–602. doi: 10.1016/j.janxdis.2004.05.003

McNally, R. J., & Clancy, S. A. (2005b). Sleep paralysis, sexual abuse, and space alien abduction. *Transcultural Psychiatry, 42*(1), 113–122. doi: 10.1177/1363461505050715

McNally, R. J., Lasko, N. B., Clancy, S. A., Macklin, M. L., Pitman, R. K., & Orr, S. P. (2004). Psychophysiological responding during script-driven imagery in people reporting abduction by space aliens. *Psychological Science, 15*(7), 493–497.

Mellman, T. A., Aigbogun, N., Graves, R. E., Lawson, W. B., & Alim, T. N. (2008). Sleep paralysis and trauma, psychiatric symptoms and disorders in an adult African American population attending primary medical care. *Depression and Anxiety*, *25*(5), 435–440. doi: 10.1002/da.20311

Michelson, L., & Ray, W. J. (1996). *Handbook of dissociation: Theoretical, empirical, and clinical perspectives*. New York: Plenum.

Neal-Barnett, A. M., & Crowther, J. H. (2000). To be female, middle class, anxious, and black. *Psychology of Women Quarterly*, *24*, 129–136.

Ohayon, M. M., & Shapiro, C. M. (2000). Sleep disturbances and psychiatric disorders associated with posttraumatic stress disorder in the general population. *Comprehensive Psychiatry*, *41*(6), 469–478.

Ohayon, M. M., Zulley, J., Guilleminault, C., & Smirne, S. (1999). Prevalence and pathologic associations of sleep paralysis in the general population. *Neurology*, *52*(6), 1194–1200.

Otto, M. W., Simon, N. M., Powers, M., Hinton, D., Zalta, A. K., & Pollack, M. H. (2006). Rates of isolated sleep paralysis in outpatients with anxiety disorders. *Journal of Anxiety Disorders*, *20*(5), 687–693. doi: 10.1016/j.janxdis.2005.07.002

Peterson, R. A., & Reiss, S. (1987). *Test mannual for the anxiety sensitivity index*. Orlando Park, IL: International Diagnostic Systems.

Plante, D. T., & Winkelman, J. W. (2008). Parasomnia: Psychiatric considerations. *Sleep Medicine Clinics*, *3*, 217–229.

Plante, D. T., & Winkelman, J. W. (2006). Parasomnias. *The Psychiatric Clinics of North America*, *29*(4), 969–987; abstract ix. doi: 10.1016/j.psc.2006.08.006

Ramsawh, H. J., Raffa, S. D., White, K. S., & Barlow, D. H. (2008). Risk factors for isolated sleep paralysis in an african american sample: A preliminary study. *Behavior Therapy*, *39*(4), 386–397. doi: 10.1016/j.beth.2007.11.002

Rapee, R. M. (1996). *Current controversies in the anxiety disorders*. New York: Guilford Press.

Rocha-Rego, V. I., Fiszman, A., Portugal, L. C., Pereira, M. G., de Oliveira, L., Mendlowicz, M. V.,...Volchan, E. (2009). Is tonic immobility the core sign among conventional peritraumatic signs and symptoms listed for PTSD? *Journal of Affective Disorders*, *115*(1), 269–273.

Sharpless, B. A., & Grom, J. L. (2013). Isolated sleep paralysis: Prevention, disruption, and hallucinations of others (poster). *American Psychological Association Annual Conference*, Honolulu, Hawaii.

Sharpless, B. A., & Barber, J. P. (2011). A clinician's guide to PTSD treatments for returning veterans. *Professional Psychology: Research and Practice*, *42*(1), 8–15. doi: 10.1037/a0022351

Sharpless, B. A., McCarthy, K. S., Chambless, D. L., Milrod, B. L., Khalsa, S. R., & Barber, J. P. (2010). Isolated sleep paralysis and fearful isolated sleep paralysis in outpatients with panic attacks. *Journal of Clinical Psychology*, *66*(12), 1292–1306. doi: 10.1002/jclp.20724

Steine, I. M., Harvey, A. G., Krystal, J. H., Milde, A. M., Gronli, J., Bjorvatn, B.,...Pallesen, S. (2012). Sleep disturbances in sexual abuse victims: A systematic review. *Sleep Medicine Reviews*, *16*(1), 15–25. doi: 10.1016/j.smrv.2011.01.006; 10.1016/j.smrv.2011.01.006

Szklo-Coxe, M., Young, T., Finn, L., & Mignot, E. (2007). Depression: Relationships to sleep paralysis and other sleep disturbances in a community sample. *Journal of Sleep Research*, *16*(3), 297–312. doi: 10.1111/j.1365-2869.2007.00600.x van der Kloet, D., Giesbrecht, T., Lynn, S. J., Merckelbach, H., & de Zutter, A. (2011). Sleep normalization and decrease in dissociative experiences: Evaluation in an inpatient sample. *Journal of Abnormal Psychology, 121*(1), 140–150.

Watson, D. (2001). Dissociations of the night: Individual differences in sleep-related experiences and their relation to dissociation and schizotypy. *Journal of Abnormal Psychology, 110*, 526–535.

Yeung, A., Xu, Y., & Chang, D. F. (2005). Prevalence and illness beliefs of sleep paralysis among Chinese psychiatric patients in China and the United States. *Transcultural Psychiatry, 42*(1), 135–143. doi: 10.1177/1363461505050725

CHAPTER 10

Theories on the Etiology of Sleep Paralysis

As with any strange phenomenon, there are many theories for the origin of sleep paralysis. The most colorful of these may be the various "folk" theories that arose outside of traditional Western scientific worldviews and frameworks. After discussing folk psychological theories, we next turn to psychological and medical theories for sleep paralysis. Finally, we summarize the most promising etiological hypotheses and contributory factors.

FOLK AND CULTURAL THEORIES ON THE ORIGIN OF SLEEP PARALYSIS

For the vast majority of human history people lacked a "scientific" and psychological understanding of sleep paralysis. Instead, readily available conceptual categories were used to make sense of these frightening nocturnal paroxysms and the hallucinations that accompany them. These conceptual categories, in many cases, involved powerful external forces. Thus, in the course of our review we were able to compile quite an extensive natural and supernatural bestiary of the agents "responsible" for attacks (see appendix A). These demons, vampires, aliens, and various animals were thought to either be real attackers or to in some way cause sleep paralysis episodes. As these beings are extensively discussed in chapter 3, we will not repeat them here, and instead focus upon other folk theories.

It is worth mentioning that "personalizing" (for lack of a better term) the cause of sleep paralysis engenders several consequences, some of which may actually be positive for a suffering individual, at least from a certain perspective. First, the act of locating the origin of the (hallucinated) attacks within a specific being, supernatural or otherwise, allows a person and/or community to discern some means of *stopping* the newly identified tormentor or, at least preventing future torment. This possibility likely reduced feelings of hopelessness/powerlessness that may otherwise manifest if no cause were able to be identified. The act of personification also means that various preventative rituals, personal supplications, or even defensive physical attacks can now be focused on the offending being (e.g., see chapter 14). And, given what we know about placebo/nocebo effects (Adler, 2011) as well as the general power of suggestion and expectancy, such "treatments" could be effective even if the mechanism of action is not quite the one that was intended by the individual.

Second, the act of personalizing the cause of sleep paralysis allows the sufferer to directly connect with available cultural narratives. Even if one is being malevolently "tormented" by demons or undergoing unwanted surgical procedures at the hands of gray extraterrestrials, there is ineluctably a sense of "specialness" that follows. After all, the demons/aliens are "choosing me to torment," and, even if this may be due to "bad" reasons (e.g., sinning), the sufferer is still special in his or her *degree of badness*.

Finally, victims of personified attacks may also benefit from denying that the cause/origin of the "attack" is an internal, endogenous process. Although there is often little personal control over whether or not one has an episode, the idea that one's own body and personal psychology generated these terrifying events may make the sufferer uncomfortable. It may be even more threatening to consider the possibility that certain behaviors (e.g., inconsistent sleep patterns, use of substances) may make episodes more likely. A less scary (and less ego dystonic) alternative may be to believe that external forces are to blame for these troubling experiences.

Although the majority of folk theories involve external agents, there are exceptions. Hinton's work with Cambodian refugees revealed that many of them attributed sleep paralysis to various culturally relevant bodily dysfunctions (Hinton, Pich, Chhean, & Pollack, 2005). For example, a weakening of the body or the presence of a "weak heart" may elicit the characteristic atonia or "freezing" (*keang*). When in these weakened states or experiencing what they term "low luck," it is believed that one is particularly vulnerable to attacks by ghosts and other supernatural beings. Thus, in the case of these refugees, a physical condition arising from *within the body* is believed to set the stage for subsequent supernatural impingements. An analogous belief in the West would be that the emotional turmoil of adolescence makes one vulnerable to demonic possession or torment by a poltergeist (Fodor, 1964).

Ness (1978) found two other etiological hypotheses when studying sufferers of the "old hag" phenomenon in rural Newfoundland. First, some believed that these attacks occurred as blood stagnates or is "standin' still" (p. 17). This sanguinary phenomenon was thought to occur as a result of sleeping in a supine position (which, coincidentally, is the most common sleeping position for sleep paralysis to occur). Other Newfoundlanders believed that excessive physical labor and pushing one's body too hard was the cause.

Specific types of *interpersonal interactions* were also thought to precede sleep paralysis. Newfoundlanders thought that an individual could be "hagged" if someone he or she knew bore ill will toward the person (Ness, 1978). This seems to be akin to a sort of "evil eye" or curse. In a sample of medical students, Penn and colleagues found that heated arguments were believed to precede sleep paralysis episodes, but additional details of the more precise causal link were not reported (Penn, Kripke, & Scharff, 1981).

Finally, several other folk hypotheses have been put forth. Some have claimed that the flu may be a proximal cause and others blamed sleep paralysis on viewing scary movies before bed (Penn et al., 1981). In our work with sufferers, we have also heard that eating the wrong kinds of foods (see also Macnish, 1834), having too much stress, repetitive nightmares, and general bad moods were to blame. Now that some of the folk theories have been discussed, we turn to more traditional psychological perspectives.

PSYCHOLOGICAL THEORIES ON THE ETIOLOGY OF SLEEP PARALYSIS

Personality Traits and Types

The search for a relationship between disorders and specific personality types/traits is an old one, and it remains a common approach in psychopathology research today. Some searches (e.g., schizoid traits in schizophrenia) have been more successful than others. The implicit and very intuitive assumption is that certain personality traits predispose individuals to manifest one or more specific types of symptoms given the right personal and environmental contingencies. For example, a man with relatively higher levels of pre-trauma dissociation may be more likely to experience dissociation during a traumatic event (i.e., peri-traumatic dissociation). Though not unanimous, studies to date have noted that individuals who experience peritraumatic dissociation are more likely to be diagnosed with subsequent post-traumatic stress disorder (as reviewed in Breh & Seidler, 2007). Similarly, higher levels of negative affect/trait neuroticism have been associated with the development of non-psychotic anxious and depressive disorders and higher overall levels of comorbidity (e.g., Andrews, 1996; Clark & Watson, 1999; Mineka, Watson, & Clark, 1998; Watson, Clark, & Care, 1988).

The search for a specific "personality type" associated with sleep paralysis has not been successful. Two studies by Ohaeiri failed to discriminate between those with and without sleep paralysis when using the *Eysenck Personality Questionnaire* and other measures (Ohaeri, Adelekan, Odejide, & Ikuesan, 1992; Ohaeri, Odejide, Ikuesan, & Adeyemi, 1989). Similarly, earlier researchers who studied individuals with sleep paralysis noted the presence of passive–aggressive personality traits (e.g., Firestone, 1985; Schneck, 1969), but we are not aware of subsequent research validating this hypothesis (e.g., Bell et al., 1984).

There have only been a small number of positive findings. Higher levels of paranoia, neuroticism, and masculinity–femininity were found in individuals with sleep paralysis when the *Minnesota Multiphasic Personality Inventory* was used (Fukuda, Inamatsu, Kuroiwa, & Miyasita, 1991). However, only the paranoia subscale remained significantly different when correcting for multiple analyses. The presence of unusual beliefs (possibly related to schizotypy) and higher levels of dissociation have been described as well (e.g., Ramsawh, Raffa, White, & Barlow, 2008; Watson, 2001). Replications of these findings would be helpful.

If we expand the research base to include individuals who have reported alien abductions, more robust findings emerge. However, even though certain researchers have established the presence of at least one sleep paralysis episode in their samples (e.g., McNally et al., 2004), others have not. Clancy summarized the empirical findings on "abductees" in general (Clancy, 2007). She found that individuals who reported abduction scenarios tended to be higher in "fantasy proneness," or the deep and vivid involvements in one's inner fantasy life. Some of these individuals may be described as having overactive imaginations, and their fantasies are typically rich in detail. Putative abductees also score higher on measures of schizotypy. Schizotypy has been considered to be a risk factor for schizophrenia, but is a dimensional construct found throughout the general population. Those high in this trait tend to have "odd" beliefs (e.g., magic, extrasensory perception, "new age" phenomena), are introverted and anhedonic, and may eschew certain social conventions (e.g., manner of dress). However, a consistent finding in reported abductees is that they do not demonstrate higher overall levels of psychopathology than non-abductees (Clancy, 2007).

Psychoanalytic Theories

"Psychoanalysis" is a broad term that encompasses a number of theories of human behavior. Derived from the original writings of Sigmund Freud, it is the earliest form of secular talk therapy and remains an important force in contemporary psychology and psychiatry (e.g., Barber, Muran, McCarthy, & Keefe, 2013; Sharpless & Barber, 2012). As with most theories that have been with us for more than 100 years, many original formulations have been modified, and there are now a number of subfields of psychodynamic psychotherapy. Given that many summaries of this literature are available elsewhere (e.g., Boswell et al., 2011; Mitchell & Black, 1995), we will not delve too deeply into this topic. However, it is important to note that psychodynamic therapies all adhere to a belief that psychopathology is situated in a developmental context, that unconscious meanings and wishes influence behavior, and that relief of distress and positive growth often arise from a better understanding of oneself and one's interactions with others (e.g., Sharpless & Barber, 2012). Symptoms are not "random" or merely the result of conditioning and happenstance, but more often than not possess a significant meaning that is not always known to the sufferer.

To the best of our knowledge, Freud himself never wrote about the Nightmare or any other synonymous term for sleep paralysis, but dreams were obviously a strong focus of his theoretical and clinical work. His most sustained discussions on dreams are found in the *Interpretation of Dreams* (Freud, 1953). Although the *Interpretation of Dreams* is a very early psychoanalytical work only published in 1900 (some argue it was the first truly psychoanalytical work), many of the core principles of psychoanalytical thought are already contained within it. These concepts were elaborated upon by subsequent theorists, but in the interests of historical primacy, we first briefly discuss relevant passages in the *Interpretation of Dreams*.

Freud provided some interesting speculations about dreams accompanied by an inability to move. They may therefore overlap somewhat with the phenomenon of sleep paralysis/isolated sleep paralysis. Freud saw this inability to move as indicative of a "conflict of will" such that a desire for some sort of action occurred in conjunction with a contrary desire to *inhibit* the action. As he noted:

> In other dreams, in which the 'not carrying out' of a movement occurs as a sensation and not simply as a situation, the sensation of the inhibition of movement gives a more forcible expression to the same contradiction—it expresses a volition which is opposed by a counter-volition. Thus the sensation of the inhibition of a movement represents a conflict of will. We shall learn later that the motor paralysis accompanying sleep is precisely one of the fundamental determinants of the psychical process during dreaming. (Freud, 1953, p. 337)

Thus, for Freud the paralysis in these dreams is the symptomatic expression of a conflict in much the same way that a neurotic or hysterical symptom represents the compromise of a conflict.

Similar constructs can be found in non-psychoanalytic theorizing as well. Some psychologists might term this an *approach-avoidance conflict* (Lewin, Adams, & Zener, 1935). A proto-existentialist thinker like Soren Kierkegaard would term this conflict a *sympathetic antipathy* or *antipathetic sympathy* or, when put into layman's terms, a desire for what one dreads, and a dread for what one desires (Kierkegaard, 1980; Sharpless, 2013). Regardless, the presence of some sort of intrapsychic conflict undergirds all of the extant psychoanalytic theorizing on sleep paralysis.

The type of conflict thought to be responsible for sleep paralysis's manifestation and particular symptomatology was a matter of some debate. As these are reviewed, the reader may be inclined to see (and/or dismiss) some of these theories as stereotypically Freudian, or even a *caricature* of Freud (i.e., focused exclusively on sex and aggression). Historical context is important to keep in mind, however, as all of these speculations were made during the heyday of classical psychoanalysis and ego psychology (i.e., 1930s to 1960s), and these were indeed some of the main theories that were available at that time. Unfortunately, we are not aware of modern analysts or psychodynamic thinkers who have formulated sleep paralysis in more contemporary terms.

Sexual Conflicts

A number of proposed theories for sleep paralysis involve sexual conflict. Jones (1949) wrote that, "the malady known as Nightmare is always an expression of intense mental conflict centering about some form of 'repressed' sexual desire" (p. 44). Perhaps not surprisingly, the majority of these conflicts were thought to be almost entirely unconscious. Liddon (1967) summarized several earlier theorists' work as conflicts over homosexual (Sperling), sadomasochistic (Sperling), or masturbatory (Deutsch) urges. These urges were thought to be repressed because they were anathema to waking conscious awareness and social norms. Freud himself noted in numerous works that both childhood sexuality and the presence of sexual and aggressive urges/acts outside of rigid societal confines were much broader than most proper Victorian ladies and gentlemen would admit (e.g., Freud's [1953] discussion of polymorphous perversity). However, the formation of complex societies required the renunciation of many of these urges (Freud, 2010). This resulted is a modicum of unavoidable human unhappiness, which served as a tithe of sorts for the safety that civil society provided those who followed prevailing social contracts. For Freud, this renunciation of certain sexual and aggressive drives did not equate to a removal of the drives, but more accurately indicated that the drives went underground, and operated without our awareness.

The speculation of some of Freud's adherents incorporated other constructs that were thought to be outside of the bounds of polite conversation. Specifically, both Schoenberger (as cited in Liddon, 1967) and Jones (1949) noted that sleep paralysis attacks may also result from witnessing the "primal scene" (i.e., parents having intercourse) in childhood. The subsequent experience of paralysis and fear during Nightmare/sleep paralysis attacks was thought to essentially be a recapitulation of these early traumatic experiences during which the child was confused, scared, and sexually overstimulated. When combined with Oedipal longings, the child who witnessed this scene was thought to have a desire to supplant one of the parents in this sexual encounter. This wish, combined with a prohibition of such behavior, led to the paralytic attack of Nightmare. From this viewpoint, the Nightmare was conceptualized to be a severe (and seemingly life-threatening) self-imposed punishment resulting from the child's unacceptable wishes. More generally, the intensity of the fear/dread during episodes was thought to be proportional to the degree to which the repressed wishes striving for discharge violated the individual's internalized sense of morality.

Interestingly, there may be some merit to sleep paralysis containing a sexual component, but not necessarily in the analysts' hypothesized manner described herein. As previous chapters demonstrate, sexuality, and especially *frightening* sexuality, has been intertwined with sleep paralysis since the earliest descriptions of the phenomenon. Episodes often involved sexual assault imagery along with various other types of personal violation. Data on the frequency of incubus and intruder experience are consistent with this as well (see chapter 6), and the thematic consistency across time and place make the connection appear to be less than coincidental.

Further, normal human variations in arousal are also likely contributors to the association between sleep paralysis and sexuality. Healthy men experience nocturnal penile tumescence (i.e., "morning wood") and healthy women experience nocturnal clitoral tumescence several times during the night. This is especially the case during rapid eye movement (REM) sleep (Chokroverty, 2010), which is the phase of sleep most associated with sleep paralysis symptomatology. Thus, individuals may be primed to experience sleep paralysis (and the attendant hallucinations) as possessing a strong sexual valence. Physical stimulation may also play a role. Variations in sleep position (with supine and prone being the most common and, coincidentally enough, the ones most often associated with sexual activity), nighttime attire, and bedding may all interact with normal sexual arousal patterns and serve to either intensify sexual arousal or lead to discomfort. Nocturnal emissions have been reported during sleep paralysis episodes (e.g., Jones, 1949; Roscher, 2007), as has genital soreness upon awakening (Ness, 1978).

Conflicts of Aggression

Aggressive conflicts have also been theorized to be a cause of sleep paralysis. Jones' incorporation of Oedipal themes into the Nightmare already contained a mixture of sex and aggression, but one can extrapolate more broadly from this very specific case. Following along similar lines as the sexual conflicts, the characteristic paralysis could be a defense against the expression of *any* frightening aggressive urges that are not consistent with a person's conscious morality. Similar to certain analysts' (e.g., see McWilliams, 2011) views that obsessive–compulsive defense mechanisms protect the individual from experiencing aggressive thoughts and behavioral urges, sleep paralysis could serve a parallel inhibitory function.

A More Contemporary Psychoanalytic Understanding of Sleep Paralysis

Psychodynamic principles and theories may still be useful for an understanding of sleep paralysis and its vicissitudes even if one does not necessarily adhere to early drive theory and classical Freudian meta-psychology.

One need only assume that the REM content of episodes is not merely random or happenstance, but has a particular "sense" (i.e., meaning) for the sufferer that is generated for a good reason (viz., the hallucinations derive from a meaningful conflict, wish, anxiety, or fear). We propose that, much like the content of any standard dreams, a great deal of clinical insight could be gained through the interpretation of these REM productions. Interestingly, the findings of contemporary neuroscientists do not disprove Freud's thoughts about dreams and their potential meaningfulness, and are actually quite consistent with his early writings (e.g., see Gabbard, 2010, for a brief review). For example, Sharpless and Grom's recent (2013) research into sleep paralysis hallucinations of others demonstrates that deceased loved ones often figure prominently in SP episodes. Though this finding is only one example, it indicates that, at least in certain cases, the REM content points toward emotionally salient topics or unfinished business. Anxiety about unfinished business (e.g., guilt and ambivalent feelings), when manifested in the bizarre imagery of dreams, may also help explain the pervasiveness of frightening figures and demonic entities during sleep paralysis (e.g., vampires, witches). Thus, a careful analysis of hallucinations may point toward important clinical material.

BIOLOGICAL AND MEDICAL THEORIES

Normal Sleep Neurophysiology

Sleep Stages

Before progressing to hypotheses more specific to sleep paralysis, we first describe sleep more broadly. From a behavioral standpoint, human sleep is a fairly simple state of existence, during which there is minimal motor activity as individuals lie down with their eyes closed. However, from an electrophysiological standpoint, sleep is highly complex, consisting of REM and non–rapid eye movement (NREM) sleep. Non–rapid eye movement sleep can be further subdivided into three stages. These stages are established through a process referred to as "polysomnography," the simultaneous monitoring and recording of multiple physiological measures during sleep. Three physiological measures define the main stages of sleep and wakefulness: Skeletal muscle tone, recorded through electromyogram (EMG); eye movements, recorded through an electro-oculogram (EOG); and brain activity, recorded through an electroencephalogram (EEG) (American Academy of Sleep Medicine, 2014). The EEG pattern of drowsy wakefulness consists of low-voltage rhythmic alpha activity (8 to

13 cycles per second [Hz]). In stage 1 of NREM sleep (N1), the low-voltage mixed frequency theta waves (4 to 8 Hz) replace the alpha rhythm of drowsy wakefulness. Slow asynchronous eye movements are seen on the EOG in the beginning of stage N1 sleep and disappear after a few minutes. Muscle activity is highest during wakefulness, but diminishes as sleep approaches. Arousal threshold is also lowest during N1 sleep.

During N2, sleep spindles (12- to 14-Hz synchronized EEG waveforms with duration of up to 1.5 seconds) and K complexes (negative, sharp wave immediately followed by a positive component standing out from the background EEG, with total duration greater than or equal to 0.5 seconds) appear. Sleep spindle waves arise as a result of synchronization of groups of thalamic neurons by a GABAergic thalamic spindle pacemaker. During N2 sleep the arousal threshold increases.

Stage N3 of NREM sleep is characterized by a synchronized high-amplitude (more than 75 mV) and slow (0.5 to 2 Hz) delta wave EEG pattern. Stage N3 is referred to as deep sleep, delta sleep, or slow-wave sleep (SWS). Slow-wave sleep is associated with an even higher arousal threshold.

During REM sleep the EEG is characterized by low voltage, and fast frequency activity (alpha or 8 to 13 Hz). Electroencephalogram waveforms are desynchronized, random-appearing wave patterns in contrast to the synchronized uniform wave pattern seen on the NREM sleep EEG. During REM sleep, the EMG displays muscle atonia and the EOG reveals presence of rapid eye movements. Rapid eye movement atonia is the product of active skeletal muscle paralysis.

Sleep typically begins with N1 and undergoes an orderly progression into NREM stages N2 and N3, followed by the first period of REM sleep after approximately 90 minutes. This first sleep cycle is followed by multiple, similar, cycles with NREM–REM cycles lasting approximately 90 to 120 minutes (Sinton & McCarley, 2004). Typically, stage N1 constitutes 2% to 5% of total sleep time, N2 45% to 55% of the total sleep time, and N3 constitutes 15% to 20% of the total sleep time. Stage 3 of NREM sleep predominates during the first third of the night. The first REM period is brief and occurs approximately 90 minutes after sleep onset, a period referred to as "REM latency." Rapid eye movement sleep episodes become longer as the night progresses, and the longest REM periods are found in the last third of the night. Non–rapid eye movement sleep accounts for 75% to 80%, and REM sleep accounts for 20% to 25% of total sleep time.

Most dreams occur during REM. In contrast to those experienced during NREM, REM sleep dreams are more complex, have more emotional valence, often have more bizarre content, and are easier to recall. Non–rapid eye movement sleep dreams are more logical and realistic, but more difficult to recall. As noted, REM activity is implicated in sleep paralysis.

Sleep Neurobiology

Arousal

Within the brain, the ascending arousal system consists of noradrenergic neurons of the ventrolateral medulla and locus coeruleus (LC), cholinergic neurons (ACh) in the pedunculopontine and laterodorsal tegmental (PPT/ LDT) nuclei, serotoninergic neurons (5-HT) in the dorsal raphe nucleus (DR), dopaminergic neurons (DA) of the ventral periaqueductal gray matter (vPAG) and histaminergic neurons (His) of the tuberomammillary nucleus (TMN). These systems produce cortical arousal via two pathways: a dorsal route through the thalamus and a ventral route through the hypothalamus and basal forebrain. The latter pathway receives contributions from the orexin and MCH neurons of the lateral hypothalamic area as well as from GABA-ergic or cholinergic neurons of the basal forebrain (Fuller, Gooley, & Saper, 2006).

Orexin neuropeptides are excitatory and also produce arousal. Orexin-A and -B (also known as hypocretin-1 and -2) are synthesized by neurons in the lateral and posterior hypothalamus and orexin neurons project widely and heavily innervate all the arousal regions described, with particularly dense innervation of the LC and TMN (Espana & Scammell, 2011). Orexins are thought to be important in maintaining wakefulness and the regulation of transitions between sleep and wakefulness. Their deficiency is thought to be the central pathophysiological event in narcolepsy; individuals with narcolepsy with cataplexy have a severe (85% to 95%) loss of the orexin neurons and very low CSF levels of orexin-A (American Academy of Sleep Medicine, 2005).

Non–rapid Eye Movement Sleep

The ventrolateral preoptic nucleus (VLPO) contains sleep-active cells that contain the inhibitory neurotransmitters GABA and galanin. The VLPO projects to all of the main components of the ascending arousal system. Inhibition of the arousal system by the VLPO during sleep is critical for the maintenance and consolidation of sleep.

Cholinergic neurons located in the LDT/PPT play a key role in the control of REM sleep and may help generate the cortical activation and atonia of REM sleep. Monoamines such as NE and 5-HT increase muscle tone by directly exciting motor neurons. Monoamines also inhibit REM sleep itself. During wakefulness, and to some degree during NREM sleep, the REM-active cholinergic neurons are inhibited by 5-HT, NE, and HA. This interaction between cholinergic and monoaminergic populations forms the foundation of the classic model explaining the alternation of NREM and REM sleep across the night (Espana & Scammell, 2011).

Etiological Hypotheses

Sleep paralysis likely represents the juxtaposition of the atonia and dream imagery (i.e., hallucinations) of REM sleep with wakefulness. As noted, the orderly progression of REM and NREM sleep stages on the one hand, and their demarcation from wakefulness on the other hand, is carefully orchestrated by a complex set of neurophysiological mechanisms. Breaches in this process can emerge at any point, and these favor the co-occurrence of REM sleep with wakefulness. The same ultimate pathway is also thought to be responsible for other phenomena commonly seen in narcolepsy, such as cataplexy and hypnagogic hallucinations. In the case of hypnagogic hallucinations, the cognitive and psychological components of REM (i.e., dreaming) predominate, whereas during both cataplexy and sleep paralysis, the motor inhibition that normally accompanies REM sleep predominates.

The temporal juxtaposition of REM sleep elements with wakefulness can, in turn, be mediated by a variety of primary causes. We note these briefly here, as many of these are discussed in detail elsewhere in this book.

(1) Sleep deprivation is a very likely factor. Rebound of REM sleep has been observed on the second night of recovery sleep following total sleep deprivation (Carskadon & Dement, 1979). Rebound of REM often manifests as a sleep-onset REM episode (SOREMP), a period of REM occurring much earlier than anticipated following sleep onset. When this coincides with partial wakefulness, it can be experienced as an episode of sleep paralysis or hypnogogic hallucination.

(2) Poor sleep quality induced by a multiplicity of potential factors can cause partial REM deprivation and promote the rebound

of REM sleep on subsequent nights and therefore induce sleep paralysis. Systematically interrupting NREM–REM cycles in normal subjects leads to subsequent episodes of sleep paralysis during SOREMPs (Takeuchi, Miyasita, Sasaki, & Inugami, 1992). In turn, multiple interruptions in sleep can be produced by a host of everyday life experiences, such as the consumption of (or withdrawal from) sleep-disruptive substances and medications, noise, temperature extremes, and stress and overwork and subsequent disruptive effects on sleep (Spanos, McNulty, DuBreuil, & Pires, 1995).

(3) Unusual sleep schedules are also contributing factors. Multiphasic sleep–wake schedules in one study were associated with an increase in rates of sleep paralysis (Takeuchi, Fukuda, Sasaki, Inugami, & Murphy, 2002). Such schedules can, in turn, result from jet lag and shift work (Snyder, 1983).

(4) Certain sleep positions (i.e., supine and prone) appear to make sleep paralysis more likely to occur, and higher body mass indexes may be related to characteristic feelings of breathlessness and suffocation (e.g., Sharpless et al., 2010)

(5) In the context of medical and neurological conditions, sleep paralysis can result from a variety of mechanisms, as noted in chapter 8.

 (a) Hypocretin deficiency appears to be the primary etiological factor in narcolepsy which, in turn, leads to the dissociation of the various elements of REM sleep (i.e., muscle paralysis and vivid dreaming occurring in the context of continuous sleep). Sleep cannot be fully maintained during REM periods, leading to the temporal juxtaposition of partial wakefulness with REM-related muscle paralysis.

 (b) Rapid eye movement sleep fragmentation appears to play a central role in the genesis of sleep paralysis in obstructive sleep apnea. Rapid eye movement sleep in patients with OSA is typically associated with an increased frequency of obstructive events that are often prolonged and accompanied with severe oxyhemoglobin desaturation. The arousal response is responsible for the termination of these events. Arousal, in the context of REM sleep, is thought to produce sleep paralysis. Alternatively, OSA treatment with continuous positive airway pressure (CPAP) may produce a REM rebound, resulting in the experience of vivid dreaming and sleep paralysis. Rapid eye movement sleep fragmentation is also thought to play an etiological role in Wilson's disease and the consumption of various substances and medications, such as alcohol, cholinomimetic medications, and withdrawal from anticholinergic medications.

(c) Dysfunctions in the tasks of the reticular formation caused by any number of factors could also lead to the characteristic inhibition of motor neurons (see chapter 6).

(6) As noted earlier in this chapter, psychological factors can enhance the vulnerability for sleep paralysis, especially those promoting vigilance levels during sleep disruption (Takeuchi et al., 2002). Daytime imaginativeness, as evidenced by standardized questionnaires, and vividness of night-time imagery, as measured by self-reported frequencies of nightmares and dream vividness, were the personality factors most predictive of sleep paralysis in a large sample of college students (Spanos et al., 1995).

(7) The mechanisms underlying the occurrence of sleep paralysis in psychiatric disorders are likely varied, and reviewed in greater detail in chapter 9. However, these include the following:

(a) Comorbidity of non-psychotic mood and anxiety disorders in general appears to be related to the experience of isolated sleep paralysis (e.g., Sharpless et al., 2010; Plante & Winkelman, 2006).

(b) A history of trauma likely plays a role. Not only do sleep paralysis episodes occur at higher levels in those with PTSD (possibly due to more general daytime/nighttime hyperarousal and hypervigilance), but sleep paralysis can itself be experienced as quite traumatic (see chapter 9).

(c) High levels of anxiety sensitivity are associated with sleep paralysis (Ramsawh, Raffa, White, & Barlow, 2008; Sharpless et al., 2010). It is currently unclear if this is a general risk factor for occurrence or is more associated with the experienced *severity* of sleep paralysis episodes (e.g., catastrophic misappraisal led to more discomfort during episodes). General levels of negative affect may play a role.

(d) Schizotypy and capacities for dissociation may also play important roles in certain specific manifestations of sleep paralysis (see chapter 6).

(e) Death distress (e.g., Arikawa, Templer, Brown, Cannon, & Thomas-Dodson, 1999) may also be a contributing factor, but more work is needed here.

(f) Hallucinatory experiences during sleep may play a role. The entire episode of sleep paralysis may represent a distorted perception in the context of schizophrenia or other psychotic conditions. However, we are not aware of elevated rates of sleep paralysis in psychotic disorders.

(g) The presence of paranormal/anomalous belief may a cause or consequence of sleep paralysis episodes (Ramsawh et al., 2008).

(h) Cognitive factors (such as those reviewed in appendix D) are likely involved in the genesis and maintenance of chronic and severe cases of recurrent isolated sleep paralysis.

(i) Cultural factors and readily available societal narratives may set the stage for experiencing particular hallucinations as well as the subsequent impact of the hallucinations.

CONCLUSIONS

In conclusion, we have presented a number of etiological hypotheses for sleep paralysis episodes. Some of these appear to be very reasonable and promising, whereas others may be perceived as mere intellectual curiosities (or more appropriately relegated to cultural anthropology). Regardless, the multitude of available explanatory mechanisms implies the important grip that sleep paralysis has held on the human imagination. Subsequent empirical findings will hopefully yield more encompassing and integrated theories of etiology.

REFERENCES

Adler, S. (2011). *Sleep paralysis: Night-mares, nocebos, and the mind-body connection.* Newark, NJ: Rutgers University Press.

American Academy of Sleep Medicine. (2005). *International classification of sleep disorders: Diagnostic & coding manual* (2nd ed.). Darien, IL: American Academy of Sleep Medicine.

American Academy of Sleep Medicine. (2014). *The AASM manual for the scoring of sleep and associated events: Rules, terminology and technical specifications, version 2.1.* Darien, IL: American Academy of Sleep Medicine.

Andrews, G. (1996). Comorbidity and the general neurotic syndrome. *British Journal of Psychiatry, 168*(Suppl 30), 76–84.

Arikawa, H., Templer, D. I., Brown, R., Cannon, W. G., & Thomas-Dodson, S. (1999). The structure and correlates of kanshibari. *The Journal of Psychology, 133*(4), 369–375.

Barber, J. P., Muran, J. C., McCarthy, K. S., & Keefe, R. J. (2013). Research on psychodynamic therapies. In M. J. Lamber (Ed.), *Bergin and Garfield's handbook of psychotherapy and behavior change* (6th ed., pp. 443–494). New York: Wiley.

Bell, C. C., Shakoor, B., Thompson, B., Dew, D., Hughley, E., Mays, R., & Shorter-Gooden, K. (1984). Prevalence of isolated sleep paralysis in black subjects. *Journal of the National Medical Association, 76*(5), 501–508.

Boswell, J. F., Sharpless, B. A., Greenberg, L. S., Heatherington, L., Huppert, J. D., Barber, J. P.,…Castonguay, L. G. (2011). *Schools of psychotherapy and the beginnings of a scientific approach.* In D. H. Barlow's (Ed.), *The Oxford Handbook of Clinical Psychology* (pp. 98–127). New York: Oxford University Press.

Breh, D. C., & Seidler, G. H. (2007). Is peritraumatic dissociation a risk factor for PTSD? *Journal of Trauma & Dissociation: The Official Journal of the International Society for the Study of Dissociation (ISSD)*, 8(1), 53–69. doi: 10.1300/J229v08n01_04 [doi]

Carskadon, M. A., & Dement, W. C. (1979). Effects of total sleep loss on sleep tendency. *Perceptual and Motor Skills*, 48(2), 495–506. doi: 10.2466/pms.1979.48.2.495 [doi]

Chokroverty, S. (2010). Overview of sleep & sleep disorders. *The Indian Journal of Medical Research*, 131, 126–140.

Clancy, S. A. (2007). *Abducted: How people come to believe they were kidnapped by aliens.* Cambridge, MA: First Harvard University Press.

Clark, L. A., & Watson, D. (1999). Temperament: A new paradigm for trait psychology. *Handbook of personality: Theory and research* (pp. 399–423). New York: Guilford Press.

Espana, R. A., & Scammell, T. E. (2011). Sleep neurobiology from a clinical perspective. *Sleep*, 34(7), 845–858. doi: 10.5665/SLEEP.1112 [doi]

Firestone, M. (1985). The "old hag": Sleep paralysis in newfoundland. *Journal of Psychoanalytic Anthropology*, 8(1), 47–66.

Fodor, N. (1964). *Between two worlds.* West Nyack, NY: Parker Publishing.

Freud, S. (1953). Three essays on the theory of sexuality. In J. Strachey (Ed.), Volume VII (J. Strachey, trans.). *Standard edition of the complete psychological works of Sigmund Freud* (pp. 125–243). London: Hogarth Press.

Freud, S. (2010). *Civilization and its discontents* [Unbehagen in der Kultur.] (J. Strachey, trans.). New York: Norton.

Fukuda, K., Inamatsu, N., Kuroiwa, M., & Miyasita, A. (1991). Personality of healthy young adults with sleep paralysis. *Perceptual and Motor Skills*, 73(3, Pt 1), 955–962. doi: 10.2466/PMS.73.7.955-962

Fuller, P. M., Gooley, J. J., & Saper, C. B. (2006). Neurobiology of the sleep-wake cycle: Sleep architecture, circadian regulation, and regulatory feedback. *Journal of Biological Rhythms*, 21(6), 482–493. doi: 21/6/482 [pii]

Gabbard, G. O. (2010). *Long-term psychodynamic psychotherapy.* Arlington, VA: American Psychiatric Publishing.

Hinton, D. E., Pich, V., Chhean, D., & Pollack, M. H. (2005). The ghost pushes you down: Sleep paralysis-type panic attacks in a Khmer refugee population. *Transcultural Psychiatry*, 42(1), 46–77. doi: 10.1177/1363461505050710

Jones, E. (1949). *On the nightmare* (2nd ed.). London: Hogarth Press and the Institute of Psycho-analysis.

Kierkegaard, S. A. (1980). In Hong H., & Hong E. (Eds.). *The concept of anxiety: A simple psychological orienting deliberation on the dogmatic issue of hereditary sin* (H. Hong, E. Hong, trans.). Princeton, NJ: Princeton University Press.

Lewin, K., Adams, D. K., & Zener, K. E. (1935). *A dynamic theory of personality; selected papers* (1st ed.). New York: McGraw-Hill.

Liddon, S. C. (1967). Sleep paralysis and hynagogic hallucinations: Their relationship to the nightmare. *Archives of General Psychiatry*, 17(1), 88–96. doi: 10.1001/archpsyc.1967.01730250090013

Macnish, R. (1834). *The philosophy of sleep* (1st American ed.). New York: D. Appleton and Company.

McNally, R. J., Lasko, N. B., Clancy, S. A., Macklin, M. L., Pitman, R. K., & Orr, S. P. (2004). Psychophysiological responding during script-driven imagery in people reporting abduction by space aliens. *Psychological Science*, 15(7), 493–497.

McWilliams, N. (2011). *Psychoanalytic diagnosis* (2nd ed.). New York: Guilford Press.

Mineka, S., Watson, D., & Clark, L. A. (1998). Comorbidity of mood and anxiety disorders. *Annual Review of Psychology, 49*, 377–412.

Mitchell, S. A., & Black, M. J. (1995). *Freud and beyond: A history of modern psychoanalytic thought*. New York: Basic Books.

Ness, R. C. (1978). The old hag phenomenon as sleep paralysis: A biocultural interpretation. *Cultural, Medicine and Psychiatry, 2*, 15.

Ohaeri, J. U., Adelekan, M. F., Odejide, A. O., & Ikuesan, B. A. (1992). The pattern of isolated sleep paralysis among Nigerian nursing students. *Journal of the National Medical Association, 84*(1), 67–70.

Ohaeri, J. U., Odejide, O. A., Ikuesan, B. A., & Adeyemi, J. D. (1989). The pattern of isolated sleep paralysis among Nigerian medical students. *Journal of the National Medical Association, 81*(7), 805–808.

Penn, N. E., Kripke, D. F., & Scharff, J. (1981). Sleep-paralysis among medical students. *Journal of Psychology: Interdisciplinary and Applied, 107*(2), 247–252. doi: 10.1080/00223980.1981.9915230

Plante, D. T., & Winkelman, J. W. (2006). Parasomnias. *The Psychiatric Clinics of North America, 29*(4), 969–987; abstract ix. doi: 10.1016/j.psc.2006.08.006

Ramsawh, H. J., Raffa, S. D., White, K. S., & Barlow, D. H. (2008). Risk factors for isolated sleep paralysis in an African American sample: A preliminary study. *Behavior Therapy, 39*(4), 386–397. doi: 10.1016/j.beth.2007.11.002

Roscher, W. H. (2007). *Ephialtes: A pathological-mythological treatise on the nightmare in classical antiquity*. [Ephialtes] (A. V. O'Brien, trans., rev ed., pp. 96–159). Putnam, CT: Spring.

Schneck, J. M. (1969). Henry Fuseli, nightmare, and sleep paralysis. *JAMA: Journal of the American Medical Association, 207*(4), 725–726. doi: 10.1001/jama.207.4.725

Sharpless, B. A. (2013). Kierkegaard's conception of psychology. *Journal of Theoretical and Philosophical Psychology, 33*(2), 90–106. doi: 10.1037/a0029099

Sharpless, B. A., & Barber, J. P. (2012). Corrective emotional experiences from a psychoadynamic perspective. In C. Hill and L. G. Castonguay's (Eds.) *Transformation in psychotherapy: Corrective experiences across cognitive behavioral, humanistic, and psychodynamic approaches* (pp. 31–49), Washington, DC: APA Press.

Sharpless, B. A., & Grom, J. L. (2013). Isolated sleep paralysis: Prevention, disruption, and hallucinations of others (poster). *American Psychological Association Annual Conference*, Honolulu, Hawaii.

Sharpless, B. A., McCarthy, K. S., Chambless, D. L., Milrod, B. L., Khalsa, S. R., & Barber, J. P. (2010). Isolated sleep paralysis and fearful isolated sleep paralysis in outpatients with panic attacks. *Journal of Clinical Psychology, 66*(12), 1292–1306. doi: 10.1002/jclp.20724

Sinton, C. M., & McCarley, R. W. (2004). Neurophysiological mechanisms of sleep and wakefulness: A question of balance. *Seminars in Neurology, 24*(3), 211–223. doi: 10.1055/s-2004-835067 [doi]

Snyder, S. (1983). Isolated sleep paralysis after rapid time zone change ("jet lag") syndrome. *Chronobiologia, 10*(4), 377–379.

Spanos, N. P., McNulty, S. A., DuBreuil, S. C., & Pires, M. (1995). The frequency and correlates of sleep paralysis in a university sample. *Journal of Research in Personality, 29*(3), 285–305. doi: 10.1006/jrpe.1995.1017

Takeuchi, T., Fukuda, K., Sasaki, Y., Inugami, M., & Murphy, T. I. (2002). Factors related to the occurrence of isolated sleep paralysis elicited during a multi-phasic sleep-wake schedule. *Sleep: Journal of Sleep and Sleep Disorders Research, 25*(1), 89–96.

Takeuchi, T., Miyasita, A., Sasaki, Y., & Inugami, M. (1992). Isolated sleep paralysis elicited by sleep interruption. *Sleep: Journal of Sleep Research & Sleep Medicine, 15*(3), 217–225.

Watson, D. (2001). Dissociations of the night: Individual differences in sleep-related experiences and their relation to dissociation and schizotypy. *Journal of Abnormal Psychology, 110,* 526–535.

Watson, D., Clark, L. A., & Care, C. (1988). Positive and negative affectivity and their relation to anxiety and depressive disorders. *Journal of Abnormal Psychology, 97,* 346–353.

CHAPTER 11

Diagnostic Criteria, Diagnostic Issues, and Possible Subtypes of Sleep Paralysis

For most of human history there has been some conception of what we would now term "disorders" or "disorderedness." However, the laser-like focus on specific symptoms and syndromes (as opposed to more global considerations of health and sickness), as well as the various attempts to clearly operationalize the "boundaries" between certain conditions and others, are both relatively modern preoccupations. In the realm of psychopathology, these foci can clearly be seen in the linear increase in the number of possible disorders found in the various editions of the *Diagnostic and Statistical Manual of Mental Disorders* and the *International Classification of Diseases*. For example, DSM-I (American Psychiatric Association, 1952) contained slightly over 100 diagnoses, whereas the more recently published DSM-5 (American Psychiatric Association, 2013) contains over 300. It is an open empirical and conceptual question as to whether this increase in the number of disorders represents conceptual progress or is indicative of a more fundamental problem in how we view psychopathology (for an example of the latter view, the interested reader is directed to Beutler & Malik, 2002).

DIAGNOSTIC CRITERIA FOR "THE NIGHTMARE"

There was no shortage of early medical descriptions of the Nightmare/sleep paralysis and speculation upon its etiology (e.g., chapter 5). Sleep paralysis was often viewed in the broader context of overall health, and was thought to be connected to factors such as diet and overall activity level. However, in reviewing these early works, the descriptions consisted primarily of clinical exemplars as opposed to the more clearly codified diagnostic criteria with which contemporary readers would be familiar. It appears possible to extract themes from these descriptions. Sharpless (2014) identified five themes that appear to be consistent across descriptions. These include 1) paralysis of the entire body except for the eyes, 2) conscious awareness of one's surroundings, 3) a feeling of weight on the chest, 4) an inability to cry out for help, and 5) extreme terror. However, these were never explicitly codified in the early writings, and were arrived at retrospectively.

In our review of the historical literature, Ernest Jones (1949) may be the first mental health professional to propose diagnostic criteria for any form of sleep paralysis. As shown in Box 11.1, he outlined a tripartite description for the *Nightmare*, or what we would today term the "incubus" subtype of sleep paralysis (Cheyne, Rueffer, & Newby-Clark, 1999).

Jones' criteria are notable in several respects. His use of the term "dread" adroitly captures the threat of non-being found in many sleep paralysis episodes. Were one to utilize this in contemporary studies, however, it would likely only allow for the most severe episodes to meet diagnostic criteria, being that it sets a higher threshold than "clinically significant fear." The second criterion is one of the main phenomenological experiences of the "incubus" subtype of sleep paralysis (Cheyne et al., 1999). Finally, the third criterion's use of the word "conviction" is interesting, as it appears to imply that the paralysis is not real in some fashion. This is in keeping with his psychoanalytic (i.e., conflict-driven) understanding of the Nightmare. Specifically, the intrapsychic conflicts thought to be at the heart of the experience of sleep paralysis are no more real than an episode of hysterical blindness or glove paralysis, and these symptoms were presumed to have

---

Box 11.1: ERNEST JONES'S CARDINAL FEATURES OF THE *NIGHTMARE*

1. Agonizing dread
2. Sense of oppression or weight at the chest which alarmingly interferes with respiration
3. Conviction of helpless paralysis

Notes: From Jones, E. (1949). On the nightmare (2nd Impression ed.). London: Hogarth Press and the Institute of Psycho-analysis.

---

no solid biological basis. This does not actually appear to be the case with sleep paralysis, however, as it involves fairly well-understood biological substrates involving rapid eye movement (REM) pathology.

CURRENT DIAGNOSTIC CRITERIA FOR SLEEP PARALYSIS

The diagnostic criteria for sleep paralysis have evolved throughout the various editions of the *International Classification of Sleep Disorders* (ICSD) and in response to empirical research findings. We will follow a temporal sequence of review. Isolated sleep paralysis was first recognized as a codable diagnosis in the revised edition of the ICSD (ICSD-R; American Academy of Sleep Medicine, 2001), but could be reached with the experience of only one episode. Severity qualifiers could be added (i.e., mild, moderate, and severe), but they were based upon episode *frequency* as opposed to other clinical considerations (e.g., distress and impairment). Duration criteria ranged from acute (one month or less) to chronic (six months or more).

The second edition of the ICSD (ICSD-2, American Academy of Sleep Medicine, 2005) made several significant modifications to the diagnostic criteria. First, it explicitly recognized that sleep paralysis needed to be "isolated" from other conditions such as narcolepsy and substance use and dubbed this condition "recurrent isolated sleep paralysis." Explicit in this new phrase was also the fact that multiple episodes were necessary for diagnosis, but it neither specified the minimum number nor included the "severity" criteria from ICSD-R. As shown in Box 11.2, ICSD-2 criteria also recognized the relative brevity of episode duration and the fact

---

Box 11.2: DIAGNOSTIC CRITERIA FOR VARIOUS
DEFINITIONS OF ISOLATED SLEEP PARALYSIS

ICSD-2 RECURRENT ISOLATED SLEEP PARALYSIS CRITERIA[1]
A. The patient complains of an inability to move the trunk and all limbs at sleep onset or on waking from sleep.
B. Each episode lasts seconds to a few minutes.
C. The sleep disturbance is not better explained by another sleep disorder (particularly narcolepsy), a medical or neurological disorder, mental disorder, medication use, or substance use disorder.

Note: Hallucinatory experiences may be present but are not essential to the diagnosis. Polysomnography, if performed, reveals the event to occur in a dissociated state with elements of REM sleep and wakefulness.

A. A recurrent inability to move the trunk and all of the limbs at sleep onset or upon awakening from sleep.

B. Each episode lasts seconds to a few minutes.

C. The episodes cause clinically significant distress including bedtime anxiety or fear of sleep.

D. The disturbance is not better explained by another sleep disorder (especially narcolepsy), mental disorder, medical condition, medication, or substance use.

FEARFUL ISOLATED SLEEP PARALYSIS EPISODE[3]

A. A period of time at sleep onset or upon awakening during which voluntary movement is not possible, yet some degree of awareness is present.

B. The episode(s) of sleep paralysis is/are accompanied by significant fear, anxiety, or dread that may be associated with either the paralysis itself or the presence of hypnogogic (sleep onset) or hypnopompic (sleep offset) hallucinations.

C. The episode(s) of sleep paralysis is/are not better accounted for by the direct physiological effects of a substance (e.g., alcohol, drug of abuse, or medications).

D. Isolated sleep paralysis is not better accounted for by a general medical condition (e.g., narcolepsy, seizure disorder, hypokalemia) or other psychiatric diagnosis (e.g., sleep terror disorder).

RECURRENT FEARFUL ISOLATED SLEEP PARALYSIS[3]

A. At least two episodes of fearful Isolated Sleep Paralysis (as defined above) taking place in the past 6 months

B. The episodes of sleep paralysis are accompanied by clinically significant distress and/or impairment.

C. The episodes of sleep paralysis are not better accounted for by the direct physiological effects of a substance (e.g., alcohol, drug of abuse, or medications).

D. The sleep paralysis episodes are not better accounted for by a general medical condition (e.g., narcolepsy, seizure disorder, hypokalemia) or other psychiatric diagnosis (e.g., sleep terror disorder).

Notes: Adapted from Sharpless (in press) and reprinted with permission from Elsevier.
[1] *= (American Academy of Sleep Medicine, 2005);* [2] *= (American Academy of Sleep Medicine, 2014);* [3] *= (Sharpless et al., 2010).*

that hallucinations may be present, but were not considered essential for diagnosis. Interestingly, ICSD-2 followed ICSD-R in not including clinical impact or episode distress in the criteria. Thus, a patient experiencing predominantly pleasant episodes of sleep paralysis (e.g., blissful vestibular-motor hallucinations of floating) could still presumably reach diagnostic threshold.

Sharpless et al. (2010) found the existing ICSD criteria somewhat limited for exploring the *clinical impact* of isolated sleep paralysis on patients, and proposed several significant changes. In general, they utilized panic disorder as an analogous condition to isolated sleep paralysis, and generated separate criteria for both individual episodes and for a "disorder" of recurrent isolated sleep paralysis (see Box 11.2). Regarding episodes, the presence of clinically significant fear was made a requirement in order to better differentiate scary from non-scary experiences (i.e., what they termed "fearful isolated sleep paralysis"). Thus, they moved a bit closer to Jones' early Nightmare formulations by emphasizing the aversive nature of the episodes. In terms of isolated sleep paralysis as a "disorder" or "diagnostic entity" they proposed criteria for *recurrent fearful isolated sleep paralysis*. This included the presence of distressing episodes (i.e., fearful ISP episodes), minimal episode frequencies over a particular period of time, and a requirement for clinically significant distress and/or impairment *as a result* of the episodes. The use of fearful isolated sleep paralysis criteria increased specificity when conducting basic psychopathology research (Sharpless et al., 2010).

Most recently, the third edition of ICSD was released (ICSD-3; American Academy of Sleep Medicine, 2014). As shown in Box 11.2, all diagnostic criteria from ICSD-2 were retained in ICSD-3, but a requirement for the presence of clinically significant distress was added. However, no requirements for impairment as a result of episodes or minimal episode thresholds were included.

In closing, much work remains to be done on the most appropriate diagnostic criteria for isolated sleep paralysis. Empirically-established thresholds are not yet available to better differentiate isolated sleep paralysis as a "disorder" versus isolated sleep paralysis as merely an unusual experience. Clearly, a not-insignificant proportion of people experience problems as a result of these episodes (e.g., Sharpless et al., 2010; Sharpless & Grom, in press). We recommend that future diagnostic systems emphasize the clinically significant impacts of isolated sleep paralysis, not only *during* episodes, but also as a result of these episodes.

REFERENCES

American Academy of Sleep Medicine. (2001). *International classification of sleep disorders*. Darien, IL: American Academy of Sleep Medicine.

American Academy of Sleep Medicine. (2005). *International classification of sleep disorders: Diagnostic & coding manual* (2nd ed.). Darien, IL: American Academy of Sleep Medicine.

American Academy of Sleep Medicine. (2014). *International classification of sleep disorders: Diagnostic and coding manual* (3rd ed.). Darien, IL: American Academy of Sleep Medicine.

American Psychiatric Association. (1952). *Diagnostic and statistical manual of mental disorders* (1st ed.). Washington, DC: American Psychiatric Association.

American Psychiatric Association. (2013). *Diagnostic and statistical manual of mental disorders: DSM-V* (5th ed.). Arlington, VA: American Psychiatric Association.

Beutler, L. E., & Malik, M. L. (2002). *Rethinking the DSM: A psychological perspective.* Washington, DC: APA Press.

Cheyne, J. A., Rueffer, S. D., & Newby-Clark, I. R. (1999). Hypnagogic and hypnopompic hallucinations during sleep paralysis: Neurological and cultural construction of the night-mare. *Consciousness and Cognition: An International Journal, 8*(3), 319–337. doi: 10.1006/ccog.1999.0404

Jones, E. (1949). *On the nightmare* (2nd Impression ed.). London: Hogarth Press and the Institute of Psycho-analysis.

Sharpless, B. A. (2014). Changing conceptions of the nightmare in medicine. *Hektoen International: A Journal of Medical Humanities (Moments in History Section).*

Sharpless, B. A., & Grom, J. L. (in press). Isolated sleep paralysis: Fear, prevention, and disruption. *Behavioral Sleep Medicine.*

Sharpless, B. A., McCarthy, K. S., Chambless, D. L., Milrod, B. L., Khalsa, S. R., & Barber, J. P. (2010). Isolated sleep paralysis and fearful isolated sleep paralysis in outpatients with panic attacks. *Journal of Clinical Psychology, 66*(12), 1292–1306. doi: 10.1002/jclp.20724

CHAPTER 12

Review of Measures Used to Assess Sleep Paralysis

Although the empirical study of sleep paralysis is still in its relative infancy, a number of assessment instruments exist. Many of these measures appear to have been created for very study-specific research purposes and were constructed in relative isolation from other instruments. Thus, there exists quite a deal of heterogeneity in terms of measure length, format, content, potential clinical utility, and reported psychometric properties.

We are not aware of any available resources that summarize these many measures. As a result, researchers and clinicians who are interested in selecting a sleep paralysis assessment instrument are faced with a complex task that may result in a large review of literature and/or a close reading of method sections. We therefore synthesize the literature below, separately reviewing self-report questionnaires and clinical interviews.

SELF-REPORT MEASURES

The vast majority of sleep paralysis measures are in a self-report format (Sharpless & Barber, 2011). Self-reports are obviously cheaper to administer than interviews, as they require little, if any, individualized face-to-face contact. Their use also eliminates requirements for trained assessors/diagnosticians and the abundant time commitments usually required to reach appropriate levels of reliability. Thus, self-reports are very well suited for mass screenings or any other large research protocols. Many could be placed online with computerized scoring and data entry. Thus, they are obviously very attractive for any number of purposes.

As shown in Table 12.1, researchers and clinicians have a number of choices available for self-report instruments. These range from extremely brief (i.e., one or two-item) screening measures to much lengthier surveys with multiple response formats (e.g., dichotomous, dimensional, open-ended questions). It may also be useful to note that self-report questionnaires are currently available in seven languages (i.e., Arabic, English, French, German, Japanese, Mandarin, and Spanish). Measure choice should obviously be dictated by the specific requirements of the study/clinical task, but we will provide some general guidance based upon our review.

If one requires an extremely brief screening instrument (e.g., a large epidemiological study not focused on sleep paralysis), the content found in the *Munich Parasomnia Screening* possesses the most psychometric evidence in favor of its use (Fulda et al., 2008). This item asks individuals to rate if (and how often) they experience: "Waking with a paralysis of the whole body (not including eyes and breathing) that can last for several seconds."

For those looking for a more in-depth assessment of sleep paralysis that remains relatively brief, researchers might consider the *Sleep Experiences Questionnaire* (McNally & Clancy, 2005) or the *Isolated Sleep Paralysis Questionnaire* (Ramsawh, Raffa, White, & Barlow, 2008). The former is derived from the *Waterloo Unusual Sleep Experiences Questionnaire* and is fairly broad in scope. In contrast, the *Isolated Sleep Paralysis Questionnaire* focuses on the intensity of physical and cognitive experiences that occur *during* episodes. The dimensional nature of this scale's items, item content, and acceptable psychometric properties may make it particularly useful as an outcome measure for clinical work or clinical trials, and the two subscales (i.e., physical and cognitive) allow for added flexibility.

For more extensive assessments of sleep paralysis and projects where it may be the primary focus, we recommend the *Waterloo Unusual Sleep Experiences Questionnaire* (Cheyne, Newby-Clark, & Rueffer, 1999) and *Unusual Sleep Experiences Questionnaire* (Paradis et al., 2009). Both contain very broad and thorough assessments of sleep paralysis and related phenomena, inquire into fear/distress, and also assess for interesting attributions of sleep paralysis phenomena. The *Waterloo* has more psychometric evidence in favor of its use and has been more widely used, but both possess excellent and usable content.

Interviews have a number of relative advantages over self-report instruments, but also bear significant burdens in terms of cost and time. Unless they are completely structured (e.g., *Sleep EVAL*), moving the format somewhat closer to self-reports, interviews require training and clinical judgment. If used for research purposes, regular inter-rater reliability checks are required as well. However, interviews allow for more assurance that interviewees are interpreting questions in a manner similar to the interviewer's intensions and also allow for better differential diagnosis (which, as shown in chapter 13, can be complicated). Thus, for clinical purposes and research projects focused on sleep paralysis, interviews are clearly preferred, although a multi-method assessment (e.g., interviews and self-reports used in conjunction) would be ideal.

Interviews for sleep paralysis can be found in Table 12.2. Seven languages are represented (i.e., English, German, Italian, Khmer, Mandarin, Portuguese, and Spanish). In general, these interviews are more extensive than many of the self-report measures and will require more time to administer. Regarding structured interviews in particular, the sleep paralysis items from the *Sleep EVAL* have been widely used, and can be administered in five different languages (Ohayon, Zulley, Guilleminault, & Smirne, 1999).

We have several recommendations for semi-structured interviews. If a very brief and "barebones" diagnostic assessment is warranted, the isolated sleep paralysis module from the *Duke Structured Interview for Sleep Disorders* is an excellent choice (Edinger et al., 2004). Criteria and prompts can be found in Box 12.1. It could also be easily modified to fit current *ICSD-3* criteria (American Academy of Sleep Medicine, 2014) if an additional fear item were added. For more extensive interviews, the various sleep paralysis measures developed by Hinton and colleagues (2005), the *Isolated Sleep Paralysis Interview* (Ramsawh et al., 2008), and the *Fearful Isolated Sleep Paralysis Interview* (Sharpless et al., 2010) all possess at least some degree of psychometric evidence in favor of their use. All would be very useful for research purposes, as they include dimensional scoring and are fairly broad. However, as the *Fearful Isolated Sleep Paralysis Interview* (appendix B) specifically focuses on many of the important clinically significant manifestations of sleep paralysis and also contains diagnostic and clinical thresholds that are consistent with current ICSD criteria (American Academy of Sleep Medicine, 2014), it may also be useful for clinical assessment work.

Table 12.1. SELF-REPORT MEASURES OF SLEEP PARALYSIS

Citation	Name	Language(s)	Population(s) Administered to	Special Features	Psychometric Properties of the Measure
Arikawa et. al. 1999	*Kanashibari Questionnaire*	Japanese	General population	Makes explicit reference to *kanashibari* and inquires into putative supernatural causes	None reported
Awadalla et al., 2004	Unnamed measure (available in article)	Arabic; English	Undergraduates	Only includes chest oppression item beyond paralysis	Arabic version was back translated.
Cheyne, Newby-Clark, & Rueffer, 1999	*Waterloo Unusual Sleep Experiences Questionnaire/Survey versions I—VIII* (available online)	English	Psychology undergraduates/ Online respondents	Assesses the frequency and vividness/intensity of SP experiences. Different versions vary on frequency descriptors. Assesses many SP hallucinations as well as certain variables that may predispose one to experience SP. One version (i.e, WUSEQ-LV) assesses for the laterality of hallucinations.	Replicated tripartite factor structure of SP hallucinations (i.e., intruder; incubus; vestibular-motor), Coefficient alpha = 0.75 for hallucinations, stability of intensity ratings ranges from 0.66-0.74 (Cheyne et al., 1999; Cheyne & Girard, 2004; Cheyne, 2005; Cheyne, Rueffer, & Newby-Clark, 1999; Cheyne & Girard, 2007)
Everett, 1963	Unnamed measure (available in article)	English	Undergraduates	Completion of questionnaire is preceded by verbal description of SP	None reported
Fukuda et al., 1987; Fukuda et al., 1991	Unnamed measure (available in article)	Japanese	Undergraduates	Explicitly notes *kanashibari* in descriptions and assesses for putative beliefs of supernatural causation	None reported

Citation	Measure	Language	Population	Description	Psychometrics
Fulda et al., 2008	*Munich Parasomnia Screening* (available in article)	German; English	Psychiatric inpatients, sleep disorder patients, and controls	Includes one item on SP and two other questions on hallucinations and choking sensations	Sensitivity for SP item = 0.75; specificity = 0.97; positive predictive value = 0.75; negative predictive value = 0.97.
Goode, 1962	Unnamed measure (available in article)	English	Undergraduates	Asks about other sleep experiences such as sleep-walking and sleep-talking	None reported
Hedman et al., 2002	Unnamed measure	English	Expecting mothers	Brief screening instrument for parasomnias, including SP	None reported
Hsieh et al., 2010	*Sleep Questionnaire for Isolated Sleep Paralysis* (available in article)	Chinese (Mandarin)	Patients with sleep disturbances	Brief measure that includes questions on hallucinations	None reported
Jimenez-Genchi et al., 2009	*Sleep Paralysis Questionnaire* (available in article)	Spanish	High school students	Brief measure that includes explicit mention of the "dead body climbed on top of me" phenomenon	None reported
Kotorii et al., 2001	Unnamed measure	Japanese	General population	Few details provided	None Reported
McNally & Clancy, 2005	*Sleep Experiences Questionnaire* (partially available in article)	English	Adults reporting sexual abuse; controls	Adapted from the Waterloo and includes questions about how individuals interpret their SP experiences.	None Reported

(Continued)

Table 12.1. CONTINUED

Citation	Name	Language(s)	Population(s) Administered to	Special Features	Psychometric Properties of the Measure
Mellman et al., 2008	*Sleep Paralysis Questionnaire* (available in article)	English	Primarily hospital patients	SR measure modeled after Bell et al., 1984. Includes open-ended descriptions of SP episodes and also assesses fear.	None reported
Munezawa et al., 2009	Unnamed measure (available in article)	Japanese	High school students	Brief questionnaire that also assesses first experiences of SP	None reported
Ohaeri et al., 1989	Unnamed measure	English	Medical students	Self-report version of Bell et al.'s, 1984 interview which also includes prompts to describe episodes in detail	None reported
Ohaeri, 1997	Unnamed measure	English	Civil servants and undergraduates	Contains items on SP and dream experiences	Content validity established by members of psychology, psychiatry, and philosophy departments.
Ohaeri et al., 2004	Unnamed measure (most items available in article)	English	General population	Items were provided from Hinton and include questions about emotional reactions and supernatural beliefs about SP experiences.	Inter-rater reliability of items over two-week interviews yielded Kappa values of 0.74-0.96. Cronbach's alpha of items was 0.66.

Citation	Measure	Language	Population	Description	Reliability
Paradis et al., 2009	*Unusual Sleep Experiences Questionnaire* (available in article)	English	Undergraduates	Broad measure of SP symptoms and correlates of the experience that also assesses catastrophic cognitions and supernatural attributions	None reported
Penn et al., 1981	Unnamed questionnaire (available in article)	English	Medical students	Brief measure that also assesses for cataplexy	None reported
Ramsawh et al., 2008	*Isolated Sleep Paralysis Questionnaire*	English	African Americans	Relatively brief measure consisting of physical and cognitive subscales.	Cronbach's alphas for subscales = 0.71 and 0.89 and the total scale = 0.88
Sherwood, 1999	Unnamed measure	English	Online Respondents	Includes one item on SP	None reported
Simard & Nielsen, 2005	*Isolated Sleep Paralysis and Sensed Presence Questionnaire*	French	Undergraduates	Includes questions on sensed presence, emotional experiences, and intensity ratings for episodes based on the Waterloo.	None reported
Spanos et al., 1995	*Sleep-Related Questionnaire*	English	Undergraduates	Assesses frequency and psychological components of SP	Factor analysis yielded personality, psychopathology, and imaginative factors. Cronbach alphas for each factor ranged from 0.66-0.95.
Takeuchi et al., 1992	Unnamed measure	Japanese	Undergraduates	Measure includes explicit reference to *kanashibari*	None reported
Wing et al., 1994; 1999	Unnamed measure	Chinese (Mandarin)	Undergraduates	Measure includes explicit reference to ghost oppression phenomena	None reported

Table 12.2. INTERVIEW MEASURES OF SLEEP PARALYSIS

Citation	Name	Language(s)	Population(s) Administered to	Special Features	Psychometrics Properties of the Measure
Bell et al., 1984; 1986	Unnamed measure administered in person or over the phone	English	African Americans	Measure begins with a description of sleep paralysis.	None reported
Dahmen et al., 2002	*Stanford Center for Narcolepsy Sleep Inventory* (adapted sections)	German	General Population (telephone)	Built upon a well-established measure	None reported
Edinger et al., 2004	*Duke Structured Interview for Sleep Disorders*	English	Suspected sleep disorder patients	Brief and mirrors ICSD criteria	None Reported
Friedman et al., 1994; Paradis et al., 1997	Unnamed measure	English	Anxiety disorder patients; community volunteers	Measure was adapted from Bell et al., 1984.	Inter-rater reliability was 100%.
Hinton et al., 2005	*Sleep Paralysis Panic Attack Questionnaire and Post-Sleep Paralysis Panic Attack Questionnaire*	Khmer	Cambodian Refugees in the US	Asks about panic attacks and panic disorder in the context of SP using *Structured Clinical Interview for DSM-IV* items.	Inter-rater reliability for *SP Panic Attack Questionnaire* = 0.91; Test-retest reliability for *Post-SP Panic Attack Questionnaire* over 2 weeks = 0.88

Citation	Measure	Language	Population	Description	Reliability/Validity
Hinton et al., 2005	*Sleep Paralysis Hallucination Interview*	Khmer	Cambodian Refugees in the US	Asks about hallucinated forms (e.g., black shapes) and descriptions of the experience.	Inter-rater reliability = 1.00.
Hinton et al., 2005	*Sleep Paralysis Questionnaire* (partially available in article)	Khmer	Cambodian Refugees in the United States	Includes frequency items and six questions related to visual hallucinations, 17 catastrophic cognition items, and descriptions relevant to Cambodian experiences of SP.	None reported
Hinton et al., 2005	*Sleep Paralysis Frequency and Duration Interview*	Khmer	Cambodian refugees in the United States	Focuses on past year SP episodes and includes free response descriptors.	Inter-rater reliability of SP diagnosis kappa = 0.93. Test-retest reliability over two weeks = 0.78.
Ohayon et al., 1999; Ohayon & Shapiro, 2000; Ohayon et al., 2002	Sleep EVAL Questionnaire (Sleep Paralysis questions available in article)	German; Italian; Portuguese; Spanish; English	General population	This measure is broad in scope and employs causal reasoning in its diagnostic system via a computerized administration.	Extensive reliability and validity reports can be found in original articles.
Pires et al., 2007	*UNIFESP Sleep Questionnaire* (Sleep Paralysis item)	Portuguese	General population	Brief	None reported

(Continued)

Table 12.2. CONTINUED

Citation	Name	Language(s)	Population(s) Administered to	Special Features	Psychometric Properties of the Measure
Ramsawh et al., 2008	*Isolated Sleep Paralysis Interview*	English	African-Americans	Partially modeled after the *Anxiety Disorders Interview Schedule*. Assesses for distress and impairment.	ICC for severity = 0.81.
Sharpless et al., 2010	*Fearful Isoalted Sleep Paralysis Interview* (appendix B)	English	Anxiety disorder patients; undergraduate students	Measure follows *Anxiety Disorders Interview Schedule* format and allows for ICSD-2 and ICSD-3 diagnoses as well as scores using a structured severity scale. Assesses the common clinical impacts of ISP as well as distress and impairment.	Internal consistencies ranged from 0.83–0.93 for structured severity scale items; kappas for various ISP diagnosis definitions ranged from 0.93–0.97 and ICCs for severity ranged from 0.95–0.99.
Wing et al., 1999	*Ghost Oppression Questionnaire*	Mandarin	General population (elderly)	Measure is derived from their earlier SR measure and also makes explicit reference to ghost oppression phenomena.	None reported

Box 12.1: DUKE STRUCTURED INTERVIEW FOR
DSM-IV-TR AND INTERNATIONAL CLASSIFICATION
OF SLEEP DISORDERS, SECOND EDITION: RECURRENT
ISOLATED SLEEP PARALYSIS PROMPTS AND
DIAGNOSTIC CRITERIA

QUESTIONS

1. Have you ever been unable to move your body or arms and legs or have you felt paralyzed while you were in bed? During these times, have you had strange sensory experiences?
2. Have such events occurred just as you were falling asleep or just after you awakened from sleep?
3. How long do these episodes last?
4. Are these events related to any medical condition or emotional problem that might cause them?

NOTE: *Verify that the sleep disorder is not better explained by another sleep disorder, medical/neurological disorder, psychiatric disorder, or medication/substance use or exposure.*

CRITERIA

1. Subject reports an inability to move the body and all limbs. Hallucinations may be present, but are not necessary for diagnosis.
2. Subject indicates events occur at sleep onset or upon awakening.
3. Subject reports each episode lasts seconds to a few minutes.
4. Subject reports no apparent medical (e.g., hypokalemia) or psychiatric (e.g., hysteria) cause. Cataplexy and narcolepsy are not present.

Edinger, J. D., Bonnet, M. H., Bootzin, R. R., Doghramji, K., Dorsey, C. M., Espie, C. A., et al. (2004). Derivation of research diagnostic criteria for insomnia: Report of an American Academy of Sleep Medicine work group. Sleep, 27(8), 1567–1596.

RECOMMENDATIONS AND FUTURE DIRECTIONS

As can be seen in the tables, there are a number of options in the current sleep paralysis assessment armamentarium. Although many choices exist, the current lack of a "gold standard" instrument may lead to some important (and possibly negative) consequences. For instance, many of these measures have not been extensively used, and the vast majority have not undergone psychometric testing. Further, the framing and operationalization of sleep paralysis phenomena can differ markedly between instruments. Although many follow *International Classification of Sleep Disorders* (ICSD; American Academy of Sleep Medicine, 2005) criteria (e.g., Ramsawh et al., 2008; Sharpless et al., 2010), some may be a bit more idiosyncratic in the way questions are asked (e.g., Bell et al.'s [1984] and Everett's [1963] presentation of paradigmatic descriptions of sleep paralysis followed by asking raters if they've experienced something similar as opposed to symptom checklists of individual criteria). The combination of these factors may be important contributors to the high variability found in sleep paralysis prevalence rate data (e.g., Sharpless & Barber, 2011).

Finally, we end this chapter with several recommendations for assessment. First, for most research purposes we would prioritize semi-structured interviews over self-report questionnaires. Along with the clear importance of accurate differential diagnosis, interviews allow researchers to gain a richer picture of sleep paralysis phenomena. Given the early stage of the research, it would be a shame if clinical conceptions of sleep paralysis and sleep paralysis phenomena became prematurely fixed and reified. Second, more psychometric work is needed. We were somewhat surprised by the lack of testing that many of these measures underwent. This may be due to the fact that many were used for only one study, but knowing the properties of these instruments is a clear *sine qua non* to more extensive programs of research. Third, measures should be clearly named in method sections. As seen in the Tables, a number of measures were not named, a factor that may lead to some confusion in journal indexing databases and will not facilitate repeated use of the same measure by different labs. Fourth, a number of the measures reviewed were actually made publically available either in print or online, and we hope that this trend continues. Finally, it is recommended that measures used for basic psychopathology research and clinical research pay more attention to *clinical impact* so that future work can determine better thresholds for problematic cases of sleep paralysis.

REFERENCES

American Academy of Sleep Medicine. (2005). *International classification of sleep disorders: Diagnostic & coding manual* (2nd ed.). Darien, IL: American Academy of Sleep Medicine.
American Academy of Sleep Medicine. (2014). *International classification of sleep disorders: Diagnostic and coding manual* (3rd ed.). Darien, IL: American Academy of Sleep Medicine.
Arikawa, H., Templer, D. I., Brown, R., Cannon, W. G., & Thomas-Dodson, S. (1999). The structure and correlates of kanshibari. *The Journal of Psychology, 133*(4), 369–375.

Awadalla, A., Al-Fayez, G., Harville, M., Arikawa, H., Tomeo, M. E., Templer, D. I., & Underwood, R. (2004). Comparative prevalence of isolated sleep paralysis in Kuwaiti, Sudanese, and American college students. *Psychological Reports, 95*(1), 317–322. doi: 10.2466/PR0.95.5.317-322

Bell, C. C., Dixie-Bell, D. D., & Thompson, B. (1986). Further studies on the prevalence of isolated sleep paralysis in black subjects. *Journal of the National Medical Association, 78*(7), 649–659.

Bell, C. C., Shakoor, B., Thompson, B., Dew, D., Hughley, E., Mays, R., & Shorter-Gooden, K. (1984). Prevalence of isolated sleep paralysis in black subjects. *Journal of the National Medical Association, 76*(5), 501–508.

Cheyne, J. A., Newby-Clark, I. R., & Rueffer, S. D. (1999). Relations among hypnagogic and hypnopompic experiences associated with sleep paralysis. *Journal of Sleep Research, 8*, 313–317.

Dahmen, N., Kasten, M., Muller, M.J., & Mittag, K. (2002). Frequency and dependence on body posture of hallucinations and sleep paralysis in a community sample. *Journal of Sleep Research, 11*, 179–180.

Edinger, J. D., Bonnet, M. H., Bootzin, R. R., Doghramji, K., Dorsey, C. M., Espie, C. A., et al. (2004). Derivation of research diagnostic criteria for insomnia: Report of an American Academy of Sleep Medicine work group. *Sleep, 27*(8), 1567–1596.

Everett, H. C. (1963). Sleep paralysis in medical students. *Journal of Nervous and Mental Disease, 136*(6), 283–287.

Friedman, S., Paradis, C. M., & Hatch, M. (1994). Characteristics of African-American and white patients with panic disorder and agoraphobia. *Hospital and Community Psychiatry, 45*(8), 778–803.

Fukuda, K., Inamatsu, N., Kuroiwa, M., & Miyasita, A. (1991). Personality of healthy young adults with sleep paralysis. *Perceptual and Motor Skills, 73*(3, Pt 1), 955–962. doi: 10.2466/PMS.73.7.955-962

Fukuda, K., Miyasita, A., Inugami, M., & Ishihara, K. (1987). High prevalence of isolated sleep paralysis: Kanashibari phenomenon in Japan. *Sleep: Journal of Sleep Research & Sleep Medicine, 10*(3), 279–286.

Fulda, S., Hornyak, M., Muller, K., Cerny, L., Beitinger, P. A., & Wetter, T. C. (2008). Development and validation of the Munich Parasomnia Screening (MUPS): A questionnaire for parasomnias and nocturnal behaviors. *Somnologie, 12*, 56–65.

Goode, G. B. (1962). Sleep paralysis. *Archives of Neurology, 6*, 228–234.

Hedman, C., Pohjasvaara, T.,Tolonen, U., Salmivaara, A., & Myllyla, V. V. (2002). Parasomnias decline during pregnancy. *Acta Neurological Scandinavica, 105*, 209–214.

Hinton, D. E., Pich, V., Chhean, D., Pollack, M. H., & McNally, R. J. (2005). Sleep paralysis among Cambodian refugees: Association with PTSD diagnosis and severity. *Depression and Anxiety, 22*(2), 47–51. doi: 10.1002/da.20084

Hsieh, S., Lai, C., Liu, C., Lan, S., & Hsu, C. (2010). Isolated sleep paralysis linked to impaired nocturnal sleep quality and health-related quality of life in Chinese-Taiwanese patients with obstructive sleep apnea. *Quality of Life Research, 19*(9), 1265–1272. doi: 10.1007/s11136-010-9695-4

Jimenez-Genchi, A., Avila-Rodriguez, V. M., Sanchez-Rojas, F., Terrez, B. E., & Nenclares-Portocarrero, A. (2009). Sleep paralysis in adolescents: The 'a dead body climbed on top of me' phenomenon in Mexico. *Psychiatry and Clinical Neurosciences, 63*(4), 546–549. doi: 10.1111/j.1440-1819.2009.01984.x [doi]

Kotorii, T., Kotorii, T., Uchimura, N., Hashizume, Y., Shirakawa, S., Satomura, T., et al. (2001). Questionnaire relating to sleep paralysis. *Psychiatry and Clinical Neurosciences*, 55(3), 265–266. doi: 10.1046/j.1440-1819.2001.00853.x

McNally, R. J., & Clancy, S. A. (2005). Sleep paralysis in adults reporting repressed, recovered, or continuous memories of childhood sexual abuse. *Journal of Anxiety Disorders*, 19(5), 595–602. doi: 10.1016/j.janxdis.2004.05.003

Mellman, T. A., Aigbogun, N., Graves. R. E., Lawson, W. B., & Alim, T. N. (2008). Sleep paralysis and trauma, psychiatric symptoms and disorders in an adult African American population attending primary medical care. *Depression and Anxiety*, 25, 435–440.

Munezawa, T., Kaneita, Y., Yokoyama, E., Suzuki, H., & Ohida, T. (2009). Epidemiological study of nightmare and sleep paralysis among Japanese adolescents. *Sleep and Biological Rhythms*, 7(3), 201–210. doi: 10.1111/j.1479-8425.2009.00404.x

Ohaeri, J. U. (1997). The prevalence of isolated sleep parlaysis among a sample of Nigerian civil servants and undergraduates. *African Journal of Medicine and Medical Sciences*, 26, 43–45.

Ohaeri, J. U., Awadalla, V. A., Maknjuola, V. A., & Ohaeri, B. M. (2004). Features of isolated sleep paralysis among Nigerians. *East African Medical Journal*, 81(10), 509–519.

Ohaeri, J. U., Odejide, O. A., Ikuesan, B. A., & Adeyemi, J. D. (1989). The pattern of isolated sleep paralysis among Nigerian medical students. *Journal of the National Medical Association*, 81(7), 805–808.

Ohayon, M. M., Priest, R. G., Zulley, J., Smirne, S., & Paiva, T. (2002). Prevalence of narcolepsy symptomatology and diagnosis in the general population. *Neurology*, 58, 1826–1833.

Ohayon, M. M., & Shapiro, C. M. (2000). Sleep disturbances and psychiatric disorders associated with posttraumatic stress disorder in the general population. *Comprehensive Psychiatry*, 41(6), 469–478.

Ohayon, M. M., Zulley, J., Guilleminault, C., & Smirne, S. (1999). Prevalence and pathologic associations of sleep paralysis in the general population. *Neurology*, 52(6), 1194–1200.

Paradis, C. M., Friedman, S., & Hatch, M. (1997). Isolated sleep paralysis in African Americans with panic disorder. *Cultural Diversity and Mental Health*, 3(1), 69–76. doi: 10.1037/1099-9809.3.1.69

Paradis, C., Friedman, S., Hinton, D. E., McNally, R. J., Solomon, L. Z., & Lyons, K. A. (2009). The assessment of the phenomenology of sleep paralysis: The unusual sleep experiences questionnaire (USEQ). *CNS Neuroscience & Therapeutics*, 15(3), 220–226. doi: 10.1111/j.1755-5949.2009.00098.x

Penn, N. E., Kripke, D. F., & Scharff, J. (1981). Sleep-paralysis among medical students. *Journal of Psychology: Interdisciplinary and Applied*, 107(2), 247–252. doi: 10.1080/00223980.1981.9915230

Ramsawh, H. J., Raffa, S. D., White, K. S., & Barlow, D. H. (2008). Risk factors for isolated sleep paralysis in an African American sample: A preliminary study. *Behavior Therapy*, 39(4), 386–397. doi: 10.1016/j.beth.2007.11.002

Sharpless, B. A., & Barber, J. P. (2011). Lifetime prevalence rates of sleep paralysis: A systematic review. *Sleep Medicine Reviews*, 15(5), 311–315. doi: 10.1016/j.smrv.2011.01.007; 10.1016/j.smrv.2011.01.007

Sharpless, B. A., McCarthy, K. S., Chambless, D. L., Milrod, B. L., Khalsa, S. R., & Barber, J. P. (2010). Isolated sleep paralysis and fearful isolated sleep paralysis in outpatients with panic attacks. *Journal of Clinical Psychology,* *66*(12), 1292–1306. doi: 10.1002/jclp.20724; 10.1002/jclp.20724

Sherwood, S. J. (1999). Relationship between childhood hypnagogic, hypnopompic, and sleep experiences, childhood fantasy proneness, and anomalous experiences and beliefs: An exploratory WWW survey. *The Journal of the American Society for Psychical Research, 93*(2), 167–197.

Simard, V., & Nielsen, T. A. (2005). Sleep paralysis-associated sensed presence as a possible manifestation of social anxiety. *Dreaming, 15*(4), 245–260. doi: 10.1037/1053-0797.15.4.245

Spanos, N. P., McNulty, S. A., DuBreuil, S. C., & Pires, M. (1995). The frequency and correlates of sleep paralysis in a university sample. *Journal of Research in Personality, 29*(3), 285–305. doi: 10.1006/jrpe.1995.1017

Takeuchi, T., Miyasita, A., Sasaki, Y., & Inugami, M. (1992). Isolated sleep paralysis elicited by sleep interruption. *Sleep: Journal of Sleep Research & Sleep Medicine, 15*(3), 217–225.

Wing, Y., Chiu, H., Leung, T., & Ng, J. (1999). Sleep paralysis in the elderly. *Journal of Sleep Research, 8*, 151–155.

Wing, Y., Lee, S. T., & Chen, C. (1994). Sleep paralysis in chinese: Ghost oppression phenomenon in Hong Kong. *Sleep: Journal of Sleep Research & Sleep Medicine, 17*(7), 609–613.

CHAPTER 13
Differential Diagnosis of Sleep Paralysis

Accurate diagnosis of sleep paralysis is difficult, possibly even more so than many other disorders. In general, arriving at an accurate patient diagnosis is much more complex than many would believe. In our experience, especially with beginning students, diagnosis can be viewed as a fairly "superficial" process that is secondary to treatment in terms of intrinsic level of interest. Thus, misdiagnoses can and do occur.

There are at least three main ways in which misdiagnosis happens. First, they can be willfully made in order to achieve certain ends. As one example, a therapist could purposefully misdiagnose a patient suffering from severe major depressive disorder as having an adjustment disorder for the purpose of keeping a third party payer (such as an insurance provider) from knowing the true extent of the patient's illness. Other examples of willful misdiagnosis have occurred for various political reasons (e.g., diagnosing political dissidents with schizophrenia, as has been documented under certain repressive regimes [e.g., Reich, 1999]).

Misdiagnoses can also be made in various non-purposeful ways. In these circumstances, the diagnostician is adequately trained and not willfully inaccurate, yet still arrives at inaccurate conclusions due to factors extrinsic to the patient. For instance, a diagnostician may become personally preoccupied with specific diagnoses as opposed to thoughtfully considering the full range of psychopathological flavors that are available. Some diagnosticians may see every patient as having post-traumatic stress disorder or sleep apnea, and are therefore not open to the full, rich panoply of diagnostic options.

Finally, misdiagnosis can occur through ignorance, and this may be particularly salient for sleep paralysis. As noted in previous chapters, there is a general lack of awareness of this condition. Many health providers do not inquire into it, and many of those who suffer from it do not volunteer their symptom unless they are directly queried. Needless, to say, misdiagnosis under these circumstances can be quite likely. Assuming that there is a general awareness of sleep paralysis as a diagnostic option, clinicians are still faced with the complex task of accurately differentiating it from other symptoms and syndromes. In this chapter, we therefore attempt to provide clinically-useful guidance in differential diagnosis.

SLEEP PARALYSIS AND OTHER SLEEP DISORDERS AND SYMPTOMS

Nightmare Disorder

Nightmare disorder, like sleep paralysis, is an REM-based parasomnia accompanied by frightening sensory experiences and acute autonomic arousal. Further, the illusory dream contents can be quite elaborate, and even grandly thematic in nature. Thus, differential diagnosis may be challenging.

In order to meet diagnostic criteria for nightmare disorder, a person must experience, "Repeated occurrences of extended, extremely dysphoric, and well-remembered dreams that usually involve efforts to avoid threats to survival, security, or physical integrity (American Academy of Sleep Medicine, 2014, p. 257)." As the person awakens from these nightmares, he or she quickly returns to alertness and is once again oriented.

In reviewing the aforementioned descriptions, crucial differences with sleep paralysis may be apparent. For one, some degree of alertness to external surroundings and, for lack of a better phrase, consensual reality, is already in effect during sleep paralysis. Thus, sleep paralysis episodes, even if they involve hallucinations, include an overlay of conscious awareness usually missing in traditional nightmares. One of the more scary aspects of sleep paralysis hallucinations is that their vividness does not always allow for easy recognition of the REM content *as* REM content. This is why some individuals may believe they were actual victims of some form of assault. This would be extremely unlikely in nightmare disorder.

Another crucial difference involves the experience of the paralysis. Certainly, we've all experienced dreams in which we either felt unable to move or moved in slow motion when in the presence of threatening dream images, but this is not the *sine qua non* for nightmares that it is for sleep paralysis. Therefore, all episodes of sleep paralysis will include the conscious experience of paralysis, whereas this will likely not be the case for the recurrent dreams found in nightmare disorder.

Sleep Terrors

Alternately termed *night terrors* or *pavor nocturnus*, sleep terrors are classified as a non-REM-based parasomnia consisting of: ". . . episodes of abrupt terror, typically beginning with an alarming vocalization such as a frightening scream. There is intense fear and signs of autonomic arousal, including such as mydriasis, tachycardia, tachypnea, and diaphoresis during an episode. (American Academy of Sleep Medicine, 2014, p. 230)." There is also a relative unresponsiveness to the efforts of others to comfort the individual during episodes.

The phenomenology of sleep terrors differs quite a bit from sleep paralysis, and clinicians are encouraged to focus on three pieces of information for differential diagnosis. First, dream imagery, if present at all in sleep terrors, is minimal, and often not remembered. Per DSM-5, this may consist of only a single remembered visual scene (American Psychiatric Association, 2013, p. 399). In contrast, hallucinatory images in sleep paralysis are well remembered and often elaborate. Second, screams are not generated during sleep paralysis. Clinical reports sometimes include strained breathing and guttural sounds (e.g., Roscher, 2007), but we are not aware of any documented cases of screaming. Another difference is that those under the sway of a night terror are unable to be soothed by others, at least during the acute phase. In contrast, clinical reports of sleep paralysis sufferers indicate that such benevolent attentions often result in a termination of episodes and some degree of "relief." Finally, upon awakening from sleep terrors, individuals are often confused and only partially responsive, whereas the latter does not appear to be as evident in sleep paralysis.

Nocturnal Panic Attacks

Panic attacks are relatively common experiences in the general population (at least 14%, as reviewed in Barlow, 2002). Attacks consist of acute rushes of fear or anxiety that are accompanied by at least four of thirteen possible symptoms ranging from physical responses (e.g., tachycardia, sweating) to catastrophic appraisals (e.g., "I'm going crazy"; "I'm dying") of the attacks (American Psychiatric Association, 2013). If an attack occurs when the individual is emerging from sleep, it is termed a nocturnal or sleep panic attack (Mellman & Uhde, 1989). Almost by definition these attacks are considered to be unexpected, and they are fairly common in individuals suffering from panic disorder (American Psychiatric Association, 2013).

As noted in chapter 6, panic disorder and sleep paralysis have been discussed together for quite some time. Rates of sleep paralysis are higher in those with panic disorder, and reports of panic attacks subsequent to sleep paralysis have been described in the literature (e.g., Gangdev, 2006). Therefore, care should obviously be taken in differential diagnosis.

In summary, differentiating nocturnal panic from sleep paralysis requires a careful questioning of the affected patient, with particular attention to their cognitive and perceptual experiences. The unexpected nature of nocturnal panic (i.e., the abrupt and unexpected fear) is quite different from the fear seen in sleep paralysis. The latter is usually secondary to the subjective appraisals of the paralysis or hallucinations as opposed to being a fear that is immediately present upon awakening. Panic attacks also lack dream imagery. This is likely due to the fact that nocturnal panic attacks seem to occur during non-REM sleep (as reviewed in Mellman & Uhde, 1989). Although sleep paralysis does not always include hallucinations, the vast majority of sufferers report them (e.g., Cheyne, Newby-Clark, & Rueffer, 1999; Sharpless, McCarthy, Chambless, Milrod, Khalsa, & Barber, 2010). Finally, those experiencing nocturnal panic are not paralyzed, and their panic symptoms are present during full conscious and waking awareness. In contrast, sleep paralysis patients seem to experience the majority of their fear *during* the paralysis, and it appears to lessen when voluntary muscle control is regained.

Exploding Head Syndrome

Exploding head syndrome is the provocative name for a parasomnia that, like sleep paralysis, elicits fear and apprehension (see Sharpless, 2014, for a recent review). Per ICSD-3 criteria (American Academy of Sleep Medicine, 2014, p. 264), exploding head syndrome is characterized by the perception of loud noises (e.g., explosions, gunshots, bells) at wake–sleep transitions or upon waking. Although not usually associated with pain, these noises cause abrupt arousal and can be quite frightening. Flashes of light and other visual phenomena are also not uncommon accompanying sensations (Pearce, 1989).

Exploding head syndrome can be differentiated from sleep paralysis fairly easily through a close analysis of the symptoms. First, although exploding head syndrome sufferers are not technically asleep but in a state of quiescent wakefulness per electroencephalogram (EEG) (e.g., Yoon, Hwang, Roh, & Shin, 2011), they do not appear to have the same degree of conscious awareness that is experienced by sleep paralysis patients. People with exploding head syndrome often have sleep state misperceptions during their episodes, and believe themselves to be jarred into wakefulness by the explosion as opposed to being already awake (Sharpless, 2014). Second, the auditory (and sometimes visual) sensations of exploding head syndrome are fairly non-distinct and inchoate. Articulate speech is not heard, and the auditory perceptions are quite brief. Further, the *visual* phenomena are undifferentiated as well. Perceptions of lightning, bright light flashes, or "visual static" (like a poorly tuned television channel) are reported in exploding head syndrome in contrast to the fairly elaborate hallucinations seen in sleep paralysis. Finally, the duration of episodes is different. In most cases, the explosions/sounds are perceived to last one to several seconds whereas the mean duration of sleep paralysis episodes is five to six minutes (e.g., Sharpless et al., 2010). It is also important to note that exploding head syndrome has been reported to be an aura for subsequent sleep paralysis episodes (Evans, 2006), so it may be important to generate a timeline of symptoms in order to disentangle the sequence.

SLEEP PARALYSIS AND OTHER PSYCHIATRIC CONDITIONS

Schizophrenia and Other Psychotic Disorders

Differential diagnosis of sleep paralysis can also be complicated by various psychotic experiences. Care must also be taken in diagnosis because comorbid sleep paralysis can occur within the context of psychotic phenomena as well, a fact potentially muddying an already murky diagnostic picture. In fact, the first author worked with a patient during graduate school where the hallucinations experienced during sleep paralysis episodes (viz., hallucinations with paralysis and a clear sensorium) actually compounded already existing difficulties in reality testing. The contents of sleep paralysis were also incorporated into normal waking hallucinations and delusions. Specifically, this gentleman (who believed that he was a minor god) felt that the paralysis he experienced was a punishment from other gods for various indiscretions. Sensed presence and "other" hallucinations during the paralysis undergirded both his waking hallucinations of myriad tormentors and his paranoid belief that he was constantly in danger.

It is perhaps not surprising to find that hypnagogic and hypnopompic hallucinations are more commonly found in psychotic disorders than the other major groups of diagnoses (Plante & Winkelman, 2008). Further, several have warned that sleep paralysis and other narcoleptic symptoms may be misdiagnosed as psychotic (e.g., Douglass, Hays, Pazderka, & Russell, 1991). This is one of the cases where psychiatric misdiagnosis can quickly (and directly) lead to serious harm, as medications helpful for one may not only be unhelpful for the other but may actually *increase* the symptoms. For instance, antipsychotics are the drugs of choice for schizophrenic patients. Should stimulants be provided instead, an intensification of psychosis is possible and indeed likely. Similarly, the use of antipsychotics with patients suffering from sleep paralysis and/or narcolepsy could intensify symptoms; presumably this would be due to their well-known sedating properties (Szucs, Janszky, Hollo, Migleczi, & Halasz, 2003). Thus, accurate diagnosis is essential, and this is predicated on a good deal of knowledge of patient history and course/type of symptoms (e.g., see the case of "Sor" in Hinton, Pich, Chhean, & Pollack, 2005).

Patients with sleep paralysis and accompanying hypnagogic/hypnopompic experiences as well as those with psychotic symptoms will report hallucinations. However, those with sleep paralysis will only describe these experiences at sleep transitions, whereas they will be more pervasive in psychosis. Similarly, there may occasionally be disturbances in reality testing in patients who are particularly troubled by, and in the acute recovery phase of, their hallucinations, but they will not maintain this disturbance at other times unless they also suffer from comorbid psychosis. The vast majority of people with sleep paralysis that we have worked with have been able to recognize hallucinations as hallucinations, whereas this is much less common in psychosis. Further, no general personality deterioration will be present in sleep paralysis, whereas this will be seen in the more severe psychotic disorders. In terms of history, records of previous treatments may prove helpful. Favorable response to antipsychotics more likely implies a psychotic disturbance, whereas favorable response to stimulants may indicate narcolepsy. An actual increase in hallucinations when using antipsychotics may provide indirect evidence of sleep paralysis.

Post-Traumatic Stress Disorder

As noted in chapter 9, several studies have linked trauma and sleep paralysis. Some common post-traumatic experiences reactions can make differential diagnosis with sleep paralysis potentially quite difficult, however. For example, individuals with PTSD experience vivid flashbacks with concurrent autonomic arousal and fear, dissociative phenomena such as out-of-body experiences, and subjective feelings of being "frozen" or paralyzed when experiencing/re-experiencing traumatic events. Needless to say, all three of these symptoms could be misdiagnosed as sleep paralysis and vice versa. Thus, care must be taken to appropriately diagnosis individuals who may have trauma histories.

As is well-known, flashbacks in PTSD are common, vivid, and frightening. Those that occur at night or in sleep transitions may be particularly hard to differentiate from sleep paralysis, but sleep paralysis hallucinations only occur at sleep–wake or wake–sleep transitions. Further, the content of PTSD flashbacks is trauma specific. This is not necessarily the case in sleep paralysis, although trauma-related themes have been reported to emerge during episodes (e.g., Hinton, Pich, Chhean, Pollack, & McNally, 2005). Third, flashbacks, when examined closely, are usually tied to a particular triggering stimulus (e.g., a woman who was raped in a parking lot experiences a flashback when entering a similar structure; a veteran experiences a flashback when passing a restaurant that serves food from the country he was stationed in). This is not as common in sleep paralysis and, again, the sleep transition element is key.

Sleep paralysis and PTSD flashbacks also differ in their particular manifestations of autonomic arousal, atonia, and out-of-body experiences. Clearly, both PTSD flashbacks and sleep paralysis hallucinations are activating events that are associated with fear-based physiological responses. In contrast to sleep paralysis, those with PTSD often have more *chronic* levels of arousal and hypervigilance. This chronicity is obviously much rarer in sleep paralysis.

Atonia can manifest in both disorders. However, atonia in PTSD is most likely to occur during very activating flashbacks, whereas it occurs during sleep paralysis regardless of the emotional valence of the hallucinations. It even occurs without the presence of any hallucinations whatsoever. Further, PTSD sufferers must be carefully questioned, as some may be so terrified that they feel *as if* they are frozen and cannot move, whereas in point of fact they could if they tried. It may be useful to ask the patients if they could move if they had too, or whether they were actually paralyzed. Those in a state of sleep paralysis are incapable of movement no matter how much will to move that they exert (i.e., in at least some cases of PTSD there may be a *misperception* of paralysis).

Finally, and similar to the above, out-of body experiences can occur in sleep paralysis regardless of the emotional valence of the hallucination.

They also appear to be a bit less emotionally "jarring" to the sufferer than out-of-body experiences during PTSD, but this is based on clinical lore, and not firm data.

Conversion Disorder

Conversion disorder, sometimes termed *functional neurological symptom disorder* (American Psychiatric Association, 2013) involves a patient experiencing altered motor or sensory functions that are incompatible with known medical conditions. For instance, a patient experiencing blindness when ocular tests appear normal would likely be suffering from conversion. The construct harkens back to the early days of psychopathology (e.g., Freud and Charcot) and the observation that psychic distress can be "converted" into anomalous physical ailments. Classic symptoms of conversion include motor weakness, but can include paralysis.

Differentiating conversion disorder (especially paralytic forms) from sleep paralysis rests upon the temporal course and context of the paralysis. The atonia found in sleep paralysis is transient, and relatively brief, whereas the paralysis of conversion is usually more chronic. The paralysis is also global (viz., over the entire body apart from eye movements), whereas the paralysis in conversion can take more specific, localized forms (e.g., "glove" paralysis). Finally, sleep paralysis only occurs during sleep–wake and wake–sleep transitions, whereas conversion symptoms are usually present during full wakefulness.

SLEEP PARALYSIS AND OTHER MEDICAL CONDITIONS

A variety of medical conditions mimic sleep paralysis and isolated sleep paralysis, yet should not be confused with either of these conditions.

Cataplexy

Cataplexy, the pathognomonic symptom of narcolepsy type 1, is also associated with a generalized paralysis of skeletal muscles (American Academy of Sleep Medicine, 2014). However, unlike sleep paralysis, cataplexy occurs in the context of wakefulness and is precipitated by strong emotional stimuli. Cataplexy and sleep paralysis may coexist in the same narcoleptic patient, and the presence of cataplexy increases the likelihood of also having sleep paralysis in a narcoleptic patient (Scammell, 2003).

Narcolepsy

As noted in chapter 8, sleep paralysis often occurs in the context of narcolepsy and is one of its associated features. It is also a central symptom in recurrent isolated sleep paralysis. However, recurrent isolated sleep paralysis lacks many of the essential clinical features of narcolepsy, such as EDS, hypnagogic hallucinations, and cataplexy. In addition polysomnographic studies in recurrent isolated sleep paralysis do not demonstrate the characteristic diagnostic findings of narcolepsy (see chapter 8).

Atonic Seizures

Atonic seizures (also referred to as drop attacks and akinetic seizures) may resemble cataplexy but, unlike sleep paralysis, occur during wakefulness. They are characterized by a loss or diminution of muscle tone, which may be confined to a specific body part (e.g., limb, jaw, head) or involve all postural muscles, leading to collapse or a slumping to the ground. However, patients remain conscious or only experience a momentary loss of consciousness. They usually last less than 15 seconds. These seizures begin in childhood but may persist into adulthood, and the diagnosis can be confirmed by electroencephalography (Zhao, Afra, & Adamolekun, 2010).

Focal Epileptic Seizures

Although focal seizures are not typically considered in the differential diagnosis of sleep paralysis, one report described a patient who met diagnostic criteria for recurrent isolated sleep paralysis. She was described as a 54-year-old woman with a longstanding history of epilepsy who reported sleep-related episodes during which she "woke and was unable to speak or perform voluntary body movements. She could subjectively move her eyes and experienced simple visual hallucinations (a diffuse 'intense light glow' involving the entire visual field and persisting on eye closure) as well as a feeling of anguish/fear" (Galimberti, Ossola, Colnaghi, & Arbasino, 2009). The onset of these symptoms coincided with the replacement of carbamazepine with primidone for seizure control (because of leukopenia associated with the former agent). A 24-hour ambulatory EEG revealed focal interictal epileptiform abnormalities, characterized by spikes or sharp waves with slow waves over the right temporal regions exclusively during non-REM sleep, and video monitoring captured stereotyped electrographic seizures over the right hemisphere. A key distinguishing feature from sleep paralysis was the observation that ictal visual hallucinations occurring during periods of immobility were elementary, repetitive, and stereotyped; as noted previously, sleep paralysis episodes are generally multimodal, variable in duration, and non-repetitive. Therefore, a history of seizure disorder, repetitive and stereotyped nature of the episodes, and documented EEG abnormalities were essential clues in distinguishing this focal seizure disorder from sleep paralysis.

Familial Periodic Paralysis

There are four forms of this disorder: Hypokalemic, hyperkalemic, thyrotoxic, and Andersen-Tawil syndrome. These are rare, autosomal dominant conditions with considerable variation in penetrance. Clinically, they manifest as episodes of flaccid paralysis with loss of deep tendon reflexes and failure of muscles to respond to electrical stimulation. Episodes may occur at rest and on awakening from sleep, so they can be confused with sleep paralysis. However, unlike sleep paralysis episodes, these typically last longer (e.g., hours to days as opposed to 5–6 minutes). The hyperkalemic variety may be the most difficult to distinguish from sleep paralysis because episodes are shorter, more frequent, and less severe than in the other disorders.

Each disorder also has characteristic clinical findings that distinguish it from sleep paralysis. For example, in hypokalemic paralysis, episodes usually follow the day after vigorous exercise and are precipitated by carbohydrate-rich meals, emotional or physical stress, alcohol ingestion, and cold exposure. Serum and urine K are decreased. Diagnosis can also be confirmed by provoking an episode by, for example, administering dextrose and insulin to cause hypokalemia or KCl to cause hyperkalemia (Porter, 2013).

Transient Compression Neuropathies

Also referred to as "entrapment neuropathies," these are caused by direct pressure on a single nerve. They can be confused with sleep paralysis since they may affect the radial, ulnar, median, or other nerves during sleep resulting in paralysis or paresis. Unlike sleep paralysis, however, symptoms usually also include a sensory component, such as pain, tingling, and numbness, and typically affect a single body part in congruence with the affected nerve. Nerve conduction studies can help to confirm the diagnosis (Stewart, 2000).

SLEEP PARALYSIS AND OTHER ASSORTED CONDITIONS AND EXPERIENCES

Actual Nocturnal Assaults

Chapter 2 summarizes some of the literature hypothesizing that nocturnal assaults, at least in some cases, may be misinterpretations of hallucinatory sleep paralysis phenomena. Sharpless and Grom (2013) found that it is not uncommon for "attackers" to be individuals known to the sufferer. Thus, the possibility exists that some reports of assault may be unintentionally spurious, although this is presumably a fairly rare occurrence. Given the profound implications, both personal and legal, that could arise from decisions made in either direction, it is important to note that this is not an area of differential diagnosis that should be undertaken lightly. Prior to this work, diagnosticians should be confident in their ability to work in these potentially forensic matters, and should otherwise refer the patient or secure competent consultation.

A thorough interview and documentation of evidence from a third party would be crucial in such a tricky case of differential diagnosis. First, and most importantly, are the descriptions of the assault consistent with the known phenomenology of sleep paralysis? Is actual paralysis present along with a clear sensorium? Further, is there any corroborating evidence that an actual assault took place? Did the perpetrator (or perpetrators) have access to the victim? Is there any physical evidence of assault (e.g., broken windows)? Another factor to consider would be the overall psychological state of the reported victim. Did they possess adequate reality testing? Do they suffer from other comorbid conditions (e.g., psychosis) that may make it possible for them to ascribe real-world veracity to sleep paralysis hallucinations? These are just a few of the questions that would need to be answered should a person wish to determine whether or not sleep paralysis may be a better explanation than nocturnal assault.

CONCLUSIONS

The preceding discussion highlights the many disorders and phenomena that can mimic sleep paralysis. Our list clearly highlights the need for a thorough psychological, medical, and psychiatric evaluation to ensure diagnostic accuracy. Diagnosticians should be aware of the limits of their competence and, if needed, refer to other appropriate specialists (e.g., when differentiating sleep paralysis from hyperkalemia).

Resources for the assessment of sleep paralysis, especially the more chronic variants, can be located in chapter 12. Appendix B contains a semi-structured interview (viz., the *Fearful Isolated Sleep Paralysis Interview*) that has been utilized with clinical and non-clinical samples (i.e., Sharpless & Grom, in press; Sharpless et al., 2010). These resources, and the recommendations made earlier in this chapter, will hopefully provide diagnostic guidance to clinicians.

REFERENCES

American Academy of Sleep Medicine. (2014). *International classification of sleep disorders: Diagnostic and coding manual* (3rd ed.). Darien, IL: American Academy of Sleep Medicine.

American Psychiatric Association. (2013). *Diagnostic and statistical manual of mental disorders: DSM-V* (5th ed.). Arlington, VA: American Psychiatric Association.

Barlow, D. H. (2002). *Anxiety and its disorders: The nature and treatment of anxiety and panic* (2nd ed.). New York: Guilford Press.

Cheyne, J. A., Newby-Clark, I. R., & Rueffer, S. D. (1999). Relations among hypnagogic and hypnopompic experiences associated with sleep paralysis. *Journal of Sleep Research, 8,* 313–317.

Douglass, A. B., Hays, P., Pazderka, F., & Russell, J. M. (1991). Florid refractory schizophrenias that turn out to be treatable variants of HLA-associated narcolepsy. *The Journal of Nervous and Mental Disease, 179*(1), 12–17.

Evans, R. W. (2006). Exploding head syndrome followed by sleep paralysis: A rare migraine aura. *Headache, 46*(4), 682–683. doi: 10.1111/j.1526-4610.2006.004 16.x

Galimberti, C. A., Ossola, M., Colnaghi, S., & Arbasino, C. (2009). Focal epileptic seizures mimicking sleep paralysis. *Epilepsy & Behavior, 14*(3), 562–564. doi: 10.1016/j.yebeh.2008.12.018

Gangdev, P. (2006). Comments on sleep paralysis. *Transcultural Psychiatry, 43*(4), 692–694. doi: 10.1177/1363461506066992

Hinton, D. E., Pich, V., Chhean, D., & Pollack, M. H. (2005). The ghost pushes you down: Sleep paralysis-type panic attacks in a Khmer refugee population. *Transcultural Psychiatry, 42*(1), 46–77. doi: 10.1177/1363461505050710

Hinton, D. E., Pich, V., Chhean, D., Pollack, M. H., & McNally, R. J. (2005). Sleep paralysis among Cambodian refugees: Association with PTSD diagnosis and severity. *Depression and Anxiety, 22*(2), 47–51. doi: 10.1002/da.20084

Mellman, T. A., & Uhde, T. W. (1989). Sleep panic attacks: New clinical findings and theoretical implications. *The American Journal of Psychiatry, 146*(9), 1204–1207.

Pearce, J. M. (1989). Clinical features of the exploding head syndrome. *Journal of Neurology, Neurosurgery, and Psychiatry, 52*(7), 907–910.

Plante, D. T., & Winkelman, J. W. (2008). Parasomnia: Psychiatric considerations. *Sleep Medicine Clinics, 3*, 217–229.

Porter, R. S. (2013) Merck manual go-to home guide for symptoms. Whitehouse Station, NJ: Merck.

Reich, W. (1999). Psychiatric diagnosis as an ethical problem. In S. Bloch, P. Chodoff & S. A. Green (Eds.), *Psychiatric ethics* (Third ed., pp. 193–224). London, UK: Oxford University Press.

Roscher, W. H. (2007). Ephialtes: A pathological-mythological treatis on the nightmare in classical antiquity. [Ephialtes] (A. V. O'Brien Trans.). (Revised ed., pp. 96–159). Putnam, CT: Spring Publishing.

Scammell, T. E. (2003). The neurobiology, diagnosis, and treatment of narcolepsy. *Annals of Neurology, 53*(2), 154–166. doi: 10.1002/ana.10444 [doi]

Sharpless, B. A. (2014). Exploding head syndrome. *Sleep Medicine Reviews, 18*(6), 489–493.

Sharpless, B. A., & Grom, J. L. (2013). Isolated sleep paralysis: Prevention, disruption, and hallucinations of others (poster). *American Psychological Association Annual Conference*, Honolulu, HI.

Sharpless, B. A., & Grom, J. L. (in press). Isolated sleep paralysis: Fear, prevention, and disruption. *Behavioral Sleep Medicine*.

Sharpless, B. A., McCarthy, K. S., Chambless, D. L., Milrod, B. L., Khalsa, S., & Barber, J. P. (2010). Isolated sleep paralysis and fearful isolated sleep paralysis in outpatients with panic attacks. *Journal of Clinical Psychology, 66*(12), 1292–1306. doi: 10.1002/jclp.20724

Stewart, J. D. (2000). *Focal peripheral neuropathies, 3rd edition*. Philadelphia: Lippincott Williams & Wilkins.

Szucs, A., Janszky, J., Hollo, A., Migleczi, G., & Halasz, P. (2003). Misleading hallucinations in unrecognized narcolepsy. *Acta Psychiatrica Scandinavica, 108*, 314–317.

Yoon, J.-E., Hwang, K. J., Roh, T.-H., & Shin, W. C. (2011). A case of exploding head syndrome: Focus on polysomnographic finding. *Journal of the Korean Sleep Research Society, 8*, 45–47.

Zhao, J., Afra, P., & Adamolekun, B. (2010). Partial epilepsy presenting as focal atonic seizure: A case report. *Seizure: The Journal of the British Epilepsy Association, 19*(6), 326–329. doi: 10.1016/j.seizure.2010.04.014 [doi]

CHAPTER 14

Folk Remedies for Sleep Paralysis

As with any phenomenon perceived to be scary or potentially dangerous, people attempt to protect themselves by taking preventative
actions and generating cures. This was (and is) certainly the case with
sleep paralysis. Irrespective of whether or not these tactics were effective in reducing episodes, they served important social and psychological
functions by providing sufferers and communities with feelings of hope
and agency (as opposed to despair and powerlessness). As will be shown,
some of these techniques used to prevent and disrupt sleep paralysis were
clever, and likely useful, whereas others appear quite strange to the contemporary reader.

Although we survey a variety of cultures and time periods, the various palliatives described in this chapter most likely represent only the
smallest fraction of the actual folk remedies used for sleep paralysis, as
most have unfortunately been lost in the mists of time. This lack of documentation is due to the unfortunate facts that: 1) certain cultures never
developed a written language system with which to document them;
2) learned individuals may not have taken folk treatments seriously, and
instead prioritized the more ostensibly scientific approaches; and 3) these
beliefs/treatments were so commonplace and apparent to everyone in
the community that no one ever thought it important to actually write
them down. Regardless of the cause(s), we are left with only a smatter-
ing of reports. We will separately discuss methods used to *prevent* and to
disrupt sleep paralysis episodes. In order to minimize reader confusion,
we use sleep paralysis in most cases instead of the more culture-specific
indigenous terms.

FOLK METHODS USED TO *PREVENT* SLEEP PARALYSIS EPISODES

Bedroom Accoutrements

Preventatives: Bed and Body

If one considers both the frequency of historical descriptions and the sheer number of distinct cultures taking part in these activities as primary criteria, then placing various objects under the pillow/bed or in the bedroom would be the most popular means of warding off sleep paralysis attacks and the creatures attributed to them. In a community that lacked a westernized, scientific understanding of sleep paralysis experiences, these activities would make intuitive sense. Sleep paralysis "attacks" happen at night when one is weak and vulnerable. Thus, according to this set of beliefs, placing charms or other helpful objects in close proximity to one's body could be an effective strategy.

A widely used means of self-protection involved placing defensive objects on one's person or under one's pillow before going to sleep. Sharp objects such as knives, razors, shears, or ulus (an all-purpose Inuit knife with a semi-circular blade) have been reported (e.g., Hufford, 1982; Law & Kirmayer, 2005). These were presumably used to ward off scary figures or provide some opportunity for self-defense. Hufford reported a case in Newfoundland where a young sufferer was instructed by an elder to lay a board on his chest with an open pocket knife on top of it. It was believed that when the Hag attacked him, she would be killed (Hufford, 1982, p. 3).

A number of religious objects have also been used in the bed and on/in the body. Proximity to these holy objects was thought to offer some means of protection to the sufferer. For instance, placing a bible under one's pillow was a common preventative (e.g., Hufford, 1982; Ness, 1978; Ohaeri, Awadalla, Maknjuola, & Ohaeri, 2004). Hanging rosary beads around one's neck or ingesting holy water have also been reported (Hufford, 1982).

Salt has been placed under pillows to ward off nocturnal attacks (Roberts, 1998). Jones noted that this practice likely related to ancient beliefs that the devil detested salt. When one considers the prized nature of salt (due to its rarity in earlier times) and its necessity for health and survival, its purported protective abilities may be easier to comprehend. A mixture of bread and salt was also used as a general "anti-witch" charm (Jones, 1949). This combination was also viewed as a physical representation of sexual fertility and, as such, may relate to certain medieval witchcraft beliefs. Specifically, it was believed even by many learned people that witches could nocturnally drain men and women of their sexual potency (e.g., Kramer & Sprenger, 1971; see also chapter 3). For every spell there is a counterspell, so a symbol of fecundity could prove an effective antidote to one that leads to barrenness and impotence. Therefore, it appears likely that this particular practice may be closely tied to "hags" and the more sexually assaultive variations of sleep paralysis hallucinations.

We should also note that keeping a light on in the bedroom has also been used preventatively (Hufford, 1982). For some adults, and a number of children, the world at night is a threatening place comprised of monsters and malevolent forces. From a practical standpoint, this may make the experience of sleep paralysis a bit easier to tolerate, as one could at least see the hallucinated threats instead of dimly viewing shadowy forms in the faint moonlight.

Preventatives: Objects in the Bedroom

Another preventative measure was to strategically place certain objects in other areas of the bedroom. For example, crucifixes, candles, and other blessed religious objects were utilized by sufferers for this purpose (e.g., Hufford, 1982; Roberts, 1998). Ancient Babylonians purportedly used a drinking bowl that depicted a man copulating with a recently decapitated vampire. This was believed to be a means to frighten Lilith and her sisters away from the bedroom (Summers, 1991). Slippers, particularly those composed of leather, were also situated in various places and orientations. Some recommended that the toes be pointed away from the bed (Firestone, 1985; Hufford, 1982). Matches and other objects connected with fire were held to be particularly effective deterrents (Firestone, 1985).

Mistletoe was thought to provide protection from attack, and this belief likely traces its origins to the Druids. Mistletoe was a sacred plant to these people, and considered to be a potent charm against the Nightmare (Jones, 1949). Interestingly, the Druids also believed horses were sacred (see chapter 3). Finally, objects such as brooms or cutlasses were placed on or by bedroom doors in order to somehow bar entry or ward off the various supernatural "causes" of sleep paralysis (Ohaeri et al., 2004)

Preventative Rituals and Prayers

Prayers (and repeating holy scripture) have also been used to prevent sleep paralysis/supernatural attacks. In order to protect oneself from oppressive *Jinn*, for instance, it has been recommended to even contemporary Muslims to read the last verse of the *Surat Kahl* (and other passages) prior to going to sleep (e.g., Jalal, Simons-Rudolph, Jalal, & Hinton, 2014). Among the Buddhist Cambodians, sufferers of sleep paralysis were encouraged to perform rituals that create "good luck" (Hinton, Pich, Chhean, Pollack, & McNally, 2005).

For Christians, prayer in general, and even faith healing of various sorts, has been advocated (e.g., Ohaeri et al., 2004). Ness reported a belief among Newfoundlanders that repeating a favorite hymn backwards may ward off night attacks (Ness, 1978). As will be shown this strategy was thought to also be helpful *during* attacks. Among Christian Inuits, going to confession and receiving various church blessings was thought to help those suffering from *uqumangirniq* (Law & Kirmayer, 2005).

Use of Strong-Smelling Substances

Some of the more unusual methods for preventing sleep paralysis involved the use of strong and/or foul-smelling substances. Interestingly, many of the beings and creatures thought to be the *causes* of what we would now term sleep paralysis (e.g., demons) were thought to be foul-smelling themselves. For instance, Summers (1987) noted that, in the Pyrenees, the word for "witch" derived from *putere*, a word signifying that one possessed a fetid odor (p. 44). Similarly, the vampire, a re-animated corpse, was also described in many sources as quite malodorous.

Jones noted that the use of pungent and strong-smelling charms was not a preventative measure limited to Nightmare alone, but was used to ward off evil more generally (Jones, 1949). Some cultures used flowers, caraway bread, and milk that had been exposed to smoke. The Greeks were reputed to have smeared pitch on houses to specifically keep vampires away from new mothers (Summers, 1991).

Reports also exist about using human waste. For instance, the indigenous treatment prescribed to a woman in Newfoundland involved collecting her urine in a bottle and placing it under her bed. Whether the preventative power of this charm was due exclusively to the urine's odor or some other mechanism is unclear. Much less ambiguous is a preventative practice described by Jones. In order to keep away the *Mara*, the Czechs would place a towel over their body that was streaked with human feces (Jones, 1949, p. 309). Presumably, the use of these substances was intended to make the sleeper a much less attractive victim.

Horses

The lengthy and complicated history connecting sleep paralysis (the Night-*mare*) and horses is briefly summarized in chapter 3. This history continues on in the attempts to prevent sleep paralysis/Nightmare, and Jones documented several examples from Scandinavian countries (Jones, 1949). At the most extreme end of this continuum, horses were buried alive in order to supplicate the female Night-Fiend. Individual body parts were similarly used. For example, horse feet were sometimes hung up in stables, with skulls placed on the rooftops of houses if people were the potential victims, or on top of the manger if horses themselves were at risk. Finally, the use of horseshoes in the house or barn, a practice still common in rural areas today, was another means of guarding against nocturnal attacks.

Encouraging Compulsive Behavior in Potential Nocturnal Tormentors

Interestingly, many of these "attackers" appear to have been compulsively driven to collect and count objects. This odd predilection was used to the advantage of potential victims who actively encouraged these behaviors as a way of staving off nocturnal assaults. For example, witches were reputedly unable to *not* count broom straws. Thus, African Americans in the rural South often slept with a broom close by their door so that their sleep would be undisturbed (Paradis & Friedman, 2005). For those in French-speaking areas of the American South, the *cauchemar* could be tricked in a similar fashion. Stones or dried beans would be placed under the bed, and the *cauchemar* would be forced to count these objects and/or the holes in screen doors prior to its malevolent pressings (Roberts, 1998).

Vampires in particular appeared to be riddled with compulsiveness. Placing piles of millet or other grains inside or outside of the home would help ensure that the vampire wasted time counting the grains, and would still be doing so by cock's crow. This would force the revenant to either leave the area immediately or be destroyed (Summers, 1991). The same source described how millet was often scattered over the graves of suspected vampires so that they would count grains and meet their true death by the morning sun instead of seeking out hapless victims. The *Longaroo* (an apparent corruption of *loupgarou*, or werewolf, but possessing many vampiric qualities) was similarly susceptible to grain counting, especially sand or rice. They too were forced to remain until they counted every grain, and would succumb to the sun.

The cross-cultural synchronicity of these compulsive behaviors is quite puzzling. It does not appear to have been discussed in contemporary source materials, and there also seems to be a lack of any clear explanations from our contemporary vantage point. Did some cultures make connections between certain observable forms of mental illness (e.g., certain obsessive-compulsive behaviors) and the odd dangerousness of these nighttime attackers? Were these compulsive behaviors the wishful fantasies of frightened victims (i.e., "I am not completely helpless, and my attackers have all-too-human weaknesses and psychological frailties")? These answers are likely unknowable. From an early psychoanalytic perspective (e.g., Freud, 1913), obsessive defenses are often conceptualized as a means of warding off unacceptable aggressive urges, and it is interesting how a parallel process may have occurred in those holding a pre-scientific view of sleep paralysis. The victims appear to wish for a cessation of hostile intentions through their attackers becoming absorbed in arithmomania.

Miscellaneous Preventatives

Various other preventative measures were advocated. For instance, dietary changes such as eating less (Golzari et al., 2012) or drinking energy-increasing beverages (Ohaeri et al., 2004) were thought to be helpful. An ancient domestic recipe to ward off Nightmare involved the ingestion of black pips of peony, an edible ornamental flower (Roscher, 2007). Avoiding foods that cause flatulence was also recommended by some of the ancients. It is reported that the famous prohibition against beans enacted by the Pythagoreans was partially due to this quality, as flatulence was associated with evil dreams and Nightmare (Roscher, 2007).

People also changed their behaviors to avoid sleep paralysis, and some of these methods were likely effective. Ness (1978) noted that some Newfoundlanders would avoid sleeping on their backs, and Hinton's group of Cambodian refugees (Hinton, Pich, Chhean, & Pollack, 2005) took pains to improve their sleep quality. Both of these efforts likely made sleep paralysis less likely. Others engaged in exercise (Ohaeri et al., 2004), a factor likely also leading to improved sleep quality, albeit indirectly. A less effective strategy was adopted by women in the West Indies who feared the return of their deceased husbands. They would reportedly spend their mourning periods in red underwear, as that particular color was thought to repel ghosts (Editors of Time-Life Books, 1988).

Congeniality was thought to be helpful in avoiding sleep paralysis/ Nightmare as well, especially among the Inuit people (Law & Kirmayer, 2005). In general, they would attempt to avoid conflicts with others, especially shamans and other powerful members of the community. It was also thought to be helpful to confess ones wrongdoings and, in general, to be respectful and kind to others. Presumably these mannerisms and social niceties made it less likely that a malevolent person or spirit would take a negative interest and choose to curse/torment you.

Finally, there were also some more radical and invasive techniques used for sleep paralysis. Drawing blood, although usually done by medical professionals, was used as a preventative strategy by laymen as well (Hufford, 1982). A traditional Nigerian method consisted of grinding together various animal parts (esp., reptiles and sometimes birds), alligator pepper (also known as *mbongo* spice), and black soap made from plantain skin and shea butter. This pungent mash was then rubbed into incisions (Ohaeri et al., 2004), but the supposed mechanism of action for this treatment was not reported.

FOLK METHODS USED TO *DISRUPT* SLEEP PARALYSIS EPISODES

Far fewer methods to *disrupt* sleep paralysis could be found in the historical literature. All of them involved movement or religious actions. Regarding the former, attempts to move individual fingers or toes have been described (e.g., Law & Kirmayer, 2005), and these techniques remain common today, albeit with mixed effectiveness (Sharpless & Grom, in press). It has also been suggested that having another individual shake the victim will disrupt episodes (Law & Kirmayer, 2005), and this is also likely to be effective.

It appears that some cultures attempted to break the paralysis so that they could engage the attacking entity more directly and stop the assault. For instance, when being attacked by a witch, it was recommended that you somehow throw a pillow onto the floor (Firestone, 1985). This would force the (compulsive) witch to sit on it and end the attack. Roscher (2007) summarized several techniques that are even more direct. The Slavic/ German *Murawa* could be made to cease her assaults if the victim touched her smallest toe. Another female Slavonic spirit, the *Pschezolnica*, could be forced to leave through gripping her finger, and a Nightmare witch could be made to vanish if one could firmly grab her hair. Of course, these techniques are quite difficult to enact given that the victim is atonic, and as with many other techniques described in this chapter, their origins are difficult to ascertain. It is possible that they were partly generated through the phenomenology of sleep paralysis itself. For example, sleep paralysis hallucinations tend to cease when movement returns. This may also explain the "vanishing" of certain creatures upon daybreak and/or the return of movement.

Specific religious actions could also disrupt attacks. Making the sign of the cross with one's tongue was thought to be an effective antidote to evil in general, and these nocturnal attacks in particular (Davies, 2003). One could also recite prayers, but not in the traditional and expected manner. Although some sources reported that saying the Lord's Prayer was a protective act (e.g., Kramer & Sprenger, 1971), the people of India believed that its recitation could actually *bring on an attack*. Similarly, the people of Newfoundland believed that its *backward* recitation would disrupt sleep paralysis. Interestingly, and somewhat paradoxically, the recitation of the Lord's Prayer backwards was a common component of the blasphemy-laden "black rites" required for becoming a witch or a werewolf (e.g., Summers, 1987). How this inversion of prayer came to be viewed as having a *positive*, protective effect is unknown and quite curious.

TECHNIQUES USED AGAINST CONTEMPORARY "ALIEN ABDUCTIONS"

Although the majority of the techniques just described were used in earlier time periods and in several pre-scientific cultures, many are still being used today but in a very different societal context. As noted in chapter 3, nocturnal alien abduction scenarios map very well onto sleep paralysis phenomenology. What is particularly striking about these contemporary narratives in contrast to earlier sleep paralysis narratives (which usually involved medieval demons or supernaturally powered beings) is the fact that most of these reports take place in the contemporary West. Thus, many "abductees" are not scientifically illiterate, or necessarily even devoutly religious people, and yet they still believe that they have been the victims of anomalous events in the absence of solid empirical evidence. It is also likely that these abductees were naïve to techniques described in the earlier nocturnal abduction narratives, although it is of course a possibility that some were not.

Methods used to ward off alien abductions were compiled in a book written by Ann Druffel (1998). She focused on first-hand accounts of individuals who believed they were *successful* in their efforts. When we reviewed these techniques, we found a striking degree of similarity with the methods described in the preceding text, even though many of the latter were described hundreds of years ago. In fact, four of her nine classes of techniques are represented in our preceding sections. Many of her "abductees" made direct reference to subjective feelings of paralysis at some point during the attempted abduction, and their techniques are briefly discussed below.

The first set of techniques (i.e., *mental struggle*) involved attempts to break off paralysis through forcing a small part of the body to move. When this occurred, the paralysis ended and the extraterrestrial visitors vanished. Second, *physical struggle* involved making defensive/offensive physical contact with aliens. This sometimes included the used of weapons. In two of Druffel's cases (viz., Morgana and Patsy), the act of touching, pushing, or throttling the alien menace resulted in dematerialization. A third set of techniques, the *appeal to spiritual personages*, consisted of seeking out the assistance of powerful gods/spirits through prayer or even just uttering a holy name. Interestingly, use of the Lord's Prayer was specifically mentioned, but spoken forward, not backward. Finally, the use of various *repellants* was described to be effective. Abductees utilized flowers, herbs, salt, iron bars, crucifixes, and magnets to repel alien attackers, and this is very consistent with earlier preventatives.

CONCLUSIONS

As can be seen from the above, people who were both temporally and geographically separated took sleep paralysis quite seriously. They viewed it to be a distressing/dangerous phenomenon that warranted the formulation of a number of preventative and defensive practices. Another observation we had when reviewing these techniques was that many of them may actually be helpful for sleep paralysis, but not necessarily in the way that the practitioners intended (viz. they may have had very different therapeutic actions in mind). Although many seem ineffective at best (e.g., throwing millet on the floor) and physically harmful at worst (e.g., rubbing ground reptile body parts into open wounds), some (e.g., changes in sleep position, attempts to move individual body parts) were oddly prescient, and likely helpful. Further, use of prayer during a scary hallucination (or any other relaxing or meditative technique) may help steady the sufferer, decrease autonomic arousal, and make the episode more tolerable. Attempting to "engage the hallucination" from a position of power may have a similar effect (see also suggested methods on "aliens" listed in LaVigne, 1995). Regardless, what is particularly striking is the repetition of techniques over huge spans of time and distance. The fact that the same techniques used by the ancients to ward off evil spirits (e.g., salt) are also used today to defend against technologically advanced aliens is a fascinating cultural artifact worthy of study in its own right beyond the present task of better understanding sleep paralysis.

REFERENCES

Davies, O. (2003). The nightmare experience, sleep paralysis and witchcraft accusations. *Folklore, 114*(2), 181.

Druffel, A. (1998). *How to defend yourself against alien abduction*. New York: Rivers Press.

Editors of Time-Life Books. (1988). *Mysteries of the unknown: Phantom encounters*. Alexandria, VA: Time-Life Books.

Firestone, M. (1985). The "old hag": Sleep paralysis in newfoundland. *Journal of Psychoanalytic Anthropology, 8*(1), 47–66.

Freud, S. (1913). The disposition to obsessional neurosis. In J. Strachey (Ed.), *The standard edition of the complete psychological works of Sigmund Freud volume XII* (J. Strachey Trans.). (pp. 67–102). London: Hogarth Press.

Golzari, S. E., Khodadoust, K., Alakbarli, F., Ghabili, K., Islambulchilar, Z., Shoja, M. M., et al. (2012). Sleep paralysis in medieval Persia—the hidayat of Akhawayni (?-983 AD). *Neuropsychiatric Disease and Treatment, 8*, 229–234. doi: 10.2147/NDT.S28231; 10.2147/NDT.S28231

Hinton, D. E., Pich, V., Chhean, D., & Pollack, M. H. (2005). The ghost pushes you down: Sleep paralysis-type panic attacks in a khmer refugee population. *Transcultural Psychiatry, 42*(1), 46–77. doi: 10.1177/1363461505050710

Hinton, D. E., Pich, V., Chhean, D., Pollack, M. H., & McNally, R. J. (2005). Sleep paralysis among cambodian refugees: Association with PTSD diagnosis and severity. *Depression and Anxiety, 22*(2), 47–51. doi: 10.1002/da.20084

Hufford, D. (1982). *The terror that comes in the night: An Experience-centered study of supernatural assault traditions*. Philadelphia, PA: University of Pennsylvania Press.

Jalal, B., Simons-Rudolph, J., Jalal, B., & Hinton, D. E. (2014). Explanations of sleep paralysis among egyptian college students and the general population in egypt and denmark. *Transcultural Psychiatry, 51*(2), 158–175. doi: 10.1177/13634615 13503378 [doi]

Jones, E. (1949). *On the nightmare* (2nd Impression ed.). London: Hogarth Press and the Institute of Psycho-analysis.

Kramer, H., & Sprenger, J. (1971). In Summers M. (Ed.), *The malleus maleficarum* (N. Summers Trans.). Mineola, NY: Dover Publications.

LaVigne, M. (1995). *The alien abduction survival guide*. Newberg, OR: Wildflower Press.

Law, S., & Kirmayer, L. J. (2005). Inuit interpretations of sleep paralysis. *Transcultural Psychiatry, 42*(1), 93–112. doi: 10.1177/1363461505050712

Ness, R. C. (1978). The old hag phenomenon as sleep paralysis: A biocultural interpretation. *Cultural, Medicine and Psychiatry, 2*, 15.

Ohaeri, J. U., Awadalla, V. A., Maknjuola, V. A., & Ohaeri, B. M. (2004). Features of isolated sleep paralysis among nigerians. *East African Medical Journal, 81*(10), 509–519.

Paradis, C. M., & Friedman, S. (2005). Sleep paralysis in african americans with panic disorder. *Transcultural Psychiatry, 42*(1), 123–134. doi: 10.1177/1363461505050720

Roberts, K. (1998). Contemporary cauchemar: Experience, belief, prevention. *Louisiana Folklore Miscellany, xiii*, 15–26.

Roscher, W. H. (2007). Ephialtes: A pathological-mythological treatis on the nightmare in classical antiquity. [Ephialtes] (A. V. O'Brien Trans.). (Revised ed., pp. 96–159). Putnam, CT: Spring Publishing.

Sharpless, B. A., & Grom, J. L. (in press). Isolated sleep paralysis: Fear, prevention, and disruption. *Behavioral Sleep Medicine.*

Summers, M. (1987). *The history of witchcraft* (First Thus ed.). NY: Dorset Press.

Summers, M. (1991). *The vampire.* New York, NY: Dorset Press.

CHAPTER 15

Psychosocial Approaches to the Treatment of Sleep Paralysis

Psychotherapeutic approaches for sleep paralysis are still in their infancy. We were unable to locate a single randomized clinical trial or published treatment manual. However, four separate psychosocial treatment approaches (viz., psychoanalysis, hypnosis, cognitive-behavioral therapy, and sleep hygiene) have been described. These are summarized as follows.

PSYCHOANALYSIS

Psychoanalysis, the oldest secular form of talk therapy, has not surprisingly tackled the phenomenon of Nightmare/sleep paralysis on several occasions (e.g., Jones, 1949). However, the majority of relevant literature was dedicated to *understanding* sleep paralysis and conceptualizing it in terms of the relevant psychodynamics (see chapter 10) as opposed to providing clear recommendations for treatment. Any discussion of treatment was a very rare occurrence, and we were only able to locate three case reports of outpatient psychoanalytic treatments. These were each described as successful (e.g., Payn, 1965; Van Der Heide & Weinberg, 1945), but no outcome data were provided, and the precise operationalization of "success" is somewhat opaque.

Few details were given about what actually transpired in session, and the reader is left to speculate on session content using the relevant author's specific case conceptualization and what is already known about general psychoanalytic approaches. This is obviously less than ideal. In general, we surmise that the analysts focused upon the specific *conflict* that they believed to be responsible for the manifest sleep paralysis symptom. Sleep paralysis, and especially the atonia of sleep paralysis, was thought to represent a *compromise* between an unacceptable wish/drive/desire becoming conscious/actually being acted upon and the forces of repression that were brought forth in order to stop this unacceptable action from taking place. Thus, in the manner of a typical psychoanalytic treatment, questions, clarifications, and confrontations were likely utilized by the therapist in order to pave the way for the use of dynamic interpretations (e.g., Langs, 1973). Interpretations are held by many analysts to be the most mutative of all therapeutic techniques because they have the most power to generate insight and remove repressions (e.g., Strachey, 1934). They link the manifest symptom (i.e., the paralysis) to the unconscious material responsible for the generation of the symptom. Thus, making the unconscious content conscious would presumably lead to a remission of the symptom and/or the ability to make better choices in relation to the formerly unacceptable wishes (e.g., Boswell et al., 2011). This has to be done with affective immediacy in order to be effective (as reviewed in Crits-Christoph, Connoly Gibblons, & Mukherjee, 2013). Again, as the case studies just described do not provide sufficient detail, our psychoanalytic treatment speculations must be viewed as tentative at best. We are also unaware of any more modern psychodynamic approaches to treating sleep paralysis, but provide some clinical suggestions in chapter 10.

HYPNOSIS

An Internet search of keywords "sleep paralysis" and "hypnosis" will yield a number of results related to treatment. However, the actual empirical literature on using hypnotic techniques to reduce sleep paralysis is quite sparse. In terms of *published* treatment articles, we were unable to locate more than one, and this article only documented the treatment of two individuals with sleep paralysis. Before proceeding to this, however, it may be useful to note that sleep paralysis and hypnotizability both appear to be risk factors for the development of anomalistic beliefs in general, but this combination may be more specifically responsible for the belief that one has been abducted by aliens (e.g., see Clancy, 2007). Indeed, many putative abductees seek out hypnotists directly as a means of "refreshing" their muddled memories of abduction events (McNally & Clancy, 2005). Thus, hypnosis may have a causative role in creating these anomalistic nocturnal experiences, but has been viewed as a means to a *cure*.

Nardi described the treatment of two individuals with sleep paralysis via hypnosis (Nardi, 1981). In the first case, involving a 25-year-old woman, the initial hypnotic induction was effected through progressive muscle relaxation combined with arm levitation, deep breathing, and counting backwards from 5 to 1. She was instructed to practice this twice daily and to refrain from "forcing" herself out of episodes should they occur. Instead, she was to take three deep breaths and purposefully engage in relaxation and to count herself out of the autohypnosis (and also the paralysis). She reported success when faced with subsequent episodes. In the second case, a 30-year-old woman, the hypnotic procedures were similar, but the patient already had experienced success using autohypnotic methods to ameliorate an airplane phobia. An application of these same techniques to sleep paralysis was again suggested, and this was reported to be successful. Interestingly, and in both cases, sleep paralysis did not remit with treatment, and the "success" referred to was a reduction in fear and anxiety during episodes. The cognitive appraisals of these women's episodes shifted from abject terror and threat to a sense of benign curiosity. One wonders, however, if this same outcome could be secured through non-hypnotic means. Clearly, a number of therapeutic modalities focus on challenging maladaptive appraisals of ambiguous phenomena, and we will now turn to one of these treatments: the cognitive-behavioral therapies.

COGNITIVE AND BEHAVIORAL THERAPIES

Some of the more well-described procedures for treating sleep paralysis derive from the behavioral and cognitive therapy traditions. These approaches are far-ranging, and often focus on very different aspects of human functioning. In general, both are intended to help patients better adapt to their surroundings. This is often done using classic and operant conditioning paradigms, especially in "purer" forms of behavior therapy (e.g., exposure-based treatments) and may include techniques to reduce anxiety and fear (e.g., progressive muscular relaxation; diaphragmatic breathing) and also limit the avoidance of feared situations (e.g., systematically exposing a patient to feared stimuli and surroundings). Thus, behavior therapists facilitate *approach* behaviors through strengthening competing responses (quiescent relaxation instead of anxiety). With the advent of Aaron Beck and Albert Ellis's cognitive therapies in the 1960s, techniques to identify, evaluate, challenge, and replace maladaptive thoughts became more prominent. For simplicity's sake, we will follow existing conventions and collapse these two modalities into the label of cognitive-behavioral therapy (CBT). Many treatment manuals have arisen from this tradition, and CBT can currently be applied to a wide range of psychiatric conditions (e.g., Allen, McHugh, & Barlow, 2008, Borkovec & Sharpless, 2004; Perlis, Jungquist, Smith, & Posner, 2005).

In our review we identified no randomized clinical trials of CBT specifically for sleep paralysis. Similarly, apart from our own CBT treatment manual (Appendix C), we are not aware of any published manuals that focus on sleep paralysis. However, descriptions of the successful application of CBT techniques and principals can be found in the literature, and these were important in the creation of our own approach. The most extensive of these are found in the work of Devon Hinton and colleagues (Hinton, Pich, Chhean, & Pollack, 2005a; Hinton, Pich, Chhean, Pollack, & McNally, 2005b).

As noted in previous chapters, Hinton worked with traumatized Cambodian refugees from the Khmer Rouge period. Extensive trauma histories were common in their samples, and these researchers often heard echoes of the trauma in the specific content of sleep paralysis hallucinations. Thus, treatment for these patients' sleep paralysis was conducted within the complicated contexts of comorbid post-traumatic stress and a very specific socio-historical context (Hinton et al., 2005a). Their approach began with questions relevant to sleep paralysis onset and symptoms, attempts at self-treatment, and other common pre-treatment inquiries. Next, attempts were made to decrease both sleep disturbances and anxiety symptoms, as both have been implicated in the onset of sleep paralysis (e.g., Stores, 1998).

As for dealing with sleep paralysis more directly, Hinton and colleagues recommended psychoeducation about the nature of attacks and decatastrophizing common thoughts (e.g., "I am having a heart attack;" "I will be paralyzed for life"). Work with any hallucinated threatening figures also took place, and appears to have been grounded in a real-world, trauma-based manner, attempting to make connections to actual events and working toward the development of a coherent narrative of these scary experiences (i.e., both real and imagined). Therapy also occasionally focused on ways to deal with post-sleep paralysis distress and autonomic arousal (e.g., breathing retraining, visualization). Other techniques were described, but these may be more relevant to this particular population of Cambodian sufferers (e.g., ways of dealing with fear of "sorcery assault"), and the interested reader is directed to the actual articles (i.e., Hinton et al., 2005a; Hinton et al., 2005b) for more details. Regardless, one can see in their approach many emblematic CBT procedures (psychoeducation, cognitive restructuring, and the reduction of physiological fear responses) that have demonstrated efficacy with other disorders. These techniques were noted to be effective.

Others have used overlapping CBT approaches. For instance, Ohaeri and colleagues also utilized psychoeducation in various forms. They specifically focused on letting patients know that supernatural attributions are common in sleep paralysis (Ohaeri, Adelekan, Odejide, & Ikuesan, 1992). These beliefs were pervasive in their Nigerian sample. This same research group also noted that increased arousal during episodes only makes matters worse, and encouraged their patients to 1) trust that the episodes would eventually abate, and 2) "will" themselves to stay calm. They also prescribed two hours of "even breathing" prior to their patients retiring to sleep. Stores' approach appears to be quite similar (Stores, 1998). As will be seen in Appendix C, we have borrowed liberally from these various thinkers' ideas as we developed our own CBT treatment approach for recurrent fearful isolated sleep paralysis.

Unfortunately, outcome data for CBT are quite limited. Hinton and colleagues reported some success with their approach. Paradis and colleagues provided some outcome data from their sample of patients with panic disorder (Paradis, Friedman, & Hatch, 1997). Specifically, 5 of 11 individuals who also suffered from sleep paralysis either experienced no sleep paralysis symptoms or went below diagnostic thresholds following a panic-focused treatment. These data are intriguing for a number of reasons. First, they may provide additional (indirect) evidence that specific pathological processes may be common between panic disorder and sleep paralysis (e.g., anxiety sensitivity and misinterpretation of bodily stimuli). Second, these results imply that it may be possible that a more "generic" CBT approach may help reduce sleep paralysis regardless of whether or not it is an actual focus of treatment (as is the case with remission of other disorders not targeted for treatment as in Borkovec, Abel, & Newman, 1995 and Brown, Antony, & Barlow, 1995). Third, this implies that significant reductions in sleep paralysis can occur even as a result of a short-term intervention. The latter two are particularly hopeful findings, as few practitioners at present are knowledgeable about this condition. It is also currently unknown how many individuals with sleep paralysis present for treatment solely with this complaint. However, we surmise that they are relatively few in number, as sleep paralysis does appear to be associated with higher levels of psychiatric comorbidity (Sharpless et al., 2010), and the other disorders are relatively better known.

SLEEP HYGIENE EDUCATION

We are also not aware of any studies on the efficacy or effectiveness of insomnia treatments for sleep paralysis. One review article on the treatment of parasomnias recommended the avoidance of sleep deprivation, but this is primarily based on the observation that sleep paralysis is more frequent in those who experience sleep disruption (e.g., those who have jet lag or those who engage in regular shift work), and not on any amount of outcome data (Attarian, 2010). Probably the easiest means to reduce sleep deprivation and insomnia is through sleep hygiene education.

For those unfamiliar with sleep hygiene education, it consists of a number of related interventions intended to improve sleep initiation and sleep maintenance. The intention is to therefore reduce sleep disruption and insomnia. It is not often utilized as a monotherapy, but is more typically used in conjunction with other techniques (e.g., sleep restriction and stimulus control in cognitive behavior therapy for insommia; e.g., Perlis, et al., 2005).

Sleep hygiene education is often conducted using handouts, but can also be done verbally in session. We have found that a specific conversation with patients about their idiosyncratic bedroom behaviors and surroundings allows for a far more thorough and patient-tailored intervention than more generic instructions and/or worksheets, although the latter can be helpful if patient contact time is an issue (e.g., short medical visits to a general practitioner). We provide some sleep hygiene education instructions in appendix C that may be particularly relevant to sleep paralysis but, in general, sleep hygiene education is fairly straightforward and intuitive. Examples of good instructions can be found in Perlis and colleagues' insomnia manual (i.e., Perlis et al., 2005, p. 18). Briefly, though, maintaining a comfortable bedroom temperature (i.e., not too hot or too cold), avoiding caffeine and/or alcohol in the evenings, and getting up the same time each day are common sleep hygiene components. These interventions are not only easy to implement, but also provide the individual with a greater sense of agency and feeling of control over their ability to sleep. Therefore, they can not only be effective but can help modify feelings of powerlessness in insomnia and other sleep disorders like sleep paralysis.

AN EMPIRICAL INVESTIGATION INTO THE UTILITY OF CONTEMPORARY FOLK TECHNIQUES

One study to date (Sharpless & Grom, in press) has assessed the self-reported effectiveness of techniques used to prevent and disrupt isolated sleep paralysis episodes. Although the sample consisted exclusively of relatively young undergraduates, it was clear that many found their experience to be troubling enough to make attempts at self-treatment. The techniques that they used and the frequencies for their effectiveness can both be found in Table 15.1. Interestingly, more individuals made attempts to *disrupt* episodes than they did to *prevent* them. The authors speculated that this may be due to the fact that sleep paralysis was a relatively infrequent occurrence for many of the subjects. This fact may make prevention efforts less effective than in more chronic cases. Regardless, the most effective of these techniques were incorporated into the treatment manual found in appendix C.

Table 15.1. FREQUENCIES OF TECHNIQUES USED
TO PREVENT AND DISRUPT ISOLATED SLEEP PARALYSIS
EPISODES AND THEIR OUTCOME

Strategy	Successful	Unsuccessful
Isolated Sleep Paralysis Prevention Strategies		
Change Sleep Position	6	1
Change Sleep Patterns	7	5
Relaxation Techniques	5	2
Change Diet	2	–
Eliminate Caffeine	1	–
Try to Stop Dreaming	2	–
Exercise	2	1
Avoid Stressful Topics	2	–
Consume Caffeine	–	1
Other	4	–
Isolated Sleep Paralysis Disruption Strategies		
Attempt to Move Extremities	18	12
Attempt to Move Other Body Parts	15	18
Calm Down	15	6
Attempting to Call Out	1	9
Change Sleeping State	9	8
Become Angry/Assertive	1	–
Engage Hallucination (i.e. talk to spirit)	–	1

NOTES: Table adapted from Sharpless & Grom (in press) and reprinted with permission from Taylor & Francis. *Changing Sleep Patterns* includes such techniques as: staying up late, eliminating naps, and attaining a more regulated sleep routine; *Stop Dreaming* includes not attempting to lucid dream and attempting to prevent dreams, *Relaxation* includes techniques such as drinking warm beverages, reading, praying, and meditating; *Other* includes: sleeping with a blanket, sleeping with a nightlight, purposefully thinking scary thoughts and noticing that "tunnel vision" was a prelude to ISP before going to sleep. *Move Other Body Parts* includes the mouth and torso; *Calm Down* includes use of reassuring self-talk, trying to "let go," regulate breathing, and the use of prayer during ISP to relax.

CONCLUSIONS

In summary, it is apparent that much more work needs to be done in the field of psychosocial interventions for sleep paralysis. Although there are certainly treatment options available (see also chapter 16), an empirical basis that could undergird an informed choice of treatment for any particular patient is sorely lacking. The practitioner who is interested in treating sleep paralysis should therefore maintain an attentive and flexible treatment stance, using the best available treatment principals and available theory in order to be maximally responsive to the patient. The treatment manual in appendix C represents an initial attempt to treat sleep paralysis using a cognitive-behavioral approach, and it is specifically based on what the empirical literature has elucidated about sleep paralysis so far. However, other reasonable psychosocial treatments could be derived from any number of other therapeutic traditions.

REFERENCES

Allen, L. B., McHugh, R. K., & Barlow, D. H. (2008). Emotional disorders: A unified protocol. In D. H. Barlow (Ed.), *Clinical handbook of psychological disorders: A step-by-step treatment manual* (4th ed., pp. 216–249). New York: Guilford Press.

Attarian, H. (2010). Treatment options for parasomnias. *Neurologic Clinics, 28*(4), 1089–1106.

Borkovec, T. D., Abel, J. L., & Newman, H. (1995). Effects of psychotherapy on comorbid conditions in generalized anxiety disorder. *Journal of Consulting and Clinical Psychology, 63*, 479–483.

Borkovec, T. D., & Sharpless, B. (2004). Generalized anxiety disorder: Bringing cognitive-behavioral therapy into the valued present. In S. Hayes, V. Follette, & M. Linehan's (Eds.), *Mindfulness and acceptance: Expanding the cognitive-behavioral tradition* (pp. 209–242). New York: Guilford Press.

Boswell, J. F., Sharpless, B. A., Greenberg, L. G., Heatherington, L., Huppert, J. D., Barber, J. P., Goldfried, M. R., & Castonguay, L. G. (2010). Schools of psychotherapy and the beginnings of a scientific approach. In D. H. Barlow's (Ed.), *The Oxford Handbook of Clinical Psychology* (pp. 98–127). New York: Oxford University Press.

Brown, T. A., Antony, M. M., & Barlow, D. H. (1995). Diagnostic comorbidity in panic disorder: Effect on treatment outcome and course of comorbid diagnoses following treatment. *Journal of Consulting and Clinical Psychology, 63*(408), 418.

Clancy, S. A. (2007). *Abducted: How people come to believe they were kidnapped by aliens.* Cambridge, MA: First Harvard University Press.

Crits-Christoph, P., Connoly Gibblons, M. B., & Mukherjee, D. (2013). Psychotherapy process outcome research. In M. J. Lambert (Ed.), *Bergin and garfield's handbook of psychotherapy and behavior change* (6th ed., pp. 298–340). Hoboken, NJ: Wiley.

Hinton, D. E., Pich, V., Chhean, D., & Pollack, M. H. (2005a). The ghost pushes you down: Sleep paralysis-type panic attacks in a Khmer refugee population. *Transcultural Psychiatry, 42*(1), 46–77. doi: 10.1177/1363461505050710

Hinton, D. E., Pich, V., Chhean, D., Pollack, M. H., & McNally, R. J. (2005b). Sleep paralysis among Cambodian refugees: Association with PTSD diagnosis and severity. *Depression and Anxiety, 22*(2), 47–51. doi: 10.1002/da.20084

Jones, E. (1949). *On the nightmare* (2nd Impression ed.). London, United Kingdom: Hogarth Press and the Institute of Psycho-analysis.

Langs, R. (1973). *The technique of psychoanalytic psychotherapy, volume 1.* New York: Jason Aronson.

McNally, R. J., & Clancy, S. A. (2005). Sleep paralysis, sexual abuse, and space alien abduction. *Transcultural Psychiatry, 42*(1), 113–122. doi: 10.1177/1363461505050715

Nardi, T. J. (1981). Treating sleep paralysis with hypnosis. *International Journal of Clinical and Experimental Hypnosis, 29*(4), 358–365. doi: 10.1080/00207148108409169

Ohaeri, J. U., Adelekan, M. F., Odejide, A. O., & Ikuesan, B. A. (1992). The pattern of isolated sleep paralysis among nigerian nursing students. *Journal of the National Medical Association, 84*(1), 67–70.

Paradis, C. M., Friedman, S., & Hatch, M. (1997). Isolated sleep paralysis in african americans with panic disorder. *Cultural Diversity and Mental Health, 3*(1), 69–76. doi: 10.1037/1099-9809.3.1.69

Payn, S. B. (1965). A psychoanalytic approach to sleep paralysis. *Journal of Nervous and Mental Disease, 140*(6), 427–433. doi: 10.1097/00005053-196506000-00005

Perlis, M. L., Jungquist, C., Smith, M. T., & Posner, D. (2005). *Cognitive behavioral treatment of insomnia: A session-by-session guide.* New York: Springer Science + Business Media, LLC.

Sharpless, B. A., & Grom, J. L. (in press). Isolated sleep paralysis: Fear, prevention, and disruption. *Behavioral Sleep Medicine.*

Sharpless, B. A., McCarthy, K. S., Chambless, D. L., Milrod, B. L., Khalsa, S., & Barber, J. P. (2010). Isolated sleep paralysis and fearful isolated sleep paralysis in outpatients with panic attacks. *Journal of Clinical Psychology, 66*(12), 1292–1306. doi: 10.1002/jclp.20724

Stores, G. (1998). Sleep paralysis and hallucinosis. *Behavioural Neurology, 11*(2), 109–112.

Strachey, J. (1934). The nature of the therapeutic action of psychoanalysis. *The International Journal of Psychoanalysis, 15*, 127–159.

Van Der Heide, C., & Weinberg, J. (1945). Sleep paralysis and combat fatigue. *Psychosomatic Medicine, 7*, 330–334.

CHAPTER 16

Psychopharmacology for Sleep Paralysis

Although sleep paralysis is a common phenomenon, it is likely that those who experience it rarely present to the medical profession for management of sleep paralysis alone. As noted in our prior discussions, most individuals regard it as a strange, and occasionally troublesome, human experience. Nevertheless, sleep paralysis has been the subject of clinical management when it occurs in the context of other disorders; the only such disorders described in the literature we have reviewed include recurrent isolated sleep paralysis and narcolepsy. In this chapter, we therefore discuss the evidence available for the psychopharmacology of sleep paralysis in the context of each of these disorders. It should be noted that no pharmacological agents are currently approved by the United States Food and Drug Administration (FDA) for the treatment of sleep paralysis or recurrent isolated sleep paralysis.

RECURRENT ISOLATED SLEEP PARALYSIS

A single case report suggests the utility of fluoxetine 40 mg in a case of sleep paralysis (Koran & Raghavan, 1993). The patient had been previously treated with maprotiline 150 mg daily, yet was experiencing one to two episodes weekly. Although the diagnosis is noted to be "isolated sleep paralysis," the patient also described a history of obsessive compulsive disorder. Following treatment with fluoxetine 60 mg for two weeks, her sleep paralysis and hypnogenic hallucinations immediately ceased. During the next 20 months, she took 60 to 80mg of fluoxetine qd and had no episodes of sleep paralysis or hypnagogic hallucination. Due to hypomania, the dose was adjusted downwards to 40 mg daily, with a dissipation of sleep paralysis for the ensuing 4 months.

NARCOLEPSY

Daytime symptoms such as excessive daytime sleepiness and cataplexy are typically the focus of treatment in narcolepsy, each usually requiring separate pharmacological strategies, although some agents address both symptoms. Pharmacological studies of narcolepsy have also focused on these two symptoms, and hypnagogic hallucinations (HH), sleep paralysis, and disrupted nocturnal sleep have generally been ignored as primary outcome measures. In addition, since HH, sleep paralysis, and cataplexy have been regarded as being REM-related phenomena, their treatment has been assumed to be the same as that of cataplexy. Clinical wisdom suggests that improvement in cataplexy is associated with a concomitant reduction in both HH and sleep paralysis, yet this has not been empirically demonstrated. The most recent American Academy of Sleep Medicine practice parameters statement on this matter noted that all the narcolepsy symptoms noted here should be addressed when they are present and troublesome in patients with narcolepsy (Morgenthaler et al., 2007). However, the highest level of recommendation that it provided for any pharmacological agent in the treatment of sleep paralysis was that of an "option." In other words, it is "a patient-care strategy that reflects uncertain clinical use. The term option implies either inconclusive or conflicting evidence or conflicting expert opinion" (p. 1706).

Sodium Oxybate

Pharmacological therapies for cataplexy are listed in Table 16.1. A randomized, double-blind, placebo-controlled study of sodium oxybate (gamma hydroxybutyrare, GHB) did not reveal differences in incidence of HH and sleep paralysis when compared with placebo, yet the primary outcome measure in that study was the incidence of cataplexy and the study was not powered to detect differences in HH or sleep paralysis. A randomized, double blind, placebo-controlled multicenter trial comparing the effects of three doses of orally administered sodium oxybate with placebo for the treatment of narcolepsy (U.S. Xyrem Multicenter Study Group, 2002). In contrast, in an uncontrolled, pilot study of 21 narcolepsy patients with nightly doses of sodium oxybate, most patients reported a

Table 16.1. PHARMACOLOGICAL THERAPIES
FOR CATAPLEXY*

Medication	Daily dose
Sodium oxybate (GHB)	6–9 g (divided in two doses)
Venlafaxine	75–300 mg
Fluoxetine	20–60 mg
Viloxazine	50–200 mg
Protriptyline	2.5–20 mg
Imipramine	25–200 mg
Clomipramine	25–200 mg
Desipramine	25–200 mg

*Only sodium oxybate is FDA-approved for the management of cataplexy in the context of narcolepsy
Note: Adapted from Guilleminault, C., & Cao, M. (2011). Narcolepsy: Diagnosis and management. In M. Kryger, T. Roth & W. C. Dement (Eds.), *Principles and practice of sleep medicine* (5th ed.). Philadelphia: Elsevier Saunders.

decrease in sleep paralysis and HH when compared with baseline, and this effect appeared to increase with increasing doses of sodium oxybate from 4.5 to 9 g (Mamelak, Black, Montplaisir, & Ristanovic, 2004).

Antidepressant Agents

Tricyclic antidepressants, which suppress REM sleep, have historically been utilized for the treatment of ancillary symptoms of narcolepsy. In an uncontrolled study utilizing imipramine and desipramine at variable doses ranging from 25 to 150 mg, Hishikawa, Ida, Nakai, and Kaneko (1966) reported that 9 out of 11 patients treated with desmethylimipramine, and 7 out of 8 patients with imipramine, achieved remission, yet outcome measures were not clearly defined. Similar results were obtained for HH and cataplexy. In another uncontrolled case series utilizing clomipramine hydrochloride, Guilleminault, Raynal, Takahashi, Carskadon, and Dement (1976) reported that 7 of the 11 patients, sleep paralysis was completely eliminated under clomipramine and in the others, reports of sleep parlaysis were reduced. No effects on HH were noted.

A randomized, double-blind cross-over trial evaluated the efficacy of femoxetine 600 mg for accessory narcolepsy symptoms (Schrader, Kayed, Bendixen Markset, & Treidene, 1986). Femoxetine, related to paroxetine, is a selective serotonin reuptake inhibitor (SSRI) that is not available in the United States, and has been utilized for the treatment of depression in

Europe (Lund, Christensen, Bechgaard, Molander, & Larsson, 1979). The study should be considered to be preliminary in nature because it included only 10 patients with narcolepsy. In comparison with placebo, femoxetine treatment resulted in a decrease in severity and frequency of cataplectic attacks. It also resulted in fewer episodes of sleep paralysis (mean values not provided), yet no effects on HH were noted. Famoxetine was also associated with a decrease in the total time spent in REM sleep.

The 2007 American Academy of Sleep Medicine practice parameters statement on the pharmacological management of narcolepsy noted that tricyclic antidepressants, SSRIs, and venlafaxine may be effective treatment for treatment of sleep paralysis and hypnagogic hallucinations, yet it noted that this recommendation is based on anectodal experience of committee members, and suggested the use of these agents when the benefits of treatment outweigh the risks (Morgenthaler et al., 2007).

SUMMARY

As is evident from the previous discussion, there are no well-established pharmacological treatments for sleep paralysis, and all the evidence available thus far is in the form of anecdotal clinical experience and anecdotal reports, uncontrolled case series, and randomized/controlled studies with methodological problems. Nevertheless, like cataplexy, sleep paralysis is regarded as a product of the dysregulation of REM sleep timing and consolidation leading, in the case of sleep paralysis, to the occurrence of muscle atonia at sleep onset or offset (see chapter 10). Inhibitory pathways involving the lower motor neurons during REM involve muscarinic cholinergic and noradrenergic systems, and many of the available antidepressants act at these receptors and are, therefore, potentially useful for the management of sleep paralysis. Another possible consideration is GHB, whose mechanism in the treatment of cataplexy is unknown.

TREATMENT CONSIDERATIONS

Although sleep paralysis can occur in isolation, individuals with sleep paralysis rarely present for treatment when this is their sole clinical complaint. Rather, in clinical settings, sleep paralysis almost always occurs in the context of other conditions. Therefore, the first step in its management involves the performance of a comprehensive clinical evaluation, with the objective of identifying, and providing specific management for, the comorbid medical or psychiatric condition. The procedures involved in the evaluation of sleep-related complaints are beyond the scope of this book. However, readers are encouraged to review other publications in this area (Doghramji, Grewal, & Markov, 2009; Doghramji & Choufani, 2010). Some examples of individualized treatments for sleep paralysis are:

(1) A 40-year-old obese man who experiences sleep paralysis once a week, who also snores and wakes up intermittently from sleep with a sense of gasping and choking, is diagnosed with severe obstructive sleep apnea syndrome following sleep laboratory testing, and proceeds to be treated with a continuous positive airway pressure device.

(2) A 27-year-old night watchman who works five nights per week, sleeping 8 a.m. to 1 p.m. on ensuing days, and who is in bed 11 p.m. to 7 a.m. on days off, complains of sleepiness while on the job at night and insomnia after returning home from work; he also experiences sleep paralysis along with vivid visual hallucinations during daytime sleep episodes. He is diagnosed with shift work disorder and is managed with melatonin 1 mg at bedtime, counseled to wear sunglasses during the commute home, advised to purchase dark shades for his bedroom, and is recommended bright light therapy after awakening from daytime sleep. He is also advised to take brief naps during night work.

(3) A 21-year-old college student is brought in for medical attention by her parents, who complain that their daughter has been falling asleep in class over the past year, has been taking prolonged naps after returning home from school, and has had a notable decrement in grades. During the interview, she complains of a "sagging feeling" in her legs when she laughs, and repeated episodes of vivid, frightening dreams, during which her body feels "stuck" during sleep. She is managed with a combination of judicious naps and longer sleep hours at night, and eventually treated with modafinil for sleepiness and venlafaxine for REM-related symptoms of cataplexy, sleep paralysis, and hypnagogic hallucinations.

(4) A 62-year-old attorney presents with the complaint of shallow and interrupted sleep following sleep onset, followed by daytime fatigue. He dreams actively all night long and has intermittent episodes of sleep paralysis, during which his dreams are particularly distressing. During nocturnal awakenings, his mind "spins." Symptoms began more than 15 years ago and were managed by multiple antidepressants in the past, none of which were particularly helpful, along with various benzodiazepine hypnotic agents for insomnia. His most recent treatment regimen is alprazolam 0.5 mg at bedtime. He has

a history of hyperlipidemia, and consumes five caffeine-containing beverages per day, the last one being consumed at dinnertime, followed by three to four alcoholic beverages nightly. He is managed by a gradual withdrawal of caffeine and alcohol, and the initiation of cognitive behavioral therapy.

These examples should not be considered to be an exhaustive list of treatment options, whose number is as abundant as the types of conditions encountered. Nevertheless, pharmacological treatment directed at sleep paralysis may be appropriate if the definitive management of the comorbid condition does not produce a successful resolution of sleep paralysis. Even in such a situation, however, direct pharmacological treatment of sleep paralysis should be considered in the context of the degree to which it affects patients' quality of sleep and wakefulness, or the extent to which it causes distress or impairment in functioning. Mild, infrequent sleep paralysis that is not associated with insomnia or daytime impairment cannot justify lifelong treatment with pharmacological agents.

TENTATIVE TREATMENT GUIDELINES

Once the decision has been made to utilize a pharmacological agent, the following selected factors may help guide clinicians in the choice of an appropriate agent for clinically significant manifestations of sleep paralysis (Laurence, 2006).

(1) Side effect profile. Older agents, such as the tricyclic antidepressants, generally have a wider array of side effects and may be best avoided in favor of the newer SSRIs and SNRIs, especially in medically vulnerable populations such as the elderly and individuals with multiple medical comorbidities.
(2) Cost
(3) Time of administration
   (i) Morning administration is preferred for activating antidepressants such as venlafaxine and protriptyline
   (ii) Bedtime administration is warranted for sodium oxybate and potentially sedating antidepressants such as imipramine and clomipramine
(4) History of substance use and abuse contraindicates the use of sodium oxybate and other controlled substances.

REFERENCES

Doghramji, K., & Choufani, D. (2010). Taking a sleep history. In J. Winkelman, & D. Plante (Eds.), *Foundations of psychiatric sleep medicine* (pp. 95–110). Cambridge, MA: Cambridge University Press.

Doghramji, K., Grewal, R., & Markov, D. (2009). Evaluation and management of insomnia in the psychiatric setting. *Focus, 8*(4), 441–454.

Guilleminault, C., Raynal, D., Takahashi, S., Carskadon, M., & Dement, W. (1976). Evaluation of short-term and long-term treatment of the narcolepsy syndrome with clomipramine hydrochloride. *Acta Neurologica Scandinavica, 54*(1), 71–87.

Hishikawa, Y., Ida, H., Nakai, K., & Kaneko, Z. (1966). Treatment of narcolepsy with imipramine (tofranil) and desmethylimipramine (pertofran). *Journal of the Neurological Sciences, 3*(5), 453–461.

Koran, L. M., & Raghavan, S. (1993). Fluoxetine for isolated sleep paralysis. *Psychosomatics: Journal of Consultation Liaison Psychiatry, 34*(2), 184–187. doi: 10.1016/S0033-3182(93)71913-1

Laurence, L. B. (Ed.). (2006). *Goodman & Gilman's the pharmacological basis of therapeutics* (11th ed.). New York: The McGraw-Hill Companies.

Lund, J., Christensen, J. A., Bechgaard, E., Molander, L., & Larsson, H. (1979). Pharmacokinetics of femoxetine in man. *Acta Pharmacologica Et Toxicologica, 44*(3), 177–184.

Mamelak, M., Black, J., Montplaisir, J., & Ristanovic, R. (2004). A pilot study on the effects of sodium oxybate on sleep architecture and daytime alertness in narcolepsy. *Sleep, 27*(7), 1327–1334.

Morgenthaler, T. I., Kapur, V. K., Brown, T., Swick, T. J., Alessi, C., Aurora, R. N., et al. (2007). Practice parameters for the treatment of narcolepsy and other hypersomnias of central origin an american academy of sleep medicine report: An american academy of sleep medicine report. *Sleep, 30*(12), 1705.

U.S. Xyrem Multicenter Study Group. (2002). A randomized, double blind, placebo-controlled multicenter trial comparing the effects of three doses of orally administered sodium oxybate with placebo for the treatment of narcolepsy. *Sleep, 25*(1), 42–49.

Schrader, H., Kayed, K., Bendixen Markset, A. C., & Treidene, H. E. (1986). The treatment of accessory symptoms in narcolepsy: A double-blind cross-over study of a selective serotonin re-uptake inhibitor (femoxetine) versus placebo. *Acta Neurologica Scandinavica, 74*(4), 297–303.

CHAPTER 17

Conclusions and Future Directions

Through the course of this book we have attempted to usefully synthesize the various literatures relevant to sleep paralysis and isolated sleep paralysis. We hope that a compelling case has been made not only for the importance of these phenomena, but also for the need to devote additional research and clinical resources to *better understanding* these phenomena. Although we have already provided suggestions for future work in preceding chapters, we summarize the main ones below.

(1) More frequent and systematic assessment/diagnosis of sleep paralysis is needed. At present, accurate prevalence rates for isolated sleep paralysis are not available due to heterogeneity among assessment instruments and a lack of consideration for differential diagnosis (see chapters 7 and 13).

(2) The relationships between the various forms of sleep paralysis (e.g., isolated, recurrent, fearful) and other medical and psychiatric conditions should be more clearly established (see chapters 8 and 9).

(3) The range and extent of clinically-significant distress and interference as a result of sleep paralysis should be clarified. This will inform both treatment selection and the creation of accurate and usable diagnostic thresholds (see chapters 6 and 11).

(4) Along with our initial attempt at a treatment (i.e., CBT-ISP as described in appendix C) and medication recommendations (chapter 16), more treatment options for chronic and severe cases of sleep paralysis are needed. Although randomized controlled trials are often thought to provide the most compelling evidence of efficacy, open trials and even intensive case studies can provide useful clinical guidance. When

testing new psychological approaches, accurate treatment integrity must be ensured through the use of adherence measures (e.g., appendix D) and independent raters (see also Perepletchkova & Kazdin, 2005; Sharpless & Barber, 2009 for additional suggestions).

(5) Sleep paralysis could potentially be a vehicle through which researchers explore the causal links between strange psychological/medical phenomena and an individual's anomalous beliefs (e.g., chapters 3, 5, and 14). The causal links between anomalous beliefs and anomalous experiences have yet to be established. Clearly, it could be a non-linear reciprocal process, but this is not yet known.

(6) Finally, sleep paralysis hallucinations could provide interesting information about cultural, geographical, and temporal differences between groups of people. As discussed in chapter 2, culturally consistent sleep paralysis hallucinations could convey important information about that culture, and even be considered cultural artifacts. Such explorations could yield information about particular desires and fears that might not be manifested in other ways or directly articulated.

CODA

The process of writing this book was interesting on a number of levels. The initial intention was to compile information relevant for researchers and clinicians. We therefore began reviewing the psychological, psychiatric, and neurological sources we were most familiar with. Very early in the process of gathering sources, however, we were taken aback by the sheer number of references that were fascinating. We ultimately decided to include this material in the chapters of this work. These sources ranged from ancient medicine, philosophy, and the fine arts to folklore, mythology, and even medieval manuals on witches and witchcraft. The consistency of the *universal* characteristics of sleep paralysis (e.g., atonia and hallucinations) in combination with more idiosyncratic interpretations across time and place (individual and cultural variability) was striking on multiple levels (see also appendix A). We hope we have convinced the reader that sleep paralysis is not only intrinsically interesting and possessing of clinical relevance, but that it also has a high degree of intellectual and cultural importance. We believe that this importance holds regardless of whether it is viewed through the lenses of history, folklore, psychology, or medicine.

In closing, we also wonder what new insights could be gained through the intensive and multidisciplinary study of *other phenomena* relevant to mental health. It is unfortunately becoming increasingly easy to live solely within the boundaries of ones' own limited areas of expertise and favorite journals (i.e., being what Nietzsche would term a "nook-dweller" [1966, p. 122]). However, reading the works of these other disciplines was not only interesting and helped to broaden our perspectives on sleep paralysis, but also led us to consider new ideas for research and treatment that might not have been otherwise apparent.

REFERENCES

Nietzsche, F.W. (1966). In W. Kaufman's (Ed. and Trans.), *Beyond good and evil: Prelude to a philosophy of the future.* NY: Vintage Books.

Perepletchkova, F., & Kazdin, A. E. (2005). Treatment integrity and therapeutic change: Issues and research recommendations. *Clinical Psychology: Science and Practice, 12,* 365–383.

Sharpless, B. A., & Barber, J. P. (2009). A conceptual and empirical review of the meaning, measurement, development, and teaching of intervention competence in clinical psychology. *Clinical Psychology Review, 29*(1), 47–56. doi: 10.1016/j.cpr.2008.09.008

APPENDIX A

Terms for Sleep Paralysis

Country/Culture/ Language	Sleep Paralysis Term	Translation	Source
Botswana	*sebeteledi*	Someone who exerts pressure/force	Mdlalani, 2009
Botswana	*setshitshama*	That which paralyses	Mdlalani, 2009
Cambodia	*khmaoch sangkat*	Ghost that pushes you down	Hinton, Pich, Chhean, & Pollack, 2005
China	*bei guai chaak*	Being pressed by the ghost	Hufford, 2005; Wing, Lee, & Chen, 1994
China	*E-meng*	"Dream of surprise" thought to closely resemble sleep paralysis	Wing et al., 1994
China	*guǐ yā chuáng*	Ghost oppression	Awadalla et al., 2004; Wing et al., 1994
China	*bèi guǐ yā*	Held by the ghost	Wing et al., 1994
Croatia, Republic of	*morica*	Nightmare	Davies, 2003
Czech Republic	*Muera*	Night-mare	Adler, 2011; Cheyne, Rueffer, & Newby-Clark, 1999
Egypt	*al-Jathoom*	From *yajthum*—sits	Adler, 2011
England—Old English	*maere or mare*	From Anglo Saxon word *Merran* = "to crush"	Cheyne et al., 1999; D. J. Hufford, 2005
England—Old English	*hagge*	A woman supposed to have dealings with Satan and the infernal world	Cheyne et al., 1999

(continued)

Country/Culture/ Language	Sleep Paralysis Term	Translation	Source
English medical literature	night palsy	A temporary numbness and paresis of an extremity caused by its compression during sleep	de Jong, 2005
English medical literature	delayed psychomotor awakening	Other term for sleep paralysis	Goode, 1962
English medical literature	cataplexy of awakening	Other term for sleep paralysis	Goode, 1962
English medical literature	post-dormital chalastic fits	Other term for sleep paralysis	Goode, 1962
England (12th Century Latin text	*intolerabili phantasia vexari*	Nightmare experience (attributed to a demon)	Davies, 2003
England (12th Century Latin text	*in somnis oppressus*	Crushed in dreams (by a demon)	Davies, 2003
England (14th Century)	night-mare	Night mare who lays on top of people at night	Davies, 2003
England (Cornwall)	*Hilla*	A large hairy thing that lays upon you with dead weight and almost stops your breathing	Davies, 2003
England	Stand Stills	Condition resulting from the spirit leaving the body when asleep and not returning upon awakening	Dahlitz & Parkes, 1993
England	Wizard-pressing	Other term for sleep paralysis	Bond, 1753
England	Witch-riding	Other term for sleep paralysis	Bond, 1753
Estonia	*luupainaja*	The one who presses your bones	Davies, 2003

Country/Culture/ Language	Sleep Paralysis Term	Translation	Source
Ethiopia	dukak	Evil spirit (or devil) who disrupts sleep and threatens individuals, and/or causes nightmares; his presence is associated with withdrawal from khat (a native plant with stimulant properties).	Berhanu, Go, Ruff, Celentano, & Bishaw, 2012
Finland	painajainen	From paniaa "to press or apply pressure"; something weighing on you	Davies, 2003; Kuhn & Reidy, 1975
Finland	unihalvaus	Sleep paralysis	Google translate
France	appesart	Derived from the verb peser, meaning "to press down upon"	Davies, 2003
France	cauchemar (macouche, couchemache, couchemal)	From caucher "to tread on"	Adler, 2011; Cheyne et al., 1999; Roberts, 1998
France—Older Medical Literature	crise de l'etat de veille	Crisis of the waking state	de Jong, 2005
German medical Literature	verzochertes psychomotorisches Erwachen	Delayed psychomotor awakening	de Jong, 2005
Germany	Alpendrücken	Alps press	de Jong, 2005
Germany	alpdrück	Elf pressure	Cheyne et al., 1999
Germany	hexendrücken	Witch pressing	Cheyne et al., 1999
Germany	Mar	To crush/male love phantom	Roscher, 2007
Germany	Mare	Female love phantom	Roscher, 2007
Germany	Mahr	Mare	Cheyne et al., 1999
Germany	nachtmahr	Old German word for nightmare	Adler, 2011
Greece	ephialtes	Hurricane, nightmare, or something thrown on you, throttling demon, ἐφάλλομαι (to spring upon)	Haga, 1989

(Continued)

Country/Culture/ Language	Sleep Paralysis Term	Translation	Source
Greece	mora/Μορμώ	Monster, ogre, spirit, old lady wearing black	Cheyne et al., 1999
Greece	pan-ephialtes	Pan who leaps upon you	Cheyne et al., 1999
Greece	Graiae/graia	Monster, ogre, spirit	Cheyne et al., 1999
Greece	pnigaleon/pgnalion	Suffocation/throttle	Aegineta, 1844; Aurelianus, 1950; Roscher, 2007
Greece	epofeles	Something climbing over one and settling upon ones chest	Stol, 1993
Guinean Fulani	kibo kibongal	Someone that strangles you	de Jong, 2005
Hawaii	Hauka'I po	Night marchers—ancient warriors believed to rise from the ground and avenge their death; often associated with heavy footsteps	Conesa, 2000
Holland	nachtmerrie	Nightmare	Davies, 2003
Hungary	lidercnyomas	Derived from nyomas—"pressing"	Davies, 2003
Hungary	boszorkany-nyomas	Witches' pressure	Davies, 2003
Hungary	lidérc	Pressing entity that often took the form of a chicken; this was sometimes a witch's familiar	Davies, 2003
Iceland	matrod	From "troda"—to press, squeeze, ride	Haga, 1989
Indonesia	dicekek	Choked or strangled	Grayman, Good, & Good, 2009
Indonesia	digeunton	Pressed on	Grayman et al., 2009
Indonesia	tindihan	Someone's weight on top of you	Conesa, 2000

Country/Culture/ Language	Sleep Paralysis Term	Translation	Source
Inuit	uquamairineq	Condition described as "hypnotic states, disturbed sleep, sleep paralysis, dissociative episodes and occasional hallucinations"	Tarnovetskaia & Cook, 2008
Inuit	uqumangirniq or Aqtuqsittiq	Paralysis resulting from attack by shamans, devils, or malevolent spirits	Law & Kirmayer, 2005
Iran	bakhtak	A type of jinn that sits on the dreamer's chest, making breathing harder and movement difficult or impossible	Druffel, 1998
Ireland	tromlui; tromlaige	Being pressed upon, often experienced as a large bird	Adler, 2011; Davies, 2003
Ireland— Old Irish	Mar/More	Nightmare	Cheyne et al., 1999
Islam	Jinn (Al-Jin)	Creatures existing in a realm between humans and angels, capable of human possession and suppressing movement and breathing when one awakes in the night	Druffel, 1998; Jalal, Simons-Rudolph, Jalal, & Hinton, 2014
Italy	Incubo	Nightmare; to lie upon	Adler, 2011
Italy	pesuarole	From pesante = "weight"	Adler, 2011
Japan	kanashibari	Bound or fastened by metal	Arikawa, Templer, Brown, Cannon, & Thomas-Dodson, 1999
Korea	ka-wi-nulita	Scissors pressed	Firestone, 1985
Kurdistan	mottaka	Ghost/evil spirit that suffocates people during the night	Lockwood, 2010

(Continued)

Country/Culture/ Language	Sleep Paralysis Term	Translation	Source
Laos	tsog tsuam	To crush, press, or smother	Adler, 1991; Adler, 2011
Laos	dab tsog	Nighttime phantom that robs you of your breath	Adler, 1991; Adler, 2011
Laos	poj ntxoog	Pressing spirits	Adler, 2011
Malaysia	kena tindih/ kentindihan	Being pressed	Lockwood, 2010
Malta	Haddiela	Attack by Hares, the wife of a poltergeist-like spiritual entity	Lockwood, 2010
Mexico	se me subio el muerto	A dead body climbed on top of me.	Jimenez-Genchi, Avila-Rodriguez, Sanchez-Rojas, Terrez, & Nenclares-Portocarrero, 2009
Mexico— Tzintzuntzenos	pesadilla	Derived from the verb peser, meaning "to press down upon"	Adler, 2011; Simard & Nielsen, 2005
Morocco—Arabic	boratat	Someone who pressures you	de Jong, 2005
Netherlands	nachtmerrie	Nightmare	Davies, 2003
Neuchâtel	tchutch-muton	Nightmare causing fairy that appears in the guise of a black sheep	Davies, 2003
Newfoundland	old hag	Witch	Friedman & Paradis, 2002; Ness, 1978
Newfoundland	ag grog or ag rog	Hag-ridden	Friedman & Paradis, 2002; Ness, 1978
New Guinea	suk ninmyo	Sacred tree of life—eats the human spirit at night so as not to disturb people in the daytime. The person being eaten is often awakened and paralyzed.	Lockwood, 2010
Nigeria—Yoruba	Ogun Oru	Demonic infiltration of the body and psyche during dreaming.	Aina & Famuyiwa, 2007

Country/Culture/ Language	Sleep Paralysis Term	Translation	Source
Nigeria/Christian Faith Healers	oppression	Other term for sleep paralysis	Awadalla et al., 2004
Norway	mareritt	Mare-ridden	Davies, 2003
Norway (old Norse)	Mara	A supernatural being usually female who lay on people's chest at night, suffocating them	Davies, 2003
Norway	Svartalfar	Black elves who paralyzed their victims with arrows (elf shot), sat on their chest, and whispered horrible things to them	Hurd, 2011
Persia, Medieval	kabus	Incubus/Nightmare	Golzari et al., 2012
Philippines	bangungut	"To rise and moan in sleep" (aftereffects of a nightmare similar to SP, also possibly related to sudden and unexplained death in sleep)	Munger & Booton, 1998
Poland (sandomier forest dwellers)	Vjek	Old man	Roscher, 2007
Poland (sandomier forest dwellers)	Gnotek	Small oppressor	Roscher, 2007
Poland	zmora	Ghoulish entity, bedroom visitor; people who are able to disturb their neighbor's sleep by making them feel an enormous weight resting on their body	Cheyne et al., 1999; Davies, 2003
Poland	strzyga	From latin striga— associated with dead people's souls	Davies, 2003
Portugal	pesadelo	From pesado = "heavy"	de Jong, 2005
Roman Italy	lamia	Demon who eats children	Cheyne et al., 1999

(Continued)

Country/Culture/ Language	Sleep Paralysis Term	Translation	Source
Roman Italy	incubus/succubus	One who presses or crushes— nocturnally- assaulting spirit/ demon	Cheyne et al., 1999
Roman Italy	ephialtes (described by Galen)	Nightmare	Davies, 2003
Russia	kikimora (кукúмора)	A legendary creature; a female house spirit	Cheyne et al., 1999
Scandinavia— Old Norse	mara	Nightmare	Cheyne et al., 1999
Serbia	mòre	Nightmare	Davies, 2003
Serbia	nocna mora	Nighttime incubus	Ignjatic et al., 2002
Serbia	zao duh	Incubus	Ignjatic et al., 2002
Slav	Murawa	Nightmare witch	Roscher, 2007
Slav	Pschezolnica	Female spirit	Roscher, 2007
Southeast Asia	dab tsog	Sudden unexpected nocturnal death syndrome	Adler, 2011; Hufford, 2005
Southern Africa— Tswana-speaking	tokoloshis	Spirits of ancestors	Gangdev, 2004
Spain	pesadilla	Derived from the verb peser, meaning "to press down upon"	Cheyne et al., 1999
Spain (Catalan)	pesanta	Enormous dog or cat that goes into people's houses and sits on their chest	Lockwood, 2010
Sri Lanka	amuku be or amuku pei	Ghost that forces you down	Lockwood, 2010
Sweden	mara	Anglo-Saxon and Old Norse term for a demon that sat on sleepers' chests, causing them to have bad dreams	Hufford, 2005
Thailand	phi um	Ghost covered	Firestone, 1985
Thailand	phi khau	Ghost possessed	Firestone, 1985
Turkey	karabasan	Dark presser/black buster	Adler, 2011; Ronnevig, 2007

Country/Culture/ Language	Sleep Paralysis Term	Translation	Source
Uganda (Syan tribe)	emisambwa	Spirits of the dead responsible for pressuring and throttling sleepers	Davies, 2003; Huntingford, 1928
United States	shadow people	Paranormal (perhaps transdimensional) entities that one generally sees at night in their peripheral vision	Vila-Rodriguez, MacEwan, & Honer, 2011
United States (Southern Black)	Ridden by the witch		Hufford, 1982
Vietnam	ma dè	Held down by a ghost	Lockwood, 2010
Vietnam	bóng dè	Held down by a shadow	Lockwood, 2010
Wales	gwrach-y-rhibyn	Dribbling hag; hag of the mist	Editors of Time-Life Books, 1988
West Indies	kokma	Spirit of a dead baby that jumps on the chest	Davies, 2003; Friedman & Paradis, 2002; Ness, 1978; Nickell, 1995
Zanzibar	popabawa	Bat wing—the dark shadow cast when the bat attacks.	Blackmore, 1998; Nickell, 1995; Walsh, 2009
Zimbabwe (Shona)	madzikirira	Witch pressing one down	Lockwood, 2010

Note: Adapted from Adler, S. (2011). Sleep paralysis: Night-mares, nocebos, and the mind-body connection. Newark, NJ: Rutgers University Press.

REFERENCES

Adler, S. (1991). Sudden unexpected nocturnal death syndrome among Hmong immigrants: Examining the role of the "nightmare." The Journal of American Folklore, 104, 54–71. doi: 10.2307/541133

Adler, S. (2011). Sleep paralysis: Night-mares, nocebos, and the mind-body connection. Newark, NJ: Rutgers University Press.

Aegineta, P. (1844). In Adams F. (Ed.), The seven books of Paulus Aegineta. Translated from the Greek with a commentary embracing a complete view of the knowledge possessed by the Greeks, Romans, and Arabians on all subjects connected with medicine and surgery. (F. Adams Trans.). London: Syndeham Society.

Aina, O. F., & Famuyiwa, O. O. (2007). Ogun oru: A traditional explanation for nocturnal neuropsychiatric disturbances among the Yoruba of southwest Nigeria. Transcultural Psychiatry, 44(1), 44–54. doi: 44/1/44 [pii]

Arikawa, H., Templer, D. I., Brown, R., Cannon, W. G., & Thomas-Dodson, S. (1999). The structure and correlates of kanshibari. *The Journal of Psychology, 133*(4), 369–375.

Aurelianus, C. (1950). In Drabkin I. E. (Ed.). *On acute diseases and chronic diseases* (I. E. Drabkin Trans.). Chicago: University of Chicago Press.

Awadalla, A., Al-Fayez, G., Harville, M., Arikawa, H., Tomeo, M. E., Templer, D. I., & Underwood, R. (2004). Comparative prevalence of isolated sleep paralysis in Kuwaiti, Sudanese, and American college students. *Psychological Reports, 95*(1), 317–322. doi: 10.2466/PR0.95.5.317-322

Berhanu, D., Go, V. F., Ruff, A., Celentano, D. D., & Bishaw, T. (2012). Khat use among HIV voluntary counselling and testing centre clients in Ethiopia. *Culture, Health & Sexuality, 14*(10), 1197–1212. doi: 10.1080/13691058.201 2.722684 [doi]

Blackmore, S. (1998). Abduction by aliens or sleep paralysis? *Skeptical Inquirer, 22*, 23–28.

Bond, J. (1753). *An essay on the incubus, or night mare.* London: D. Wilson and T. Durham.

Cheyne, J. A., Rueffer, S. D., & Newby-Clark, I. R. (1999). Hypnagogic and hypnopompic hallucinations during sleep paralysis: Neurological and cultural construction of the night-mare. *Consciousness and Cognition: An International Journal, 8*(3), 319–337. doi: 10.1006/ccog.1999.0404

Conesa, J. (2000). Geomagnetic, cross-cultural and occupational faces of sleep paralysis: An ecological perspective. *Sleep and Hypnosis, 2*(3), 105–111.

Dahlitz, M., & Parkes, J. D. (1993). Sleep paralysis. *The Lancet, 341*, 406–407.

Davies, O. (2003). The nightmare experience, sleep paralysis and witchcraft accusations. *Folklore, 114*(2), 181.

de Jong, J. T. V. M. (2005). Cultural variation in the clinical presentation of sleep paralysis. *Transcultural Psychiatry, 42*(1), 78–92. doi: 10.1177/1363461505050711

Druffel, A. (1998). *How to defend yourself against alien abduction.* New York: Rivers Press.

Editors of Time-Life Books. (1988). *Mysteries of the unknown: Phantom encounters.* Alexandria, VA: Time-Life Books.

Firestone, M. (1985). The "old hag": Sleep paralysis in Newfoundland. *Journal of Psychoanalytic Anthropology, 8*(1), 47–66.

Friedman, S., & Paradis, C. (2002). Panic disorder in African Americans: Symptomatology and isolated sleep paralysis. *Culture, Medicine and Psychiatry, 26*(2), 179–198. doi: 10.1023/A:1016307515418

Gangdev, P. (2004). Relevance of sleep paralysis and hypnic hallucinations to psychiatry. *Australasian Psychiatry, 12*(1), 77–80. doi: 10.1046/j.1039-8562.2003.0206 5.x

Golzari, S. E., Khodadoust, K., Alakbarli, F., Ghabili, K., Islambulchilar, Z., Shoja, M. M., et al. (2012). Sleep paralysis in medieval Persia—the hidayat of Akhawayni (?-983 AD). *Neuropsychiatric Disease and Treatment, 8*, 229–234. doi: 10.2147/ NDT.S28231; 10.2147/NDT.S28231

Goode, G. B. (1962). Sleep paralysis. *Archives of Neurology, 6*, 228–234.

Grayman, J. H., Good, M. J., & Good, B. J. (2009). Conflict nightmares and trauma in aceh. *Culture, Medicine and Psychiatry, 33*(2), 290–312. doi: 10.1007/ s11013-009-9132-8 [doi]

Haga, E. (1989). The nightmare—A riding ghost with sexual connotations. *Nordisk Psykiatrisk Tidsskrift. Nordic Journal of Psychiatry, 43*(6), 515–520.

Hinton, D. E., Pich, V., Chhean, D., & Pollack, M. H. (2005). The ghost pushes you down: Sleep paralysis-type panic attacks in a Khmer refugee population. *Transcultural Psychiatry, 42*(1), 46–77. doi: 10.1177/1363461505050710

Hufford, D. J. (2005). Sleep paralysis as spiritual experience. *Transcultural Psychiatry*, *42*(1), 11–45. doi: 10.1177/1363461505050709

Hufford, D. (1982). *The terror that comes in the night: An experience-centered study of supernatural assault traditions*. Philadelphia, PA: University of Pennsylvania Press.

Huntingford, G. (1928). Ghosts and devils in east Africa. *Royal Anthropological Institute of Great Britain and Ireland*, *28*, 76–78. doi: 10.2307/2789197

Hurd, R. (2011). *Sleep paralysis: A guide to hypnagogic visions and visitors of the night*. Los Altos, CA: Hyena Press.

Ignjatic, Z., Jelena Kovacevic, K., Meseldzija, B., Vartabedijan, D., Vrtacnik, V., Vuckovic, P., et al. (2002). *English-Serbian & Serbian-English dictionary & grammar* (Multilingual ed.). Beograd, Serbia: Izdavec Instiutu Za Strane Jezike.

Jalal, B., Simons-Rudolph, J., Jalal, B., & Hinton, D. E. (2014). Explanations of sleep paralysis among egyptian college students and the general population in Egypt and Denmark. *Transcultural Psychiatry*, *51*(2), 158–175. doi: 10.1177/13634615 13503378 [doi]

Jimenez-Genchi, A., Avila-Rodriguez, V. M., Sanchez-Rojas, F., Terrez, B. E., & Nenclares-Portocarrero, A. (2009). Sleep paralysis in adolescents: The 'a dead body climbed on top of me' phenomenon in mexico. *Psychiatry and Clinical Neurosciences*, *63*(4), 546–549. doi: 10.1111/j.1440-1819.2009.01984.x [doi]

Kuhn, S., & Reidy, J. (1975). *Middle English dictionary*. Ann Arbor, MI: University of Michigan Press.

Law, S., & Kirmayer, L. J. (2005). Inuit interpretations of sleep paralysis. *Transcultural Psychiatry*, *42*(1), 93–112. doi: 10.1177/1363461505050712

Lockwood, J. (2010). *The maverick ghost hunter*. Capulin, CO: Xlibris Corporation.

Mdlalani, A. (2009). A sleep disorder worse than a nightmare. *Sunday Standard*. http://www.sundaystandard.info/article.php?newsID=6543&GroupID=2

Munger, R. G., & Booton, E. A. (1998). Bangungut in Manila: Sudden and unexplained death in sleep of adult Filipinos. *International Journal of Epidemiology*, *27*(4), 677–684.

Ness, R. C. (1978). The old hag phenomenon as sleep paralysis: A biocultural interpretation. *Cultural, Medicine and Psychiatry*, *2*, 15.

Nickell, J. (1995). The skeptic-raping demon of Zanzibar. *Skeptical Briefs*, *5*(4), 7.

Roberts, K. (1998). Contemporary cauchemar: Experience, belief, prevention. *Louisiana Folklore Miscellany*, *xiii*, 15–26.

Ronnevig, G. M. (2007). Toward an explanation of the "abduction epidemic": The ritualization of alien abduction mythology in therapeutic settings. In D. G. Tumminia (Ed.), *Alien worlds: Social and religious dimensions of extraterrestrial contact* (pp. 99–127). Syracuse, NY: Syracuse University Press.

Roscher, W. H. (2007). Ephialtes: A pathological-mythological treatise on the nightmare in classical antiquity. [Ephialtes] (A. V. O'Brien Trans.). (Revised ed., pp. 96–159). Putnam, CT: Spring Publishing.

Simard, V., & Nielsen, T. A. (2005). Sleep paralysis-associated sensed presence as a possible manifestation of social anxiety. *Dreaming*, *15*(4), 245–260. doi: 10.1037/1053-0797.15.4.245

Stol, M. (1993). *Epilepsy in Babylonia*. Groningen, The Netherlands: STYX Publications.

Tarnovetskaia, A., & Cook, L. (2008). The impact of cultural values, family involvement and health services on mental health and mental illness. *Canadian Journal of Family and Youth*, *1*(2), 113–126.

Vila-Rodriguez, F., MacEwan, G. W., & Honer, W. G. (2011). Methamphetamine, perceptual disturbances, and the peripheral drift illusion. *The American Journal on

Addictions, 20(5), 490. Epub 2011 Jul 18. doi: 10.1111/j.1521-0391.2011.001
61.x [doi]

Walsh, M. (2009). The politicisation of popobawa: Changing explanations of a collec-
tive panic in Zanzibar. *Journal of Humanities, 1*(1), 23–33.

Wing, Y., Lee, S. T., & Chen, C. (1994). Sleep paralysis in Chinese: Ghost oppression
phenomenon in Hong Kong. *Sleep: Journal of Sleep Research & Sleep Medicine,*
17(7), 609–613.

Fearful Isolated Sleep Paralysis Interview

I. INITIAL INQUIRIES

1a. Have you ever had periods of time when you woke in the morning or after a nap and found yourself unable to move (paralyzed), yet you were still aware of your surroundings (i.e., it did not feel like you are completely asleep)?

Yes _____ No _____

1b. Have you ever had periods of time when you found yourself unable to move (paralyzed), yet were still aware of your surroundings just as you were falling asleep or starting to nap?

Yes _____ No _____

If NO to 1a–1b, skip to **NEXT MODULE**, otherwise continue to 2.

2. How afraid are you *during* a typical episode of this paralysis?

0 ------ 1 ------ 2 ------ 3 -------- 4 -------- 5 ------ 6 ------ 7 ------ 8

None	Mild	Moderate	Severe	Very severe

3. If endorsing fear ask: **In your own words, please describe what occurs during these episodes that makes you afraid** (record verbatim, and note any idiosyncratic hallucinatory experiences in "other" symptom ratings in section II):

_____

_____

4. When was the most recent time this occurred?

_____

5. How long does this period of paralysis and fear usually last? _____ minutes

6. What position are you usually sleeping in when this occurs?

_____

7. What do you believe is the cause of these episodes (assess for paranormal beliefs as appropriate)?

_____

_____

8a. Do you do anything to try to prevent these episodes?

Yes _____ No _____

If yes, What do you do? Do you believe this works?

Yes _____ No _____

If yes, What % of the time does this work?

_____%

_____

_____

8b. Do you do anything to try to stop these episodes when they occur?

Yes _____ No _____

If yes, What do you do? Do you believe this works?

Yes _____ No _____

If yes, What % of the time does this work?

_____%

_____

_____

II. SYMPTOM RATINGS

Rate the severity of each symptom that is typical of episodes of isolated sleep paralysis. If a symptom is experienced during only some attacks (i.e., does not typically occur during an episode of sleep paralysis), enclose the rating in parentheses.

Use the following inquiry when rating symptoms:

1. **During an episode of sleep paralysis, do you usually _____?**
   (Keep reminding the patient that you are not referring to panic attacks, but

sleep paralysis, reassuring him/her that it is not an uncommon phenomenon if necessary.)

2. **How distressing/severe is the symptom to you?** If there is any doubt about whether the symptom is typical, ask: **Do you experience this nearly every time you have an episode?**

0 ------ 1 ------ 2 ------ 3 -------- 4 --------5 ------ 6 ------ 7 ------ 8

| None | Mild | Moderate | Severe | Very severe |

		Rating	Comments
a.	Try to speak or call out to someone, but feel unable to do so	_____	_____
b1.	Feel pressure on your chest (or other body part)	_____	_____
b2.	Feel that you are smothering	_____	_____
c.	Feel that you got out of bed or moved a part of your body only to discover that you had not moved at all	_____	_____
d1.	Hear unusual sounds	_____	_____
	Specify _____		
d2.	Hear footsteps	_____	_____
d3.	Hear unclear speech or gibbering	_____	_____
e1.	Feel numbness	_____	_____
e2.	Feel vibrating sensations	_____	_____
e3.	Feel tingling sensations	_____	_____
f1.	Feel like you temporarily leave your body	_____	_____
f2.	Feel that you can see your body from the outside	_____	_____
g.	Feel a presence in the room (not necessarily seeing, but just *feeling* a presence) _____		
	What do you think it is?	_____	_____
h1.	Imagine that you see a shape in the room with you	_____	_____
	What do you see? _____		
h2.	Imagine that you see a person in the room with you	_____	_____
	Who is it? _____		
h3.	Imagine that you see a being in the room with you	_____	_____
	What is it? _____		

i1. Feel like your body is falling   _____   _____
i2. Feel like your body is flying   _____   _____
i3. Feel like your body is floating   _____   _____
i4. Feel like your body is spinning   _____   _____
i5. Feel like your body is turning   _____   _____
j.   Feel like you might die   _____   _____
k.   Feel pain   _____   _____
l.   Feel cold   _____   _____
m.   Feel erotic/sexual feelings   _____   _____
n.   Feel like you're being strangled   _____   _____
o.   Feel like you're being physically touched   _____   _____
p.   Other symptom   _____   _____
q.   Other symptom   _____   _____

3. **Do these symptoms or the paralysis cause more fear?**

   Select answer   Hallucinations

                                    Paralysis

4. **How afraid are you just due to the paralysis alone?** _____

   0 ------ 1 ------ 2 ------ 3 -------- 4 -------- 5 ------ 6 ------ 7 -----8

   None   Mild   Moderate   Severe   Very
                                                        severe

5. **How afraid are you due to the symptoms described above?** (use hallucination examples) _____

   0 ------ 1 ------ 2 ------ 3 -------- 4 -------- 5 ------ 6 ------ 7------ 8

   None   Mild   Moderate   Severe   Very
                                                        severe

III. CURRENT EPISODE

1a. **How many episodes of sleep paralysis have you had in the past month?**

                                               _____

1b. **How many episodes of sleep paralysis have you had in the past six months?**

                                               _____

1c. **How many episodes of sleep paralysis have you had in the past year?**

                                               _____

1d. **How many episodes of sleep paralysis have you had in your life?**

                                               _____

2a. In what ways has sleep paralysis interfered with your life (e.g., daily routine, job, social activities)? How much are you bothered about having these episodes?

_____

_____

_____

2b. How much have episodes of sleep paralysis interfered with your life?

Interference: _____

2c. How much distress have these episodes have caused you?

Distress: _____

0 ------1 ------ 2 ------ 3 -------- 4 -------- 5 ------ 6 ------ 7 -----8

None   Mild   Moderate   Severe   Very severe

3a. Prior to your first episode (list age here _____), do you recall anything unusual going on in your life?

Specify: _____

_____

3b. Just prior to or since these episodes began, have you been regularly taking any types of drugs or alcohol?

Yes_____ No _____

Specify if was likely to have caused sleep paralysis and how:

_____

_____

3c. Just prior to or since these episodes began, have you had any physical condition such as narcolepsy, sleep apnea, cataplexy, seizure disorders, hypokalemia, or fibromyalgia?

Yes_____ No _____

Specify (type; date of onset/remission):

_____

3d. Just prior to or since these episodes began, have you ever had any surgeries?   Yes_____ No _____

Have you had surgeries as a child?   Yes_____ No _____

Were you anesthetized during the surgery?

Yes_____ No _____

Specify:

_____

4a. Some people see connections between things that go on in their life and the dreams they have when they're asleep (not paralyzed). Do you?

Yes_____ No _____

4b. Do you see any links between your experiences during these episodes when you're paralyzed and any current/past life concerns?

Yes_____ No _____

Specify: _____

_____

IV. DIAGNOSTIC SUMMARY

Isolated Sleep Paralysis Episode   Yes_____ No _____

Fearful Isolated Sleep Paralysis Episode   Yes_____ No _____

Recurrent Fearful Isolated Sleep Paralysis   Yes_____ No _____

0 ------1 ------2 ------3 -------- 4 -------- 5 ------- 6 ------- 7 ------8

| None | Mild | Moderate | Severe | Very severe |

Overall Episode Severity (0–8)   _____

ISP Frequency (0–4)   _____

Episode Distress (0–4)   _____

Overall ISP Distress (0–4)   _____

Overall ISP Interference (0–4)   _____

Overall Recurrent FISP Clinical Severity Rating (0–16):   _____

Standardized Scoring for Fearful Isolated Sleep Paralysis Episodes and Recurrent Fearful Isolated Sleep Paralysis

1. Fearful ISP frequency in the past six months
   0 = No episodes
   1 = At least one episode in the past six months, but less than one episode per month
   2 = One to three episodes per month
   3 = At least four episodes per month, but on average no more than one per week
   4 = More than one episode per week

2. Overall fear/distress experienced during fearful ISP episodes in the past six months
   0 = No fear/distress
   1 = Mild fear/distress
   2 = Moderate fear/distress
   3 = Severe fear/distress
   4 = Very severe fear/distress

3. Overall fear/distress from having ISP episodes in the past six months (i.e., DSM distress)
   0 = No fear/distress
   1 = Mild fear/distress
   2 = Moderate fear/distress
   3 = Severe fear/distress
   4 = Very severe fear/distress

4. Interference from fearful ISP episodes in the past six months
   0 = No interference
   1 = Mild, slight interference—Patient feels as if at least one aspect of his/her life has been negatively affected or impaired, but only to a very limited degree.
   2 = Moderate interference—ISP symptoms cause a definite and noticeable interference in at least one area of functioning, but these areas remain, overall, manageable. Overall functioning is not impaired.
   3 = Severe interference—ISP symptoms cause either impairment in two or more areas, or a greater than moderate degree of impairment in one specific area. Patient may feel less able to manage required affairs or, following ISP episodes, may be unable to function for a time or try to avoid sleep. This may or may not involve a belief in paranormal/supernatural explanations of hypnagogic/hypnopompic experiences that are not culturally normative and may have some degree of rigidity.
   4 = Very severe interference—ISP symptoms cause impairment in multiple areas of functioning, and patient may experience a greater degree difficulty to manage required affairs than a "3" or, following ISP episodes, may be unable to function for a time or try to avoid sleep. This may or not verge on a psychotic level of belief in the veracity of the hypnagogic or hypnopompic content.

Total Score Range: 0–16

A Cognitive Behavioral Treatment Manual for Recurrent Isolated Sleep Paralysis: CBT-ISP

WHY CBT-ISP?

As noted in chapters 15 and 16, there are no empirically supported treatments currently available for the more chronic and severe cases of isolated sleep paralysis. This is in spite of the fact that some individuals are very troubled by episodes. We therefore wanted to synthesize the limited information for practitioners who hope to treat these individuals. However, given the scant resources that are available, it is inevitable that our approach will either miss important treatment components and/or include parts which may be superfluous or ineffective. Regardless, it is important that a treatment begin somewhere, and future researchers will hopefully fine-tune this manual to make it more consistent with advances in basic science.

After reviewing the literature documented in earlier sections of this book, this material seemed to lend itself most readily to a brief (i.e., 5-session) cognitive behavioral approach. By drafting this manual, we by no means imply that this is the best or only way to treat isolated sleep paralysis. Being primarily psychodynamic therapists who also value CBT, and also methodological pluralists (e.g., Feyerabend, 2010), we instead assume that principals derived from other theoretical orientations and modalities (e.g., psychopharmacology; psychodynamic therapies) may be quite useful.

For certain sections, we do not provide only one preferred technique, but instead present several options that clinicians can responsively choose from based upon the idiosyncrasies of their patient. Should one not work, we encourage therapists to model flexibility (Borkovec & Sharpless, 2004), engage in effective problem solving, and choose their supplemental approaches in collaboration with their patient.

WHICH PATIENTS ARE APPROPRIATE FOR CBT-ISP

As with all manualized treatments, great care should be taken when selecting patients. First, prospective patients should meet diagnostic criteria for either *recurrent fearful isolated sleep paralysis* (see Sharpless et al., 2010 and chapter 11) or *recurrent isolated sleep paralysis* (American Academy of Sleep Medicine, 2014). Obviously, the presence of significant distress as a result of episodes and/or significant life interruption would be prerequisites. Second, since this treatment assumes that episodes are at least partially brought on through sleep patterns and sleep positions, potential patients must be willing to modify these behaviors on a consistent basis. Third, and related to the first, this approach presumes that episodes are not better accounted for by other factors (e.g., substance use, hypokalemia) that would be better modified through other means. Fourth, comorbid conditions, if present, should neither interfere with the application of CBT-ISP (e.g., presence of a severe depressive episode to an extent that the patient lacks the energy or motivation to complete the treatment protocol) nor imply that the patient would be better served by receiving immediate treatment for these other conditions. In the absence of empirical evidence, we are fairly agnostic as to whether or not CBT-ISP can be used concurrently with other treatment modalities and manuals. From our perspective, CBT-ISP could be readily integrated into another CBT treatment as a "special module." The directiveness of CBT-ISP may make wholesale integration into a primarily psychodynamic approach difficult, but individual components could certainly be woven into a more exploratory therapeutic framework.

WHO IS APPROPRIATE TO CONDUCT CBT-ISP

Application of CBT-ISP would not differ markedly from other CBT manuals. However, determination of a patient's appropriateness requires a specific knowledge of sleep paralysis and differential diagnosis that is beyond what most practitioners acquire during their graduate training. This information can be found in relevant sections of this book. When in doubt, a diagnostic consultation with a sleep expert is recommended. The minimal criteria we envision for treatment *application* would be that 1) therapists have experience conducting manual-based CBT in general and 2) have also had some exposure to behavioral sleep medicine. Experience conducting one of the major CBT protocols for insomnia (e.g., Edinger et al., 2004; Edinger & Carney, 2008; Perlis, Jungquist, Smith, & Posner, 2005a) would be preferred. In the absence of these educational prerequisites, we recommend that supervision under a behavioral sleep medicine expert commence.

We should also note that the length of time between sessions can be flexible. For patients with a very low frequency of episodes, it may be advisable for sessions two and onward to be conducted on a twice-monthly basis (as opposed to weekly sessions) so long as the therapist is confident that patient adherence is strong and consistent between sessions.

SESSION 1: 60 TO 120 MINUTES

Summary: By the end of this initial session, the therapist should 1) establish a rudimentary therapeutic alliance, 2) compile accurate diagnostic information for isolated sleep paralysis, 3) administer several questionnaires of relevant phenomena (i.e., insomnia, anxiety sensitivity) in order to facilitate treatment planning, 3) summarize preliminary diagnostic findings to the patient and, if warranted, 4) begin a two-week period of self-monitoring of symptoms.

Orientation to Session and Rapport Building

After greeting the patient, time should be spent establishing a rudimentary assessment-based working alliance (which will help set the stage for the subsequent therapeutic working alliance). The working alliance consists of three components: 1) agreement on goals, 2) agreement on the therapeutic/assessment tasks used to reach those goals, and 3) the creation of a personal bond strong enough to tolerate the hard work required to achieve the other components (see Sharpless, Muran, & Barber, 2010 for a review of factors associated with stronger and weaker alliances). In the context of CBT-ISP, reaching agreement on the goals for the session (i.e., determining the presence and severity of recurrent isolated sleep paralysis and also associated features that may modify the specifics of the treatment approach) and the tasks used to reach them (i.e., a semi-structured interview and the completion of several surveys) merely entails a brief, yet sufficient explanation.

Given the complexity of accurately diagnosing isolated sleep paralysis (chapter 13), we recommend the use of a semi-structured clinical interview (e.g., those described in chapter 12 and Appendix B) as the primary means of determining appropriateness for CBT-ISP. Specifically, use of an interview that assesses episode frequency, severity, levels of distress/impairment, and competing conditions is required. Interviewers should also note the presence and nature of hallucinations during sleep paralysis as well as the patients' reactions to the various symptoms.

The assessment of isolated sleep paralysis is best conducted within the context of a broader consideration of other psychological and medical conditions. We recommend using one of the better semi-structured diagnostic interviews (e.g., the *Anxiety and Related Disorders Interview Schedule* (Brown & Barlow, 2014) or the *Structured Clinical Interview for DSM-5 Disorders* (First, Williams, Karg, & Spitzer, in press). Both of these also assess many of the common psychiatric and medical conditions that will assist in determining appropriateness for treatment.

Several other areas should be assessed, as they will indicate whether the use of any additional treatment techniques or modules is warranted. Levels of sleep disruption/insomnia will determine the extent to which traditional sleep hygiene and stimulus control techniques are utilized. If levels are severe enough, use of sleep restriction (e.g., Perlis et al., 2005) to increase overall sleep time and sleep efficiency may be a reasonable prerequisite to CBT-ISP. There are many insomnia assessment measures available, but the *Insomnia Severity Index* (Bastien, Vallieres, & Morin, 2001) is a brief, psychometrically sound, and clinically-useful measure that also allows patients to be placed into three categories of severity. Should a patient be in the moderate or above range of insomnia (viz., a raw score of 15 or above), clinical judgment should be used to determine if the use of the additional modules or a full insomnia protocol is warranted.

Given the replicated relationship between sleep paralysis and anxiety sensitivity, we recommend administering the *Anxiety Sensitivity Index* (Peterson & Reiss, 1987). Higher scores (e.g., 25 or above when using the 16-item version as described in Peterson & Plehn, 1999) may warrant the dedication of additional session time to both relaxation techniques and cognitive restructuring/decatastrophizing.

Self-Monitoring

Toward the end of this session, the therapist should summarize assessment findings, make treatment recommendations (i.e., continue CBT-ISP or refer elsewhere), and if CBT-ISP is indeed indicated, briefly describe the process of self-monitoring and outline what will happen in subsequent sessions.

An explanation and justification for self-monitoring should occur. This standard part of any CBT treatment not only helps patients become more aware of their symptoms, but also facilitates these symptoms becoming an object of inquiry and observation as opposed to just an "experience that happens" (viz., what classical psychoanalytic therapy would term fostering the split between the observing and experiencing ego as in Langs, 1973). Self-monitoring should also establish a baseline so that treatment progress can be tracked over time. It also potentially allows for a better discernment of triggers for sleep paralysis episodes and an exploration of their consequences (e.g., avoidance behaviors).

Modification of any preferred sleep diary can take place so long as the following components are included: episode frequency, levels of fear during episodes, presence of hallucinations, reactions to hallucinations (i.e., fear levels), potential triggers of episodes and/or avoidance behaviors (e.g., "what did you do in the two hours before bedtime?"), presence of any catastrophic thoughts, nightly sleep quality and quantity, time to sleep, time awakening, sleep efficiency, and sleep position.

SESSION 2: 45 TO 60 MINUTES

Summary: By the end of this session, the therapist should: 1) review sleep diaries from the previous two weeks, 2) complete basic psychoeducation on isolated sleep paralysis tailored to the patient's unique symptomatic experiences, 3) provide a brief explanation of the CBT model for isolated sleep paralysis, 4) provide ISP-specific sleep hygiene instruction, 5) instruct patients in the use of diaphragmatic breathing (or other form of relaxation) as both a potential preventative and a way to reduce the intensity of episodes, 6) summarize the session, and 7) assign homework.

Review of Sleep Diaries

Prior to the psychoeducation components of this session, the therapist should review the sleep diaries with the patient while keeping in mind general patterns that were previously identified in Session 1. Attention should be focused on identifying patterns that are consistent with the cognitive model described below in order to help make the psychoeducation more personally relevant. These patterns may also indicate certain techniques over others for subsequent sessions.

As with all forms of CBT, positive feedback should be provided when patients successfully and diligently complete assignments, and problem solving of difficulties should take place when assignments are neglected or given short shrift. Regarding the latter, therapists should be sensitive to potential alliance factors/ruptures and cognitive distortions that may interfere with treatment (e.g., "I'll never get better, so why should I bother").

Psychoeducation

Psychoeducation not only provides patients with information about their disorder, but also helps to normalize their symptoms. The approach for describing sleep paralysis should be tailored to, and appropriate for, the level of education of the patient. For some, a brief description of the relatively high prevalence rates for experiencing at least one episode of sleep paralysis over the course of one's life (see chapter 7), characteristic symptoms that may or may not be present in the patient (as in chapter 6), and ways that it can impact on sufferers (chapter 6) may be sufficient. For those who also experience the hallucinatory content, a discussion of the different manifestations of hallucinations across cultures may help normalize the experiences and make them not feel like they are "crazy." Mention should also be made of the fact that although the experiences are scary, they are not dangerous, and there are no known cases of the paralysis becoming permanent. The therapist should also ensure that there is adequate time left to field idiosyncratic patient questions.

Present the CBT Model for ISP

Patients will obviously be curious as to *why* they get sleep paralysis episodes and the means through which therapy will attempt to reduce their occurrence and impact. A clear presentation of both will foster the alliance and help patients anticipate their role in the treatment.

As with the general psychoeducation about ISP, the presentation of the CBT model should be appropriate to the level of patient understanding. With regard to the *why*, mention should be made of three predisposing factors (i.e., biological, behavioral, and cognitive). The patient should be informed that there appear to be biological factors at play in sleep paralysis (Denis et al., in press), as it likely runs in families and may affect certain groups of people more than others. However, the therapist should more strongly emphasize the importance of *behavioral* and *cognitive* factors over the biological. Patients should be informed that there are many variables that are directly under the patients' control that may make sleep paralysis more likely to occur (e.g., sleep habits, use of certain substances, the presence of other psychiatric symptoms and syndromes), and that the focus of treatment will be to identify and ameliorate them. Therapists should also emphasize that some behaviors used to ostensibly *prevent* sleep paralysis may actually make it more likely to occur (e.g., drinking before bed to facilitate sleep; engaging in avoidance behaviors that may further disrupt sleep).

Further, the importance of the various cognitive *interpretations and appraisals* of sleep paralysis episodes should be emphasized. As one example, temporary paralysis in and of itself is fairly neutral and innocuous, and some people might experience it as merely "odd," or even "interesting." It is only when the more catastrophic appraisals of the paralysis come to the fore that fear starts to rise and intensify (e.g., "I'm completely helpless" or "I'll never be able to move again"). Examples should be given of different people going through an identical experience who have completely different appraisals (e.g., using television characters). This will set the stage for cognitive work in later sessions.

Patients should be informed that: 1) sleep paralysis episodes are viewed in CBT as occurring in a "sequence," 2) that there are various ways to prevent or disrupt this sequence, and 3) that session time will be devoted to figuring out the best way to accomplish both prevention and disruption. For therapists who are more familiar with CBT approaches for panic disorder than isolated sleep paralysis, it may help to view episodes as analogous to panic attacks. In a similar vein, the ultimate goal of CBT-ISP must be a "realistic" one. Just as in panic disorder, it is somewhat unreasonable to expect that the patient will never have another panic attack. However, the frequencies can be markedly reduced and, when attacks occur, they can be viewed as expectedly annoying, yet no longer catastrophic in their implications for personal health or sanity. The goal of CBT-ISP is the same. Also similar to panic attacks, *prevention* of ISP episodes is preferred, but disruption is also useful. With practice, episodes can be disrupted earlier and earlier in the sequence. Therapists should also model flexibility by noting that even if a particular approach is not effective, there are other techniques that can be tried.

As for the sequence of sleep paralysis itself, patients should be informed that the sequence appears to be fairly typical and consistent across sufferers. First, there is conscious awareness followed by conscious awareness of the paralysis. This awareness then leads very quickly to catastrophic appraisals of the paralysis. At this point the appraisals lead to increased sympathetic nervous system activation as well as increased discomfort during the episode (e.g., shallow breathing may intensify normal sensations of pressure on the chest and smothering sensations; increased activation may lead to unpleasant feelings of cold or numbness in the patient's extremities). Then, an increased focus on the body will intensify the catastrophic thoughts and unpleasant sensations which, through a vicious circle, lead to an intensification of both.

ISP-Specific Sleep Hygiene

Once it is clear that patients have a good enough understanding of isolated sleep paralysis and the CBT model, work on sleep hygiene should commence. Using a combination of open-ended questions (e.g., "tell me about how you typically go to sleep"; "describe your bedtime ritual") and information gleaned from the diaries, the therapist should identify problems in the patient's sleep hygiene. At *minimum*, the therapist should recommend modifying sleep behaviors so that the patient will have more appropriate sleep patterns, sleep positions, and use of substances. Clinical judgment and ISI scores will help determine if sleep hygiene training should be conducted in a more traditional, in depth manner.

Regarding sleep patterns, the patient should be instructed to go to sleep and wake up at the same time each day. For some patients (e.g., irregular shift workers, college students), this may take some collaborative problem-solving, but the ideal of daily sleep-wake consistency should be approximated as closely as possible. Efforts should also be made to avoid any unnecessary sleep disruptions (e.g., through using blackout curtains, turning off phones at night). Therapists should note that people with certain types of jobs (e.g., nurses) may be more likely to have sleep paralysis, and that this is likely due to the sleep disruption that results from their irregular work shifts.

Given that empirical work indicates that sleep paralysis is most likely to occur when sleeping on one's back (supine) or stomach (prone), patients should be instructed to always sleep on their *sides*. For patients who need to switch sleep positions during the night (e.g., to avoid muscle cramping or discomfort), they should be instructed to switch to their other side only. If the patient has a partner, it may be helpful to enlist the partner's aid to remind the patient of the appropriate sleep positions.

Time should be spent discussing the importance of avoiding certain substances before bed. Patients should not be using caffeine or alcohol within four to six hours of bedtime and, in general, they should work to reduce their general intake if either of these substances is used often. For more educated patients, it may be helpful to discuss how REM rebound effects can result from alcohol and benzodiazepines, and that this will make sleep paralysis episodes more likely to occur. Regarding other drugs, research is not clear. We have interviewed individuals who noted that they are more likely to have sleep paralysis episodes when they take marijuana, but this is purely anecdotal. We should also note that discontinuation of SSRIs and tricyclic antidepressants can result in an REM-rebound effect, and this should be discerned during intake.

Beyond these three sleep hygiene areas, the therapist's clinical judgment should determine if additional sleep modification is required to regulate sleep and/or reduce insomnia (e.g., stimulus control and sleep restriction as in Edinger et al., 2004; Perlis, Jungquist, Smith, & Posner, 2005).

Instruction in Diaphragmatic Breathing

Usually, CBT provides at least one tool during the first session of active therapy. We recommend that patients be instructed in diaphragmatic breathing (DB) for three specific reasons. First, it is easy to do throughout the day (at least four times per day, but more generally when they notice that they may be feeling tense and/or their breathing is shallow). This will help lower anxiety in general and may also reduce sleep disruption either directly or indirectly. Second, DB can be applied *during* isolated sleep paralysis episodes. Even if it does not effectively disrupt the episode, it may distract the patient from the scariness of the symptoms (which will hopefully lessen their intensity and decrease arousal). Finally, having at least one tool to use *during* episodes will help reduce feelings of powerlessness during paralysis.

Other forms of relaxation can be applied instead of DB, so long as they are relatively quick to teach and easy to use. This could include various forms of mindfulness and "centering" techniques. Some patients may be more comfortable with meditation or the use of prayer. Care should be taken with the latter, though, especially if the patient is experiencing hallucinations with prominent religious themes.

Review and Homework

After a brief review of the important session contents, the therapist should assign homework. This involves continuing the daily diaries with an addition of DB/other relaxation techniques.

SESSION 3: 45 TO 60 MINUTES

Summary: By the end of this session, the therapist should: 1) review sleep diaries from the previous week, modifying relaxation approaches if needed; 2) assign at least one sleep paralysis disruption technique; 3) practice the disruption technique using imaginary rehearsal; 4) summarize the session; and 5) assign homework.

Review of Sleep Diaries

As in Session 2, the therapist should review the sleep diaries with the patient, noting and resolving any difficulties in understanding or applying the previous session's content. Special attention should be paid to the novel component (i.e., DB) and the impact of this on the patient's isolated sleep paralysis and/or overall functioning. Should DB not be effective or well tolerated, session time should be devoted to instructing the patient in another brief technique (practiced four times per day) or fine-tuning the administration of DB. If warranted by high levels of anxiety and/or anxiety sensitivity, the therapist should consider guiding the patient in a progressive muscular relaxation (PMR) induction (e.g., Bernstein, Borkovec, & Hazlett-Stevens, 2000). Patients should be instructed to practice PMR at least twice per day along with DB. Given time constraints, if PMR is utilized, assigning a new disruption technique and practicing imaginary rehearsal should be delayed until Session 4.

Assign at Least One ISP Disruption Technique

Along with use of DB/other relaxation methods, patients in Session 3 should be assigned at least one other specific disruption technique. Although we are aware of only one empirical study assessing the means through with isolated sleep paralysis-sufferers attempt to disrupt their episodes (Sharpless & Grom, in press), some of these techniques appear to be promising (see Table 15.1). The most effective strategies for disruption include attempts to move parts of the body and various strategies to "calm down" and cease the episode. However, therapists should be creative and open to other disruption techniques that may not be found here.

Attempting to move during sleep paralysis appears to be a fairly effective strategy, but it is not yet known how it works (i.e., whether it is a means to directly disrupt the episode or whether this exertion of will power is a helpful distraction from the experience that leads to a quicker episode resolution). Of the people we've interviewed, attempting to move fingers, wiggle one's toes, and move other extremities were reported to be the most effective, followed by attempts to move the torso and other body parts (e.g., one's mouth or head). Patients should be directed to immediately focus their attention on the targeted body part as soon as they are aware of the paralysis. They should also be instructed to focus their attention regardless of other sleep paralysis–related experiences that may be occurring. Some may find it helpful to use mental commands to maintain their focus on the task. Patients should be informed that it is not expected that one single attempt to move will be effective, but that *repeated and persistent attempts* have been found to result in dissolution of episodes. Although not reported in the empirical literature, attempting to cough oneself out of an episode has been advocated in the lay literature (e.g., Hurd, 2011). Given that breathing is under some degree of conscious control, this approach also appears promising.

Techniques to "calm down" can take many forms, and have been described in the popular literature on sleep paralysis. We specifically recommend the use of reassuring self-talk (e.g., "I'm having a sleep paralysis episode, which is not dangerous, and it will eventually be over") during episodes. Trying to "let go" and "go along with the paralysis" has also been reported to disrupt episodes (e.g., Ohaeri, Adelekan, Odejide, & Ikuesan, 1992), and for some religious individuals soothing prayer has helped to get through the episode more quickly. Although the limited empirical literature indicates calming down to be more effective than getting upset/angry/assertive (Sharpless & Grom, in press), some laypersons have advocated these techniques as a way to end episodes (e.g., Druffel, 1998). Again, the mechanism through which any of these techniques might effect a change in sleep paralysis episodes is currently unknown.

Practice Disruption in Session Using Imaginary Rehearsal

Following adequate discussion of the use of disruptive techniques, the therapist and patient should practice it in session using imaginary rehearsal. Imaginary rehearsal in an isolated sleep paralysis context involves the patient recreating a typical (and highly fear-laden) episode in session. This episode should be as vivid and anxiety-provoking as possible, replete with imagined sounds, physical sensations, and hallucinations. However, in contrast to the usual resolution to the episode, the patient instead imagines the application of disruptive techniques (e.g., DB, attempting to move a finger) and achieves a successful (and less threatening) outcome. Along with helping to practice the techniques during a simulated sleep paralysis episode (thus building habit strength), imaginary rehearsal also pairs the utilization of the technique with a successful outcome (viz., positive coping). A secondary intention of imaginary rehearsal is to add flexibility to a potentially rigid cognitive system (e.g., "I can't do anything to get out of these episodes") and shift perspectives.

In order to lend as much real-world veracity to this exercise, several steps should be taken. First, it is *strongly* recommended that the imaginary rehearsal take place while the patient is reclining on a large couch or chaise lounge. This will more closely approximate the bedroom and thus provide similar sensory stimuli and visual perspectives. Second, the therapist should assist the patient in visualizing the sleep paralysis episode through use of narratives and specific details provided in earlier sessions (especially the intake). As the patient narrates her/his experience, care should be taken to ensure this is not merely a "cognitive" exercise. This can be accomplished by the therapist encouraging the expression of not just perceptions, but reactions, both physical and emotional. This may be difficult for some patients. Thus, it may be helpful to audio record the patient's narrative of a scary sleep paralysis episode and play it back (possibly along with helpful additions from the therapist) until the patient is sufficiently (and viscerally) absorbed in the sleep paralysis experience. At this point, the tape should be stopped, and imaginal application of the disruptive technique should take place. Third, care should be taken to accurately capture the pre-, peri-, and post-sleep paralysis episode happenings. This will help to better ensure a more authentic experience for the patient.

Imaginary rehearsal should be conducted at least twice in this session, with instructions to practice this exercise (varying the specifics of the episode to facilitate generalization) once per day. For those with somewhat limited imaginative abilities, use of audio recordings could be used initially with the expectation that they will be discontinued after several days of assisted practice. Patients should be instructed to practice these techniques in their bedroom and in relative darkness.

Patients should be directed to apply these techniques during their next episode immediately upon awareness of the paralysis (i.e., as early in the sequence of the episode as is possible). Remind them that practice of these techniques will likely allow them to more quickly and effectively disrupt episodes, and that they should not become demoralized should they not be immediately effective.

Review and Homework

After a brief review of the important session contents, the therapist should assign homework. This involves continuing the daily diaries, DB, and daily practice of imaginary rehearsal of the disruption techniques.

SESSION 4: 30 TO 60 MINUTES

Summary: By the end of this session, the therapist should: 1) review sleep diaries from the previous week, modifying relaxation and disruption approaches if needed; 2) begin disputing catastrophic thoughts (or imaginary rehearsal if PMR was conducted in the previous session); 3) if warranted, begin work on reducing the impact of hallucinations; 4) summarize the session; and 5) assign homework.

Review of Sleep Diaries

As in previous sessions, the therapist should review the sleep diaries with the patient, noting and resolving any difficulties in understanding or applying the previous week's content. Special attention should be paid to imaginary rehearsal and the impact of this on the patient's isolated sleep paralysis and/or overall functioning. Should the disruption techniques not be effective, session time should be devoted to instructing the patient in another technique or fine-tuning its application. The therapist should also encourage the patient to continue varying the scenes used during imaginary rehearsals.

Dispute Catastrophic Thoughts

In our work with patients suffering from isolated sleep paralysis, we have found that many possess a number of catastrophic thoughts that are associated with episodes. They may range widely in the *amount* of distortion and their impact on patients' lives, but the majority of individuals that we have assessed possess at least one. Patients fear that they are going crazy, believe that the episodes are indicative of something more serious (e.g., brain tumor, seizure activity), or may fear that the paralysis will someday be permanent. There are many ways to address these thoughts, and we have found that comparing probability estimates is helpful. For those familiar with the more traditional Socratic techniques to manage catastrophic cognitions, these can of course be substituted. Needless to say, a more thorough knowledge of general cognitive therapy is required to competently practice that approach.

Examples of how to conduct clinical probability estimates can be found in several sources, but we are particularly fond of Perlis et al.'s approach and their vivid clinical examples for insomnia (Perlis et al., 2005, pp. 90–96). For the sake of brevity, the clinical use of probability estimates essentially consists of calculating the number of episodes of sleep paralysis the patient has experienced, identifying and recording at least two catastrophic sleep paralysis-related cognitions, assessing the *patient's* probability estimates for the occurrence of the catastrophic events, calculating the *actual* occurrence of the catastrophic events, comparing the two estimates for each cognition, and discussing the differences between them. This alone will hopefully reassure the patient. However, it is important for the therapist to also suggest using more accurate thoughts to "counter" the catastrophic ones (e.g., "it's not at all likely that I would be permanently paralyzed by sleep paralysis").

Patients should then be instructed to practice identifying and challenging their catastrophic cognitions in their daily diary whenever they experience sleep paralysis.

Ways to Cope with Hallucinations (Optional Module)

For patients with pronounced hallucinations, especially those that manifest in a threatening manner (e.g., "intruder" or "incubus" subtypes), therapists should consider using this optional module. This is especially the case if previous techniques have not yet sufficiently reduced episodes or proved effective in early disruption. Of course, disrupting sleep paralysis as early as possible is preferred (preferably before the hallucinations begin). However, some patients may very quickly sense (or "see") disturbing hallucinations during the sequence of their episodes. This, and the high levels of distress that accompany these hallucinations, may make early disruption difficult (if not impossible) to effect. In these cases, we recommend the following additional work.

First, patients should be provided with psychoeducation about sleep paralysis hallucinations. Specifically, they should be informed that there is another sequence that appears to occur in the hallucinations themselves.

This sequence usually begins with a *sensed* presence/feeling of being watched that is initially noted and focused upon, and which is obviously disconcerting. This sensed presence is usually followed shortly thereafter by *seeing* shadowy forms that coalesce into clearer and more frightening images such as demons, aliens, or other malevolent beings (e.g., Cheyne & Girard, 2007). These images then often move toward, touch, climb on, or assault the helpless patient. Of course, not every patient will experience these sequences in the same way, but in our experience and review of the literature, they do appear to be fairly consistent being *sensed, seen,* and then *felt*. Further, all stages of this sequence may make the patient feel ill at ease, or even terrified.

Following psychoeducation, patients should be instructed in a slightly different variant of imaginary rehearsal with in-session practice. As before, emphasis should be on creating a vivid and paradigmatic episode of sleep paralysis in session, but with a slight modification to emphasis. Specifically, as soon as the patient begins to *sense* the presence (viz., before seeing the "entity"), the patient should be instructed to immediately begin DB/relaxation (which creates a calming effect) followed by assertive self-talk. This should be done prior to application of any other disruption technique. Regarding the self-talk, patients should note to themselves that they are experiencing the incipient symptoms of what could become a very scary hallucination, but that this is just a product of their mind trying to organize ambiguous stimuli in a mood-congruent manner. Thus, instead of being scared, they should keep breathing deeply (DB) and either ignore the presence (viz., distracting oneself from the presence and attempting to resolve the sleep paralysis episode) or experience it as an interesting (e.g., "having a waking dream is a strange experience" or "the way the mind works is amazing") or even humorous curiosity ("Am I *really* seeing an extraterrestrial in my bedroom right now? This is ridiculous, and probably going to get interesting...") instead of experiencing the presence with dread and anxiety. Use of humor or finding interest in the hallucinatory content would technically be considered an *approach* behavior as opposed to *distraction* or an unhealthy *avoidance* behavior.

Next, when the patient feels a bit more in control, he/she should apply the other disruption techniques (e.g., attempting to wiggle a toe) and be instructed to successfully resolve the imagined episode in a relatively effective and peaceful manner. The patient should also be provided with homework instructions for this new variant of imaginary rehearsal (viz. once daily practice and actual application should an episode arise).

Along with disrupting the episodes, and therefore reducing patient distress, another goal for this approach is to reduce the overall duration of sleep paralysis episodes over time. Patients should be instructed to move the disruption earlier and earlier in the sequence of the hallucinations/

isolated sleep paralysis episode (i.e., reducing the latency between sensing the presence/paralysis and applying the disruption techniques) as they practice. Therefore, additional sessions may be needed.

We should note that another, contradictory approach for dealing with hallucinations has been described in the literature. As opposed to calming oneself in the presence of hallucinations or ignoring them to focus on disruption techniques, some have reported success in *engaging the hallucination* by expressing righteous anger at the putative violation of personal rights to safety and a restful sleep. Some have taken this to the extreme of either (mentally) yelling at, or even mentally attacking, the hallucinated figures (e.g., Druffel, 1998). Similarly, instead of relaxing and modifying one's breathing, some (e.g., Beloved, 2012) have recommended *temporarily suspending* one's respiration (as opposed to deep, relaxing breathing) in order to break the paralysis/dissolve the hallucination. Although we have no data on whether or not these approaches are less effective than the ones described previously, we recommend beginning with the less aggressive approaches, as they are more in keeping with traditional CBT techniques.

Review and Homework

After a brief review of the important session contents, the therapist should assign homework. This involves continuing the daily diaries, continued daily practice of imaginary rehearsal of disruption techniques, reduction of catastrophic thoughts, and the incorporation of hallucination techniques if warranted.

ADDITIONAL SESSIONS (IF NEEDED): 30 TO 60 MINUTES

Summary: Should significant sleep paralysis symptoms remain, or if it appears clinically warranted to continue fine-tuning CBT-ISP techniques, one or more additional sessions should take place before termination. They should each begin with 1) a review of the diaries and homework; 2) assessing the efficacy of the prevention/disruption techniques with fine-tuning/substitution of techniques, if necessary; 3) briefly reviewing session content; and 4) assigning homework.

Review of Sleep Diaries

As in previous sessions, the therapist should review the sleep diaries with the patient, noting and resolving any difficulties in understanding or applying the previous week's content. Special attention should be paid to the impact of techniques on the patient's isolated sleep paralysis and/or overall functioning. The therapist should also encourage the patient to continue varying the scenes used during imaginary rehearsals.

Fine-Tuning of Prevention/Disruption Techniques

Along with the techniques described in previous sessions, there remain other options for helping patients ameliorate their symptoms. Some of these other options can be found in Table 15.1 and other sections of this book (e.g., chapters 14, 15, and 16). For many of these techniques, practicing in session first using imaginary rehearsal is recommended along with assigning appropriate homework.

After reasonably exhausting available techniques with no (or limited) change, the therapist should consider referring the patient for another provider. This may include a psychiatric or sleep medicine consult and the provision of REM-suppressing medications (see chapter 16) or another treatment approach.

TERMINATION SESSION (60 TO 90 MINUTES)

Summary: By the end of this session, the CBT-ISP therapist should 1) review homework and diaries, 2) administer the initially used isolated sleep paralysis diagnostic instrument, 3) administer questionnaires used in the intake (i.e., insomnia, anxiety sensitivity), 4) review progress (or lack of progress), 5) summarize final diagnostic findings, 6) describe relapse-prevention strategies, and 7) make general inquiries into the patient's experience of treatment and feelings about terminating.

Assessment and Review of Treatment Progress

In this final session, the therapist should at a minimum re-administer the isolated sleep paralysis diagnostic instrument, *Insomnia Severity Index*, and *Anxiety Sensitivity Index*. If time allows or if clinically warranted, the broader assessment battery could be used as well.

Following this "formal" assessment, the patient should be prompted to describe her/his own perception of change (or lack of change). The therapist will then discuss the battery findings as well as the changes indicated by the patient's daily diaries. These diaries contain a wealth of information (e.g., sleeping changes, sleep paralysis frequency changes, emotional reaction changes), and it is up to the therapist to select those variables most important to chart for the patient.

Relapse Prevention

As noted previously, we adopt a coping approach that does not presume a complete remission of symptoms. Thus, patients should be informed that, although they may be doing quite well, a recrudescence of symptoms could occur. They should be instructed to not only note this as soon as they have an episode, but quickly take steps to alter this state of affairs. This may include returning to a stricter adherence to sleep hygiene, recommencing DB, or recommencing imaginary rehearsal. Patients should be encouraged to contact the therapist if they do not feel that their efforts are helpful.

Saying Goodbye

Toward the end of session, the therapist should leave some time to make general inquiries about the nature of the patient's experience in therapy. Every patient is different, and some are more open than others, but all patients should at least be asked to reflect upon the treatment process more generally. This not only allows them to construct a helpful narrative (e.g., "If I pay close attention to myself and work hard trying new things, I can change things that were formerly very troubling to me"), but may also set the stage for the patient feeling comfortable in seeking out additional therapeutic help if needed.

We recommend explicitly reminding patients that treatment was not something that was "done to them," but was instead a process of joint creation between the two parties. Techniques are useless without the patient's will to use them and the hard work that was expended in applying them. Of course, comments such as this must accurately correspond to the actual course of treatment, and the dialogue would be different with patients who were less compliant.

REFERENCES

American Academy of Sleep Medicine. (2014). *International classification of sleep disorders: Diagnostic and coding manual* (3rd ed.). Darien, IL: American Academy of Sleep Medicine.
Bastien, C. H., Vallieres, A., & Morin, C. M. (2001). Validation of the insomnia severity index as an outcome measure for insomnia research. *Sleep Medicine, 2*, 297–307.

Beloved, M. (2012). *Sleep paralysis*. Pembroke Pines, FL: Self-published.

Bernstein, D. A., Borkovec, T. D., & Hazlett-Stevens, H. (2000). *New directions in progressive relaxation training: A guide for helping professionals*. Westport, CT: Praeger.

Borkovec, T. D., & Sharpless, B. (2004). Generalized anxiety disorder: Bringing cognitive-behavioral therapy into the valued present. In S. Hayes, V. Follette, & M. Linehan's (Eds.), *Mindfulness and acceptance: Expanding the cognitive-behavioral tradition* (pp. 209–242). New York: Guilford Press.

Brown, T. A., & Barlow, D. H. (2014). *Anxiety and related disorders inverview schedule for DSM-5: Lifetime version*. New York: Oxford University Press.

Cheyne, J. A., & Girard, T. A. (2007). Paranoid delusions and threatening hallucinations: A prospective study of sleep paralysis experiences. *Consciousness and Cognition: An International Journal*, 16(4), 959–974.

Denis, D., French, C. C., Rowe, R., Zavos, H. M. S., Parsons, M. J., Nolan, P. M., & Gregory, A. M. (in press). A twin and molecular genetics study of sleep paralysis and associated factors. *Journal of Sleep Research*.

Druffel, A. (1998). *How to defend yourself against alien abduction*. New York: Rivers Press.

Edinger, J. D., Bonnet, M. H., Bootzin, R. R., Doghramji, K., Dorsey, C. M., Espie, C. A., et al. (2004). Derivation of research diagnostic criteria for insomnia: Report of an American Academy of Sleep Medicine work group. *Sleep*, 27(8), 1567–1596.

Edinger, J. D., & Carney, C. E. (2008). *Overcoming insomnia: A cognitive-behavioral therapy approach*. New York: Oxford University Press.

Feyerabend, P. K. (2010). *Against method* (4th ed.). NY: Verso Books.

First, M. B., Williams, J. B. W., Karg, R. S., & Spitzer, R. L. (in press). *Structured clinical interview for DSM-5 disorders: Patient edition*. New York: Biometrics Research Department.

Hurd, R. (2011). *Sleep paralysis: A guide to hypnagogic visions and visitors of the night*. Los Altos, CA: Hyena Press.

Langs, R. (1973). *The technique of psychoanalytic psychotherapy, volume 1*. NY: Jason Aronson.

Ohaeri, J. U., Adelekan, M. F., Odejide, A. O., & Ikuesan, B. A. (1992). The pattern of isolated sleep paralysis among nigerian nursing students. *Journal of the National Medical Association*, 84(1), 67–70.

Perlis, M. L., Jungquist, C., Smith, M. T., & Posner, D. (2005). *Cognitive behavioral treatment of insomnia A session-by-session guide*. New York, NY: Springer Science + Business Media, LLC.

Peterson, R.A., & Plehn, K. (1999). Measuring anxiety sensitivity. In S. Taylor's (Ed.), *Anxiety sensitivity: Theory, research, and treatment of the fear of anxiety*. Mahwa, NJ: Erlbaum.

Peterson, R. A., & Reiss, S. (1987). *Test manual for the anxiety sensitivity index*. Orlando Park, IL: International Diagnostic Systems.

Sharpless, B. A., & Grom, J. L. (in press). Isolated sleep paralysis: Fear, prevention, and disruption. *Behavioral Sleep Medicine*.

Sharpless, B. A., McCarthy, K. S., Chambless, D. L., Milrod, B. L., Khalsa, S. R., & Barber, J. P. (2010). Isolated sleep paralysis and fearful isolated sleep paralysis in outpatients with panic attacks. *Journal of Clinical Psychology*, 66(12), 1292–1306. doi: 10.1002/jclp.20724

Sharpless, B. A., Muran, J. C., & Barber, J. P. (2010). Coda: Recommendations for practice and training. In J. C. Muran, & J. P. Barber (Eds.), *The therapeutic alliance: An evidence-based approach to practice* (pp. 341–354). New York: Guilford Press.

APPENDIX D

An Adherence Measure for Cognitive Behavioral Treatment of Isolated Sleep Paralysis

GENERAL NOTES TO ADHERENCE RATERS

(Adapted from Chambless & Sharpless, unpublished manuscript)

The purpose of the ratings found on this scale is to quantify the therapist's adherence to the CBT-ISP treatment manual. *Adherence* to a treatment manual is conceptually different from the *competence* with which the techniques are delivered (or not delivered). Sharpless & Barber (2009) argued that the difference between adherence and competence hinges on the type of knowledge that each respectively demonstrates. Specifically, adherence demonstrates a technical, rule-governed knowledge that can be used to complete a task. This is not to say that it does not take creativity, but the ultimate goal of the technical activity is known in advance and also has a fixed endpoint (e.g., being able to teach a patient to engage in diaphragmatic breathing or challenge maladaptive cognitions). Competence, on the other hand, is more responsive, context-dependent, driven by values (which act as regulative ideals which help guide behavior), and reliant upon good judgment (e.g., knowing *when* and *when not* to intervene during a session). Conceptual confusion may result if these distinctions are not kept in mind (e.g., see Barber, Sharpless, Klostermann, & McCarthy, 2007; Sharpless & Barber, 2009). Both are important to ensure that good treatment results, but ensuring adequate adherence levels is critical to establishing a treatment's potential efficacy.

Competence and adherence can certainly go together (and hopefully do so often), but they need not necessarily do so. There are many situations where the desire to do both is impossible for the therapist due to conflicting demands. For example, one could imagine a scenario where a female patient arrives for therapy in an acute crisis because her husband just served her with divorce papers. In this scenario, it would be incompetent for the therapist to ignore this fact and maintain a high adherence to the CBT-ISP manual. However, if the therapist does not engage in the prescribed treatment behaviors, the therapist is not adherent and should be rated accordingly.

It is important to note that raters of adherence should watch the entirety of the session and make their individual item ratings accordingly. In order to do this properly, viewing video recordings (as opposed to audio recordings) is a requirement. Video allows for a more nuanced assessment of what the therapist does and the patient's responses to treatment.

Order of interventions is not important for rating, although it is conventional CBT procedure to review homework first and review session material/provide homework assignments last. Some patients may be particularly "quick studies" or have some background knowledge of the disorder or its treatment. So, for example, if a patient describes an important piece of psychoeducation before the therapist actually details it, the therapist should not be penalized when rating adherence, and should instead be given full credit.

Therapists should also not be penalized on their ratings if patient behaviors circumvent the possibility for adherence. Thus, a patient who does not complete self-monitoring makes a thorough review of this assignment impossible. In this case, a therapist would be rated on attempts to recreate the past week's activities and through addressing the non-compliance issue.

Note that from Session 3 onward, the treatment protocol will differ depending on whether or not certain procedures were utilized (e.g., progressive muscle relaxation in Session 3 or hallucination-specific work in Session 4). Therefore, therapists not using these particular procedures for a patient should not be rated on these items, and their total scores should be modified accordingly. All items should be scored using whole numbers (or not applicable), with an average (1–7) score calculated using all the relevant items for each individual session.

Client Initials or Number _____ Rater ID _____ Therapist ID _____

1. The therapist obtained at least a rudimentary therapeutic alliance with the patient by discussing the goals and tasks of this session, allowing questions, and listening attentively.

1 -------- 2 --------- 3 --------- 4 --------- 5 --------- 6 -------- 7

Not at all	Somewhat	Quite	Very
descriptive	descriptive	descriptive	descriptive

2. The therapist obtained a thorough description of the patient's isolated sleep paralysis (ISP) history and symptoms using a semi-structured clinical interview.

> *Note: Scoring this item requires not only watching the video, but also a reading of the therapist's intake report.*

1 -------- 2 --------- 3 --------- 4 --------- 5 --------- 6 -------- 7

Not at all	Somewhat	Quite	Very
descriptive	descriptive	descriptive	descriptive

3. If the client seems focused on other problems beyond ISP, the therapist spent time clarifying these issues and made sure that the client understands and agrees with the treatment focus on ISP. If this was not an issue in the session, select "not applicable."

1 -------- 2 --------- 3 --------- 4 --------- 5 --------- 6 -------- 7

Not at all	Somewhat	Quite	Very
descriptive	descriptive	descriptive	descriptive

*Not applicable

4. The therapist administered a broader diagnostic interview to assess for comorbid conditions and also to rule out alternative diagnostic possibilities. When comorbid disorders were discussed/identified, the therapist briefly reviewed these with the client, explained that treatment would not be focused on these other matters, and also asked

that the patient keep the therapist informed of any worsening in these comorbid conditions. If comorbid disorders were not present, select "not applicable."

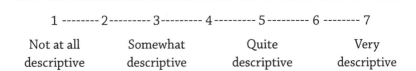

1 ------- 2 --------- 3 --------- 4 --------- 5 --------- 6 -------- 7

| Not at all | Somewhat | Quite | Very |
| descriptive | descriptive | descriptive | descriptive |

*Not applicable

5. The therapist administered, at minimum, self-report measures of insomnia and anxiety sensitivity and reviewed these results with the patient.

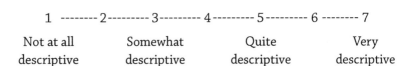

1 ------- 2 --------- 3 --------- 4 --------- 5 --------- 6 -------- 7

| Not at all | Somewhat | Quite | Very |
| descriptive | descriptive | descriptive | descriptive |

6. The therapist determined the client's goals and expectations for treatment and, if necessary, corrected those that were unreasonable and/or unrealistic (e.g., to never experience ISP episodes again).

1 ------- 2 --------- 3 --------- 4 --------- 5 --------- 6 -------- 7

| Not at all | Somewhat | Quite | Very |
| descriptive | descriptive | descriptive | descriptive |

7. The therapist described the nature of the treatment (including content and length and frequency of sessions), the fact that this will be an active treatment involving a commitment to homework, as well as work during sessions. The therapist noted that people who put more effort into homework would likely improve more.

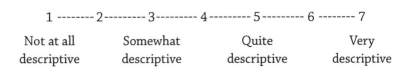

1 ------- 2 --------- 3 --------- 4 --------- 5 --------- 6 -------- 7

| Not at all | Somewhat | Quite | Very |
| descriptive | descriptive | descriptive | descriptive |

8. The therapist described the importance and use of diaries, and instructed the client to monitor symptoms on a daily basis for at least two weeks.

1 -------- 2 --------- 3 --------- 4 --------- 5 --------- 6 -------- 7

| Not at all | Somewhat | Quite | Very |
| descriptive | descriptive | descriptive | descriptive |

Notes:

CBT-ISP SESSION 2

Client Initials or Number _____ Rater ID _____ Therapist ID _____

1. The therapist reviewed sleep diaries and, if the client reported any ISP episodes, the therapist assessed the circumstances and consequences.

1 -------- 2 --------- 3 --------- 4 --------- 5 --------- 6 -------- 7

No	Some	Moderately	Complete
Review	Review	Complete	Review
		Review	

2. The therapist introduced the psychoeducational component of the session with an emphasis on normalizing ISP (e.g., the therapist discussed how ISP episodes are very common for all types of people under stress, how approximately 8% of people in the United States have had at least one episode of ISP with higher rates in students and psychiatric patients, at some time in their lives, and/or how the patient may knowingly or unknowingly be acquainted with people suffering from the same problem). The therapist also noted characteristic symptoms and the ways that ISP episodes and the consequences of episodes can impact on sufferers. If hallucinations were reported by the patient, the therapist should note that the content varies across time and place, but is a very common experience in ISP.

1 -------- 2 --------- 3 --------- 4 --------- 5 --------- 6 -------- 7

| Not at all | Somewhat | Quite | Very |
| descriptive | descriptive | descriptive | descriptive |

3. The therapist presented the cognitive model of ISP, noted biological, behavioral, and cognitive etiological factors and provided specific examples of at least the latter two (e.g., how catastrophic appraisals of the paralysis may actually intensify discomfort). The therapist described ISP as a *sequence* that can be potentially interrupted. The therapist also noted how some behaviors intended to prevent ISP may actually make episodes more likely to occur (e.g., drinking alcohol to facilitate deeper sleep).

1 -------- 2--------- 3--------- 4--------- 5--------- 6 -------- 7

| Not at all descriptive | Somewhat descriptive | Quite descriptive | Very descriptive |

4. If possible, the therapist connected relevant parts of the patient's sleep diary contents with relevant psychoeducational and/or CBT-ISP model components (e.g., noting how the patient's catatstrophic misappraisals of ISP episodes are common experiences; noting that the ISP episodes seem to occur when patient sleeps in a supine position).

1 -------- 2--------- 3--------- 4--------- 5--------- 6 -------- 7

| Not at all descriptive | Somewhat descriptive | Quite descriptive | Very descriptive |

*Not applicable

5. The therapist described the goals of CBT-ISP (i.e., reduction of ISP episodes, their severity, and their duration). The therapist noted the "realistic" goal of treatment and informed the patient that, even with successful treatment, ISP episodes may still occasionally occur and that this is to be expected.

1 -------- 2--------- 3--------- 4--------- 5--------- 6 -------- 7

| Not at all descriptive | Somewhat descriptive | Quite descriptive | Very descriptive |

6. The therapist instructed the patient in ISP-specific sleep hygiene (i.e., at minimum, discussed the importance of making changes in sleep patterns, sleep positions, minimization of sleep disruptions, and appropriate use of substances prior to bed).

Note: Some patients, due to information gleaned during intake, may be instructed on sleep hygiene techniques that go beyond these "mimimum" requirements. Raters should focus their scores on the above-mentioned minimal areas.

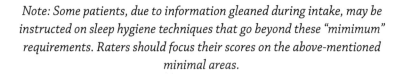

1 -------- 2 --------- 3 --------- 4 --------- 5 --------- 6 -------- 7
Not at all   Somewhat   Quite   Very
descriptive   descriptive   descriptive   descriptive

7. The therapist instructed the patient in diaphragmatic breathing (or another brief relaxation method), demonstrated to the patient how this is done, practices in session, and noted how DB should be used throughout the day and also during episodes.

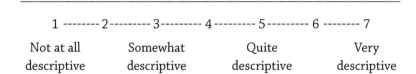

1 -------- 2 --------- 3 --------- 4 --------- 5 --------- 6 -------- 7
Not at all   Somewhat   Quite   Very
descriptive   descriptive   descriptive   descriptive

8. Overall, this psychoeducational session was more of a dialogue than a one-sided lecture on isolated sleep paralysis. That is, the therapist was open to, and responded to questions, personalized the description to this client, and attempted to make the psychoeducation interactive.

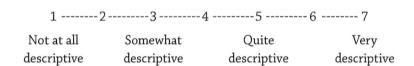

1 -------- 2 --------- 3 --------- 4 --------- 5 --------- 6 -------- 7
Not at all   Somewhat   Quite   Very
descriptive   descriptive   descriptive   descriptive

9. The therapist explained and assigned homework (including the diaphragmatic breathing/other form of relaxation, ISP-specific sleep hygiene, and completion of the panic diaries).

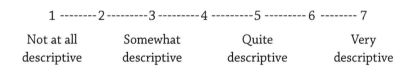

1 -------- 2 --------- 3 --------- 4 --------- 5 --------- 6 -------- 7
Not at all   Somewhat   Quite   Very
descriptive   descriptive   descriptive   descriptive

Notes:

Client Initials or Number _____ Rater ID _____ Therapist ID _____

1. The therapist reviewed sleep diaries and, if the client reported at least one ISP episode, the therapist assessed the circumstances and consequences.

1 -------- 2 --------- 3 --------- 4 --------- 5 --------- 6 -------- 7

| No Review | Some Review | Moderately Complete Review | Complete Review |

2. The therapist asked/reminded patient to continue to monitor his/her sleep and ISP episodes and provided justifications for this (e.g., a) monitor progress; b) help them approach their ISP episodes as an observing scientist, not a passive victim; c) become more accurate in recollections of what happened; d) recognize that with hindsight, events can become more awful than they actually were; and e) identify the conditions when ISP is likely to occur).

1 -------- 2 --------- 3 --------- 4 --------- 5 --------- 6 -------- 7

| Not at all descriptive | Somewhat descriptive | Quite descriptive | Very descriptive |

3. The therapist reviewed the potential effect of the previously assigned relaxation technique for the patient. If ISP occurred since the last session, the efficacy of its application to the episode was discussed.

Note: Therapists may suggest a different relaxation technique here, including progressive muscular relaxation. If this is the case, the new technique was described, practiced during session, and homework assigned (see manual for frequencies). Ratings for the new technique should be made in this same item.

1 -------- 2 --------- 3 --------- 4 --------- 5 --------- 6 -------- 7

| Not at all descriptive | Somewhat descriptive | Quite descriptive | Very descriptive |

4. The therapist instructed the patient in at least one new ISP disruption technique and discussed its potential application during an ISP episode.

*Not applicable

5. The therapist introduced imaginary rehearsal and provided a justification for its use, including the importance of daily practice in bed. The therapist then guided the patient in an in-session imaginary rehearsal, encouraged the patient to verbalize an ISP experience, instructed the patient to apply the disruption technique, and facilitated a good resolution (i.e., disruption of the episode).

Note: For patients who were instructed in progressive muscle relaxation, questions 4 and 5 will be answered in Session 4, please mark "not applicable" here. Further, some patients may require the use of a recording and/or more active encouragement during imaginary rehearsal, and therapists should not be penalized for this so long as they are encouraging practice in session.

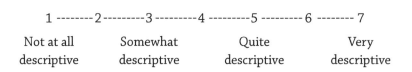

1 -------- 2 --------- 3 --------- 4 --------- 5 --------- 6 -------- 7			
Not at all descriptive	Somewhat descriptive	Quite descriptive	Very descriptive

*Not applicable

6. The therapist assigned homework (including the diaphragmatic breathing/other form of relaxation, imaginary rehearsal, at least one disruption technique if applicable) and completion of the diaries.

1 -------- 2 --------- 3 --------- 4 --------- 5 --------- 6 -------- 7			
Not at all descriptive	Somewhat descriptive	Quite descriptive	Very descriptive

Notes:

Client Initials or Number _____ Rater ID_____ Therapist ID_____

Note: For this session, some patients may not yet have been instructed in imaginary exposure due to the introduction of PMR. In these cases, rate the items from Session 3 in this section.

For these patients, cognitive work will begin in Session 5. In these cases, therapists should not be penalized in their scores.

1. The therapist reviewed sleep diaries and, if the client reported at least one ISP episode, the therapist assessed the circumstances and consequences. The therapist also reviewed assigned homework (e.g., DB or other relaxation, imaginary rehearsal of disruption) and the impact, if any, on patient functioning.

    Note: Therapists may choose to modify the relaxation or disruption techniques, and this should not be counted against their score for this item.

---

1 -------- 2 --------- 3 --------- 4 --------- 5 --------- 6 -------- 7

No Review	Some Review	Moderately Complete Review	Complete Review

2. The therapist assisted the patient in the identification of at least two catastrophic cognitions. The therapist instructed the patient on how to evaluate and challenge these cognitions (e.g., through calculating probability estimates, Socratic dialoguing)

---

1 -------- 2 --------- 3 --------- 4 --------- 5 --------- 6 -------- 7

Not at all descriptive	Somewhat descriptive	Quite descriptive	Very descriptive

*Not applicable

3. The therapist worked with the patient to develop thoughts to "counter" each of the catastrophic cognitions and instructed patients to use these when they experience ISP.

1 -------- 2 --------- 3 --------- 4 --------- 5 --------- 6 ------- 7

| Not at all descriptive | Somewhat descriptive | Quite descriptive | Very descriptive |

*Not applicable

4. (Optional) The therapist provided psychoeducation about the nature of ISP hallucinations and described the "sensed, felt, and seen" sequence. Therapist fielded patient questions.

1 -------- 2 --------- 3 --------- 4 --------- 5 --------- 6 ------- 7

| Not at all descriptive | Somewhat descriptive | Quite descriptive | Very descriptive |

*Not applicable

5. (Optional) The therapist provided a justification for the use of imaginary rehearsal for disrupting ISP hallucinations and noted the importance of daily practice in bed. The therapist then guided the patient in an in-session imaginary rehearsal, encouraged the patient to verbalize an ISP episode with prominent hallucinations, instructed the patient to apply the disruption techniques, and facilitated a good resolution (i.e., successful disruption of the episode).

1 -------- 2 --------- 3 --------- 4 --------- 5 --------- 6 ------- 7

| Not at all descriptive | Somewhat descriptive | Quite descriptive | Very descriptive |

*Not applicable

6. (Optional) The therapist described the importance of relaxation and self-talk during ISP hallucinations prior to using disruption techniques. The therapist, with the help of the patient, generated at least two examples of self-talk to use during ISP episodes.

1 -------- 2 --------- 3 --------- 4 --------- 5 --------- 6 ------- 7

Not at all	Somewhat	Quite	Very
descriptive	descriptive	descriptive	descriptive

*Not applicable

7. The therapist assigned and/or continued homework and daily completion of the diaries.

1 -------- 2 --------- 3 --------- 4 --------- 5 --------- 6 ------- 7

Not at all	Somewhat	Quite	Very
descriptive	descriptive	descriptive	descriptive

Notes:

CBT-ISP ADDITIONAL SESSIONS PRIOR TO TERMINATION SESSION

Client Initials or Number _____ Rater ID_____ Therapist ID_____

Note: Some patients may require additional sessions prior to termination. For instance, a patient who was instructed in PMR and also had prominent hallucinations would have had little ability to practice certain skills and would be somewhat "behind." In these cases, or where patients are modifying their ISP behaviors at slower than expected rates, additional sessions would be needed and should be rated as below. Therapists should, at minimum, be rated on these two items, but items from previous sessions can be rated as well.

1. The therapist reviewed sleep diaries and, if the client reported at least one ISP episode, the therapist assessed the circumstances and consequences. The therapist also reviewed assigned homework (e.g., DB or other relaxation, imaginary rehearsal of disruption) and the impact, if any, on patient functioning.

   Note: Therapists may choose to modify the relaxation or disruption techniques, and this should not be counted against their score for this item.

   1 -------- 2 --------- 3 --------- 4 --------- 5 --------- 6 -------- 7

No Review	Some Review	Moderately Complete Review	Complete Review

2. The therapist assigned and/or continued homework and daily completion of the diaries.

   _____

   1 -------- 2 --------- 3 --------- 4 --------- 5 --------- 6 -------- 7

Not at all descriptive	Somewhat descriptive	Quite descriptive	Very descriptive

   Notes:

CBT-ISP TERMINATION SESSION

Client Initials or Number _____ Rater ID_____ Therapist ID_____

1. The therapist reviewed sleep diaries and, if the client reported at least one ISP episode, the therapist assessed the circumstances and consequences. The therapist also reviewed assigned homework (e.g., DB or other relaxation, imaginary rehearsal of disruption) and the impact, if any, on patient functioning.

   _____

   1 -------- 2 --------- 3 --------- 4 --------- 5 --------- 6 -------- 7

No Review	Some Review	Moderately Complete Review	Complete Review

2. Therapist obtained a thorough description of the patient's current ISP symptoms, if any, using the same semi-structured clinical interview administered at intake.

   Note: Scoring this item requires not only watching the video, but also a reading of the therapist's termination report.

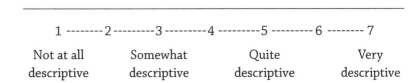

1 --------2---------3 ---------4 ---------5 --------- 6 -------- 7

| Not at all | Somewhat | Quite | Very |
| descriptive | descriptive | descriptive | descriptive |

3. (Optional) The therapist administered a broader diagnostic interview to assess for comorbid conditions and also to rule out alternative diagnostic possibilities. When comorbid disorders are discussed/identified, the therapist should briefly review these with the client, providing referrals for additional treatment if patient is interested.

1 --------2---------3 ---------4 ---------5 --------- 6 -------- 7

| Not at all | Somewhat | Quite | Very |
| descriptive | descriptive | descriptive | descriptive |

*Not applicable

4. The therapist re-administered, at minimum, the self-report measures of insomnia and anxiety sensitivity administered at intake and reviewed the results with the patient.

1 --------2---------3 ---------4 ---------5 --------- 6 -------- 7

| Not at all | Somewhat | Quite | Very |
| descriptive | descriptive | descriptive | descriptive |

5. The therapist reviewed, and invited the patient to review, the patient's overall progress (or lack of progress) in treatment. The therapist presented an overall diagnostic picture of the patient's current level of ISP symptoms (i.e., clinical severity, sub-clinical severity, early remission).

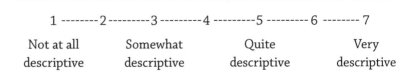

1 --------2---------3 ---------4 ---------5 --------- 6 -------- 7

| Not at all | Somewhat | Quite | Very |
| descriptive | descriptive | descriptive | descriptive |

6. The therapist discussed the likelihood of a return of ISP, and noted that this is especially likely if the is undergoing stressful times or experiences a return to maladaptive pre-treatment behaviors (e.g., sleeping regularly in a supine position). The therapist emphasizes that a lapse is not a relapse, and the recurrence of ISP is only a problem if the patient does not address it promptly.

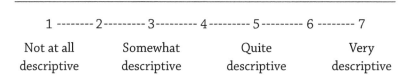

1 -------- 2--------- 3--------- 4--------- 5--------- 6 -------- 7

| Not at all descriptive | Somewhat descriptive | Quite descriptive | Very descriptive |

7. The therapist described relapse prevention strategies with the patient, and emphasized the importance of: a) quickly identifying symptoms when they return through regular self-monitoring, b) reapplying techniques that were helpful during treatment (e.g., relaxation, disruption, imaginary rehearsal), and c) seeking out additional treatment if needed.

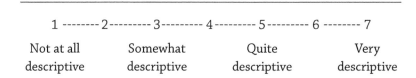

1 -------- 2--------- 3--------- 4--------- 5--------- 6 -------- 7

| Not at all descriptive | Somewhat descriptive | Quite descriptive | Very descriptive |

8. The therapist inquired into the patient's feelings about ending therapy. For example, the therapist may have asked if the patient was concerned that gains will be lost without the presence of the therapist. The therapist also emphasizes the nature of the treatment program in terms of training the patient to be his/her own therapist.

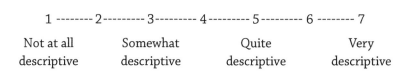

1 -------- 2--------- 3--------- 4--------- 5--------- 6 -------- 7

| Not at all descriptive | Somewhat descriptive | Quite descriptive | Very descriptive |

Notes:

REFERENCES

Barber, J. P., Sharpless, B. A., Klostermann, S., & McCarthy, K. S. (2007). Assessing intervention competence and its relation to therapy outcome: A selected review derived from the outcome literature. *Professional Psychology: Research and Practice, 38*(5), 493–500. doi: 10.1037/0735-7028.38.5.493

Chambless, D. L., & Sharpless, B. A. (unpublished manuscript). Adherence Ratings for the Panic Control Therapy Protocol for Psychotherapies for Panic Disorder Study. Philadelphia: University of Pennsylvania Center for Psychotherapy Research.

Sharpless, B. A., & Barber, J. P. (2009). A conceptual and empirical review of the meaning, measurement, development, and teaching of intervention competence in clinical psychology. *Clinical Psychology Review, 29*(1), 47–56. doi: 10.1016/j.cpr.2008.09.008; 10.1016/j.cpr.2008.09.008ss

INDEX

b denotes box; *f* denotes figure; *t* denotes table

Fearful Isolated Sleep Paralysis
Interview, 71, 155, 162*t*, 229–235
fearful paralysis, 34
females, rate of intense incubus
episodes in, 84
female sexuality, Nightmare and, 63–64
femoxetine, 207–208
Fitzgerald, F. Scott, sleep paralysis in
writing of, 50
5-HT (serotoninergic neurons), 139, 140
flashbacks, 79, 118, 120, 175
flatulence
association of with evil dreams and
Nightmare, 188
Nightmare attacks as preceded by, 62
floating, 84, 151
flowers
as prevention technique, 186
as technique against alien
abduction, 191
fluoxetine, 205, 207*t*
flying/flying abilities/flying dreams,
34, 78, 84
focal epileptic seizures, 177–178
folklore, history of sleep paralysis
in, 17–40
folk remedies/techniques/methods
for disruption of sleep paralysis,
189–190
empirical investigation into utility of,
200–201
for prevention of sleep paralysis,
184–189
folk theories, on origin of sleep paralysis,
129–131
foods, as proximal cause of sleep
paralysis, 60
freezing/frozen, 130, 175. *See also* cold
Freud, Sigmund, 57*f*, 133, 135, 137
fugue state, 121
functional neurological symptom
disorder, 176
Fuseli, Henri, sleep paralysis in the
paintings of, 21, 29, 45, 52, 84
future directions, 213–215

GABA, 139
GABA-ergic neurons of basal
forebrain, 139
galanin, 139

Galen, 56*f*, 59, 62, 66
gamma hydroxybutyrare (GHB),
206, 207*t*
gastric disturbances, as cause for sleep
paralysis, 60
Gelineau, 57*f*
gender, prevalence rates by, 97
general population, lifetime prevalence
rates of sleep paralysis in, 96*t*, 97*t*
genital soreness, 34, 136
genitals shrinking/receding, 65. *See
also koro*
Ghost Oppression Questionnaire, 162*t*,
ghosts, 30–31, 83
gluttony, as cause for sleep paralysis, 63
grains, as prevention technique, 187
Greece
prevention techniques, 186
tale of Zeus and Lycaon, 29
vampire myths in, 25
Grenada, *longaroo* (creature), 28
guilt, as cause for sleep paralysis, 62
guttural moans and groans, 75

hag, 31, 33, 185
hagge, 31
hallucinations
auditory hallucinations. *See* auditory
hallucinations
compared to delusions, 81–82
engagement of as disruption
technique, 201*t*,
as expression/intrusive symptom of
trauma, 120
factor structure of, 83–84
frequency and severity of, 75*t*,
hypnagogic. *See* hypnagogic
hallucinations (HH)
hypnopompic. *See* hypnopompic
hallucinations
inanimate hallucinations, 80
incubus subtype, 12
kinesthetic/tactile hallucinations,
75*t*, 78–79
prevalence of, 76
range of in sleep paralysis as
broad, 76
role of in sleep paralysis, 142
seen as real-world happenings, 119
sleep related, 107

out-of-body experiences, 74, 76, 78–79, 84, 122, 175, 176

Pan (Greek god), 22–23, 122
panic, prevalence of presentations of, 12
panic attacks, 12, 23, 88, 123, 124, 171–172
panic disorder, 12, 86, 94, 96, 109, 115, 122–123, 124, 151, 172, 199, 243
Paracelsus, 57f
Paradis, C. M., 199
paranormal/anomalous belief, as cause or consequence of sleep paralysis, 143
paranormal beliefs, role of sleep paralysis in explanation of, 11
parasomnia
  classification of, 4–5
  as decreasing during pregnancy, 64
  exploding head syndrome. See exploding head syndrome
  nightmare disorder, 4, 5, 170–171
  as often experienced in wake of trauma, 118
  origin of term, 4
  sleep terrors, 171
Parkes, J. D., 60, 85
patients with panic disorder, lifetime prevalence rates of sleep paralysis in, 96t, 97t
pavor nocturnus, 171
pedunculopontine and laterodorsal tegmental (PPT/LDT) nuclei, 139, 140
penile tumescence, 136
perceptual biases, in sleep paralysis hallucinations, 79
peri-episode fear, 86
peri-traumatic dissociation, 121, 131, 132
peri-traumatic dissociative symptoms, 79
peri-traumatic tonic immobility, 121
personality traits and types, impacts of on sleep paralysis, 131–133
personalizing/personification (cause of sleep paralysis), 129–130
pgnalion (throttle), 59
pH balance, as cause for sleep paralysis, 60

physical oppression, associated with Nightmare, 21
physical struggle, as technique against alien abduction, 191
Pittsburgh Sleep Quality Index, 108
playing dead/"playing possum," 121
plethora hypothesis, as cause for sleep paralysis, 62
PMR (progressive muscle relaxation), 246
Polidori, John William, 67
poltergeists, 31, 131
polysomnography, 106, 137
Pope Innocent III, 2
porphyria, 26, 30
possession, as referring to Devil's attack from within, 23
post-death existence, 26
post-episode confusion, 47
Post-Sleep Paralysis Panic Attack Questionnaire, 160t,
post-traumatic stress disorder (PTSD), 9, 79, 117–121, 174–176
powerlessness, 17, 52, 74, 130, 183, 200, 245
PPT/LDT (pedunculopontine and laterodorsal tegmental) nuclei, 139, 140
prayer
  as disruption technique, 190
  as prevention technique, 185–186
  use of, 245, 247
prazosin, 120
pregnancy, association of with sleep paralysis, 64
premature burials, 27
pressure
  as defining characteristic of classic Nightmare, 78. See also chest pressure
  feelings of, 24
prevention techniques
  in CBT-ISP, 253
  folk remedies, 184–189
  frequencies of techniques used to prevent and disrupt isolated sleep paralysis episodes and their outcome, 201t,
primal scene, witnessing of, 135

CPSIA information can be obtained
at www.ICGtesting.com
Printed in the USA
BVHW032146160822
644776BV00010B/225